SIRTFOOD DIET

2 Books in 1: Sirtfood Diet for Beginners + Sirtfood Diet Cookbook. Discover the Power of Sirtuins, Lose Weight Fast and Activate the Metabolism with 302 Recipes and a 21 Days Meal Plan

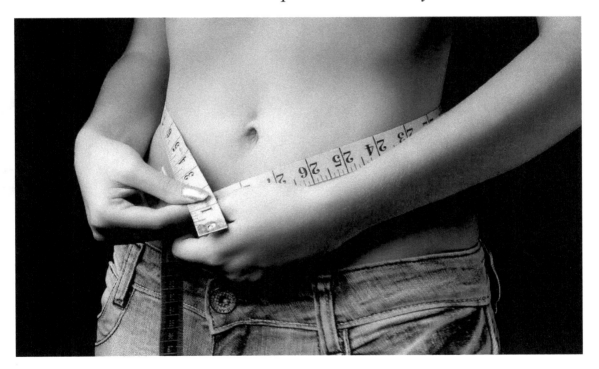

Lara Burns

Table of Contents

BOOK 2) SIRTFOOD DIET COOKBOOK

302 Quick and Healthy Sirtfood Diet Recipes to Use in Your Meal Plan. Discover the Power of Sirtuins: Activate the Metabolism, Eat Delicious Dishes and Lose Weight Quickly

SIRTFOOD DIET FOR BEGINNERS

A 21 Days Meal Plan to Stimulate Skinny Genes and Lose Weight Fast while Eating Delicious Foods. Practical Diet Book for Women and Men to Activate Metabolism and Sirtuins

Lara Burns

Introduction

Losing weight and developing a perfect body are some of the most common aspirations among individuals from different cultures, backgrounds, social classes, and genders around the world. Virtually everyone wants to lose weight and look trim and attractive.

All foods certified as sirtfood have all been extensively analyzed to understand their compositions and their effects on the body. One thing that has been found in all sirtfoods is that they contain a couple of compounds known collectively as polyphenols. The first sirtfood was analyzed in the 20th century, and it was the skin of red grapes used in making red wine. During the analysis of these skins, it was found out that these skins contained a polyphenol known as resveratrol. It had been noted earlier that unlike people who drink heavily alcoholic drinks, people who drink red wine do not tend to get unhealthy or overweight. Instead, red wine drinkers seemed to be svelte, fit, and naturally energetic.

Scientists dug further into how resveratrol, one of the most active compounds in red wine, could be affecting the burning of fat deposits and the maintenance of a trim body figure with a moderate muscle mass within the body. Their findings were nothing short of revolutionary. In their studies, these scientists found out that there are a set of genes located in our bodies known as sirtuins. There are seven sirtuins in total, and they all work together in a system. Each sirtuin is named in a simple manner. The first sirtuin gene is named SIRT 1, the second; SIRT 2, and the numbering goes on like that, reaching SIRT 7. SIRT 1 and SIRT 3 have been found out to be the most active genes in the family of the sirtuins.

The Sirt diet is loved by stars because it makes you lose weight without too many sacrifices, thanks to the foods that contain sirtuins. The Sirt diet is the diet that makes you lose weight without giving up the pleasures of the table. This type of low-calorie diet is based on the consumption of foods rich in sirtuins, a category of proteins with enzymatic activity that would be able to accelerate the metabolism, activating the so-called "lean gene," and was conceived by the two nutritionists Aidan Goggins and Glen Matten, authors of the book Sirt, the lean gene diet.

The Sirt diet is a food protocol that, through the intake of certain foods, promises to activate sirtuins, the so-called "thinness" genes. These "super metabolic regulators" can naturally set the metabolism in motion and, therefore, to burn fat and increase muscle mass. They also manage to modulate the sense of hunger and therefore help to eat less.

The Sirt diet, also known as Sirtfood, is the new way to lose weight without a radical diet by activating the same " lean gene " pathways usually induced by exercise and fasting. Some foods contain chemicals called polyphenols that exert slight stress on our cells, thus activating genes that mimic the effects of fasting and physical activity.

Foods rich in polyphenols, including cabbage, dark chocolate, and red wine, trigger sirtuins, special proteins that affect metabolism, aging, and mood. A diet rich in these foods starts weight loss without sacrificing muscles, maintaining optimal health. Thanks to this simple process, the Sirt diet is now in fashion, also used by celebrities and show business personalities.

Chapter 1: What Are Sirtuins

To know exactly how the sirtfood diet works, it is imperative to understand the role of sirtuins in the human body. In fact, sirtuins are known for playing an important metabolic role in most living organisms. This is why the production, utilization, and stimulation of sirtuins is now considered healthy.

In simple words, sirtuins by their composition are a type of protein present in various parts of the human cell from the nucleus to mitochondria. They are part of the genetic makeup and help in DNA repair and other cell regulation activities.

Sirtuins are also often called the "skinny genes" because of the role they can play in reducing human weight. But how these genes can make that magic happen is an important question. Biological sciences are no magic, it's all about understanding your body better and then meeting the body's needs to help boost its natural healthy activities. Similarly, when we boost the formation and stimulation of sirtuins in the cell, it automatically aids metabolism, prevents aging, and puts the body on a fast track.

Not every person is obese due to lack of exercise or the food they eat—some people have a naturally low metabolic rate and it makes it almost impossible for them to get out of the trap of obesity. By stimulating the sirtuins, we can put the body on track and make burning calories faster and use them effectively.

Sirtuins are a group of genes known as inducible genes. There are several other genes located throughout the body that work using a similar mechanism as the sirtuins. They stay, relatively hidden and unnoticed within the body. However, when a condition arises that necessitates them to swing into action, inducible genes become activated. They do not just become activated magically, however. They are activated in response to the situation that necessities their attention. You can think of them like firefighters. Firefighters do not just drive their trucks and come to your house. Your house has to be on fire, and you need to call their attention to the fire. The signal that is sent to the firemen in the form of your phone call or that of your neighbors then forces the firemen to spring into action to come and put out the fire – the incident that led to them getting invited in the first place. This analogy works very well with the sirtuins. The sirtuins remain dormant over the lives of most people because they are not activated. However, when they are activated with the right signals, sirtuins perform an extremely wonderful function – they put the entire body in survival mode and aim to save the body, just like firefighters saving a house. To help the body have as much energy as possible to survive the 'perilous' times that the sirtuins believe the body is in, these genes burn up stores of fat within the body to provide energy. The deploy mechanisms to repair and rejuvenate damaged cells, and they boost the abilities of the body's immune system, making the body even more resistant to disease.

Sirtuins manage a wide scope of procedures, including interpretation, digestion, fat assembly, neurodegeneration and maturing. The different elements of these proteins have been to a great extent attributed to their capacity to catalyze the expulsion of acetyl bunches from the lysine amino-corrosive deposits of different proteins through their deacetylase movement. However, the definite natural activity of sirtuins stays vague. For example, one sirtuin, SIRT6, which has been ensnared in genome strength, irritation, malignant growth cell digestion and even lifespan, is an extremely powerless deacetylase1. On page 110 of this issue, Jiang et al.2 report the astounding revelation that SIRT6 heartily evacuates a myristoyl gathering — a long-chain greasy acyl gathering — from lysine deposits, and that this biochemical action empowers the chemical to manage the emission of TNF-α, a cytokine protein discharged from cells during irritation.

Proteins experience and assorted cluster of compound modifications that adjust their movement. The catalysts that include and evacuate these modifications are therefore key chiefs in flagging falls. The lysine side chains of proteins can be modified by connection of a little acyl bunch called acetyl, which is one of the most widely recognized administrative modifications and is most popular for its job in controlling interpretation. Other, bigger acyl modifications of lysine buildups have been distinguished, in spite of the fact that their natural jobs are to a great extent obscure.

The greater part of the seven human sirtuins (SIRT1–7) show this run of the mill movement, albeit a few, including SIRT6, have either powerless or no deacetylase action. For example, SIRT5 specially ties to and expels succinyl and malonyl modifications from lysine3. These acyl bunches are bigger than acetyls and, in contrast to them, are adversely charged, yet they are connected to lysine by a similar sort of compound bond and are evacuated in the equivalent NAD+-subordinate enzymatic response as that catalyzed by different sirtuins.

Sirtuins are referred to go about as deacetylase proteins. (Nicotinamide is a side-effect of the response.) Jiang et al.2 report that SIRT6 specially evacuates a different, long-chain acyl gathering (myristoyl) from proteins — a finding that, together with past information, require a reclassification of sirtuins as deacylases.

The SIRT5 point of reference incited Jiang et al. to research whether the obviously powerless deacetylase action of SIRT6 likewise mirrors an inclination for other acyl-lysine substrates. Their pursuit started in vitro with the utilization of synthetically blended peptides bearing lysine modified with different acyl bunches that are known to happen in cells. The outcome was clear: SIRT6 was undeniably increasingly dynamic in evacuating the long-chain greasy acyl myristoyl and palmitoyl bunches than little acyl modifications, including acetyl gatherings.

Together with past basic studies 3,4,5 indicating how different sirtuins can suit different acyl modifications, including succinyl, malonyl and propionyl lysine, it presently appears to be certain that auxiliary highlights in the sirtuins' dynamic locales oversee the inclination of everyone for expelling a specific kind of acyl modification.

In vivo, SIRT6 is known to direct the degrees of TNF-α, which traverses the cell film and is cut by a layer related protease compound, bringing about the emission of this current cytokine's extracellular area. The cytoplasmic area of TNF-α contains two myristoylated lysine. This quickly brings up two issues: does SIRT6 expel these myristoyl modifications and, if things being what they are, is this enzymatic action by one way or another associated with TNF-α guideline?

Without a doubt, Jiang et al. discovered that the myristylation level of TNF-α in refined cells relied upon the enzymatic movement of SIRT6. Emission of TNF-α likewise required SIRT6, demonstrating that expulsion of its myristoyl bunches is a key advance in this procedure. It will be intriguing to perceive how myristylation manages emission, and whether expulsion of the myristoyl bunches causes a conformational revamp in TNF-α that permits its cleavage by the layer related protease.

Jiang and associates' discoveries set up for a few new headings wherein to explore the job of greasy acyl modifications and their guideline by sirtuins. The paper ought to be the last driving force for reclassifying sirtuins as lysine deacylases5, and not just deacetylases, to mirror the broader nature of their enzymatic movement.

Significantly, it presently appears that sirtuins differ from each other in the kind of acyl modification they specially expel from substrates, albeit current discoveries do not decide out the likelihood that a given sirtuin can evacuate a few sorts of acyl modification in vivo. This is maybe the situation for SIRT6. In spite of the fact that the compound specially expels long-chain greasy acyl modifications, its deacetylase movement has been implicated6 in modification of the DNA-related histone H3 protein. It may be the case that, in vivo, the feeble deacetylase action of SIRT6 is confined to specific substrates (as has been shown6), to exact subcellular restrictions or to specific flagging pathways. The way that SIRT6 can expel a more extensive range of acyl modifications should make it conceivable to coax out the overall commitments of these biochemical exercises to this current chemical's capacity.

It has for quite some time been a riddle why sirtuins expend the vivaciously exorbitant NAD+ cofactor, as opposed to — like different classes of deacetylase — utilizing basic hydrolysis to deacetylate substrates. Clarifications summoned incorporate the administrative ramifications of coupling sirtuin movement to the phone's metabolic state, in which NAD+ is included, or the conceivable flagging job of the O-acetyl ADP-ribose item (Fig. 1). Another clarification might be the need to create a nucleotide bearer for the leaving acyl gathering. The O-myristoyl ADP-ribose conjugation additionally forestalls myristate from getting lengthened by further enzymatic response to frame another unsaturated fat, palmitate, along these lines safeguarding the accessible pool of myristate.

O-Acetyl ADP-ribose is separated by a few enzymes7, and it is not yet clear which of them control the degrees of other O-acyl ADP-ribose items or move them to different bearers, and whether these exercises influence or even drive upstream pathways engaged with creating these metabolites. Until further notice, the disclosure of SIRT6-interceded demyristoylation opens an energizing section in the account of the seven human sirtuins and their natural action."

Sirtuins, Fasting, and Metabolic Activities

SIRT1, just like other SIRTUINS family, is protein NAD+ dependent deacetylases that are associated with cellular metabolism. All sirtuins, including SIRT1 important for sensing energy status and in protection against metabolic stress. They coordinate cellular response towards Caloric Restriction (CR) in an organism. SIRT1 diverse location and allows cells to easily sense changes in the level of energy anywhere in the mitochondria, nucleus, and cytoplasm. Associated with metabolic health through deacetylation of several target proteins such as muscles, liver, endothelium, heart, and adipose tissue.

SIRT1, SIRT6, and SIRT7 are localized in the nucleus where they take part in the deacetylation of customers to influence gene expression epigenetically. SIRT2 is located in the cytosol, while SIRT3, SIRT4, and SIRT5 are located in the mitochondria where they regulate metabolic enzyme activities as well as moderate oxidative stress.

SIRT1, as most studies with regards to metabolism, aid in mediating the physiological adaptation to diets. Several studies have shown the impact of sirtuins on Caloric Restriction. Sirtuins deacetylase non-histone proteins that define pathways involved during the metabolic adaptation when there are metabolic restrictions. Caloric Restriction, on the other hand, causes the induction of expression of SIRT1 in humans. Mutations that lead to loss of function in some sirtuins genes can lead to a reduction in the outputs of caloric restrictions. Therefore, sirtuins have the following metabolic functions: Regulation In The Liver

The Liver regulates the body glucose homeostasis. During fasting or caloric restriction, glucose level becomes low, resulting in a sudden shift in hepatic metabolism to glycogen breakdown and then to gluconeogenesis to maintain glucose supply as well as ketone body production to mediate the deficit in energy. Also, during caloric restriction or fasting, there is muscle activation and liver oxidation of fatty acids produced during lipolysis in white adipose tissue. For this switch to occur, there are several transcription factors involved to adapt to energy deprivation. SIRT1 intervenes during the metabolic switch to see the energy deficit.

At the initial stage of the fasting that is the post glycogen breakdown phase, there is the production of glucagon by the pancreatic alpha cells to active gluconeogenesis in the Liver through the cyclic amp response element-binding protein (CREB), and CREB regulated transcription coactivator 2 (CRTC2), the coactivator. Is the fasting gets prolonged, the effect is cancelled out and is being replaced by SIRT1 mediated CRTC2 deacetylase resulting in targeting of the coactivator for ubiquitin/ proteasome-mediated destruction? SIRT1, on the other hand, initiates the next stage of gluconeogenesis through acetylation and activation of peroxisome proliferator-activated receptor coactivator one alpha, which is the coactivator necessary for fork head box O1. In addition to the ability of SIRT1 to support gluconeogenesis, coactivator one alpha is required during the mitochondrial biogenesis necessary for the liver to accommodate the reduction in energy status. SIRT1 also activates fatty acid oxidation through deacetylation and activation of the nuclear receptor to increase energy production. SIRT1, when involved in acetylation and repression of glycolytic enzymes such as phosphoglycerate mutate 1, can lead to shutting down of the production of energy through glycolysis. SIRT6, on the other hand, can be served as a co-repressor for hypoxia-inducible Factor 1 Alpha to repress glycolysis. Since SIRT6 can transcriptionally be induced by SIRT1, sirtuins can coordinate the duration of time for each fasting phase.

Aside from glucose homeostasis, the liver also overtakes in lipid and cholesterol homeostasis during fasting. When there are caloric restrictions, the synthesis of fat and cholesterol in the liver is turned off, while lipolysis in the white adipose tissue commences. The SIRT1, upon fasting, causes acetylation of steroid regulatory element-binding protein (SREBP) and targets the protein to destroy the ubiquitin-professor system. The result is that fat cholesterol synthesis will repress. During the regulation of cholesterol homeostasis, SIRT1 regulates oxysterol receptor, thereby, assisting the reversal of cholesterol transport from peripheral tissue through upregulation of the oxysterol receptor target gene ATP-binding cassette transporter A1 (ABCA1).

Further modulation of the cholesterol regulatory loop can be achieved via bile acid receptor, that's necessary for the biosynthesis of cholesterol catabolic and bile acid pathways. SIRT6 also participates in the regulation of cholesterol levels by repressing the expression and post-translational cleavage of SREBP1/2, into the active form. Furthermore, in the circadian regulation of metabolism, SIRT1 participates through the regulation of cell circadian clock.

Mitochondrial SIRT3 is crucial in the oxidation of fatty acid in mitochondria. Fasting or caloric restrictions can result in upregulation of activities and levels of SIRT3 to aid fatty acid oxidation through deacetylation of long-chain specific acyl-CoA dehydrogenase. SIRT3 can also cause activation of ketogenesis and the urea cycle in the liver.

SIRT1 also Add it in the metabolic regulation in the muscle and white adipose tissue. Fasting causes an increase in the level of SIRT1, leading to deacetylation of coactivator one alpha, which in turn causes genes responsible for fat oxidation to get activated. The reduction in energy level also activates AMPK, which will activate the expression of coactivator one alpha. The combined effects of the two processes will give rise to increased mitochondrial biogenesis together with fatty acid oxidation in the muscle.

Chapter 2: Why the Sirtfood Diet Works

It is important to understand how and why it works however, so that you can appreciate the value of what you are doing. It is important to also know why these sirtuin rich foods help to help you maintain fidelity to your diet plan. Otherwise, you may throw something in your meal with less nutrition that would defeat the purpose of planning for one rich in sirtuins. Most importantly, this is not a dietary fad, and as you will see, there is much wisdom contained in how humans have used natural foods even for medicinal purposes, over thousands of years.

To understand how the Sirtfood diet works, and why these particular foods are necessary, we will look at the role they play in the human body.

Sirtuin activity was first researched in yeast, where a mutation caused an extension in the yeast's lifespan. Sirtuins were also shown to slow aging in laboratory mice, fruit flies, and nematodes. As research on Sirtuins proved to transfer to mammals, they were examined for their use in diet and slowing the aging process. The sirtuins in humans are different in the typing but they essentially work in the same ways and reasons.

There are seven "members" that make up the sirtuin family. It is believed that sirtuins play a big role in regulating certain functions of cells including proliferation reproduction and growth of cells), apoptosis death of cells). They promote survival and resist stress to increase longevity.

They are also seen to block neurodegeneration loss or function of the nerve cells in the brain). They conduct their housekeeping functions by cleaning out toxic proteins and supporting the brain's ability to change and adapt to different conditions, or to recuperate i.e., brain plasticity). As part of this they also help reduce chronic inflammation and reduce something called oxidative stress. Oxidative stress is when there are too many cell-damaging free radicals circulating in the body, and the body cannot catch up by combating them with antioxidants. These factors are related to age-related illness and weight as well, which again, brings us back to a discussion of how they actually work.

You will see labels in Sirtuins that start with "SIR," which represents "Silence Information Regulator" genes. They do exactly that, silence or regulate, as part of their functions. The seven sirtuins that humans work with are: SIRT1, SIRT2, SIRT3, SIRT4, SIRT 5, SIRT6 and SIRT7. Each of these types is responsible for different areas of protecting cells. They work by either stimulating or turning on certain gene expressions, or by reducing and turning off other gene expressions. This essentially means that they can influence genes to do more or less of something, most of which they are already programmed to do.

Through enzyme reactions, each of the SIRT types affect different areas of cells that are responsible for the metabolic processes that help to maintain life. This is also related to what organs and functions they will affect.

For example, the SIRT6 causes an expression of genes in humans that affect skeletal muscle, fat tissue, brain, and heart. SIRT 3 would cause an expression of genes that affect the kidneys, liver, brain and heart.

If we tie these concepts together, you can see that the Sirtuin proteins can change the expression of genes, and in the case of the Sirtfood diet we care about how sirtuins can turn off those genes that are responsible for speeding up aging and for weight management.

The other aspect to this conversation of sirtuins is the function and the power of calorie restriction on the human body. Calorie restriction is simply eating less calories. This coupled with exercise and reducing stress is usually a combination for weight loss. Calorie restriction has also proven across much research in animals and humans to increase one's lifespan.

We can look further at the role of sirtuins with calorie restriction and using the SIRT3 protein which has a role in metabolism and aging. Amongst all of the effects of the protein on gene expression, such as preventing cells from dying, reducing tumors from growing, etc.)

The SIRT3 has high expression in those metabolically active tissues as we stated earlier, and its ability to express itself increases with caloric restriction, fasting, and exercise. On the contrary, it will express itself less when the body has a high fat, high calorie-riddled diet.

The last few highlights of sirtuins are their role in regulating telomeres and reducing inflammation which also help with staving off disease and aging.

Telomeres are sequences of proteins at the ends of chromosomes. When cells divide these get shorter. As we age, they get shorter, and other stressors to the body also will contribute to this. Maintaining these longer telomeres is the key to slower aging. In addition, proper diet, along with exercise and other variables can lengthen telomeres. SIRT6 is one of the sirtuins that, if activated, can help with DNA damage, inflammation and oxidative stress. SIRT1 also helps with inflammatory response cycles that are related to many age-related diseases.

Calories restriction can extend life to some degree. Since this, as well as fasting, is a stressor, these factors will stimulate the SIRT3 proteins to kick in and protect the body from the stressors and excess free radicals. Again, the telomere length is affected as well.

Having laid this all out before you, you should be able to appreciate how and why these miraculous compounds work in your favor, to keep you youthful, healthy, and lean If they are working hard for you, don't you feel that you should do something too?

Why Eat Sirtfoods?

People are just starting to realize the great value of sirtuins, and they include them in their diets and meal plans. The sirtuin activators can have a huge impact on your health, and they also are effective when it comes to suppressing your appetite and building more muscle.

As previously mentioned, sirtuins represent a certain group of proteins that can be found in various foods, mostly in fruits and vegetables. Most of us can agree that you can't go wrong with eating fruits and veggies. They are a great source of minerals, vitamins, and proteins. Now, there are plenty of people who also consider the fact that these proteins are not enough to maintain your muscle mass and for your body to function properly, and I'm afraid I need to agree with them. Thus, most adults consider adding meat to their meals.

If you ask bodybuilders what they eat in order to get the required protein intake for growing their muscle mass, they will say meat, eggs, milk, and cheese. These are the food types with the highest concentration of proteins. However, proteins are very diverse and can be found in plenty of other sources, including plants, vegetables, and fruits. The sirtfood diet doesn't encourage people to consume just foods or ingredients with a high concentration of sirtuins. The founders of this diet, Aidan Goggins and Glen Matten, believe that no food should be left behind. Therefore, if sirtuins can only be found in fruits and veggies, this doesn't mean you have to become a vegetarian.

It is all about getting the right balance of ingredients and foods. You can still eat anything you want, but you need to lower the quantity of more harmful food (carbs, processed meat, and so on). As we all know, carbs can cause addiction. So why stuff ourselves with these food types? The sirtfood diet suggests replacing carbs with a special kind of protein (the sirtuin). You will notice that you will no longer become hungry (so easily), as this diet is designed to suppress your appetite. Therefore, your body will no longer crave calories from carbs, and you can easily control your calorie intake. Calorie deprivation and appetite suppression lead to weight loss, plus it leads to lower blood sugar and insulin level.

You already know that most health problems (e.g., diabetes, inflammation, and different types of cancer) are caused by poor nutrition, especially the accumulation of sugar in your blood. By consuming food rich in sirtuins, you don't have to worry about increasing your blood sugar or insulin level. Truth be told — most people are judging diets by its results in terms of weight loss. However, a diet can only be sustained for as long as it has health benefits to your body. It is pointless to stick to a radical diet if you lose a lot of weight very fast but jeopardize your health. This is why you need to seek long-term results and make the sirtfood diet your default eating habit. Basically, it has to become part of your lifestyle. We're not talking about a radical diet, as this one is pretty easy to stick to. No food is left behind, remember? You might be willing to give it a try but still not sure what to eat when following this diet. Well, you don't have to worry about this, as this book will provide you plenty of recipes and even a meal plan you can stick to.

Is It Effective?

The creators of the Sirtfood Diet make extreme cases, including that the eating routine can super-charge weight reduction, turn on your "thin quality" and forestall illnesses. The issue is there isn't a lot of verification to back them. Up until this point, there's no persuading proof that the Sirtfood Diet has a more significant impact on weight reduction than some other calorie-confined eating routine.

What's more, albeit a large number of these nourishments have fortifying properties, there have not been any long-haul human examinations to decide if eating an eating routine rich in sirtfoods has any substantial medical advantages. By the by, the Sirtfood Diet book reports the aftereffects of a pilot study led by the writers and including 39 members from their wellness place. Notwithstanding, the aftereffects of this examination show up not to have been distributed anyplace else.

For multi-week, the members followed the eating regimen and practiced day by day. Toward the week's end, members lost a normal of 7 pounds (3.2 kg) and kept up or even picked up the bulk. However, these outcomes are not astonishing. Confining your calorie admission to 1,000 calories and practicing simultaneously will almost consistently cause weight reduction. In any case, this sort of brisk weight reduction is neither certifiable nor dependable, and this examination didn't follow members after the first week to check whether they recovered any of the weight, which is regularly the situation.

At the point when your body is vitality denied, it goes through its crisis vitality stores, or glycogen, notwithstanding consuming fat and muscle. Every atom of glycogen requires 3–4 particles of water to be put away. At the point when your body goes through glycogen, it disposes of this water also. It's known as "water weight." In the first seven day stretch of outrageous calorie limitation, just around 33% of the weight reduction originates from fat, while the other 66% originates from water, muscle and glycogen. When your calorie admission expands, your body recharges its glycogen stores, and the weight returns right.

The sirtfood for Weight loss

Research conducted by Aidan Goggins and Glen Martin showed that 7 pounds of weight was lost on average in seven days on the Sirt food diet after taking note of muscle gain. Sirtuins' diet has not promised only weight loss; instead, good health as well. An increase in the level of body sirtuins has been proven to cause weight loss. The best way of increasing body leptin is still through fasting and exercise. Also, one of the best ways of enhancing body sirtuins is by consumption of sirtuin foods. All of the seas will affect the body metabolism, which we will treat in the next chapter.

Furthermore, hypothalamic SIRT1 has been proven to help in weight loss. The hypothalamus is the central weight and energy balance controller. It modulates energy intake and energy consumption by neural inputs from the periphery as well as direct humor inputs, which senses the energy status of the body. An adipokine, leptin, is one of the factors that signal that sufficient energy is stored on the periphery. Leptin plasma levels are positive for adiposity, suppressing energy intake, and stimulating energy spending. A prolonged increase in the level of plasma leptin in obese can cause leptin resistance. Leptin resistance, in turn, can affect the hypothalamus from having access to leptin, which also reduces leptin signals transduction in the hypothalamic neurons. Reduced peripheral energy-sensing by leptin can lead to a positive energy balance and incremental weight gain and adiposity improvements, which further exacerbate leptin resistance. Leptin resistance causes an increase in adiposity, just like weight gain are all associated with aging. Similar observations occur in central insulin resistance. The improvement of the action of humoral factors in the hypothalamus can, therefore, prevent progressive weight gains, especially among middle-aged individuals. SIRT1 is a protein deacetylase, NAD+ dependent, that has many substrates, such as transcription factors, histones, co-factors, and various enzymes. SIRT1 improves the sensitivity to leptin and insulin by decreasing the levels of several molecules that impair the transduction of leptin and insulin signals. The hypothalamic SIRT1 and NAD+ levels decrease with age. Increased in the level of SIRT1 has shown to improve kept in level in mice and so prevents age-related weight gain. By preventing the loss of age dependent SIRT1 hypothalamus role, there will be a boost in the activity of humoral factors in the hypothalamus and the central energy balance control.

Sirtfood for building muscle

sirtuins are a group of proteins with different effects. Sirt-1 is the protein responsible for causing the body to burn fat rather than muscle for energy, which is obviously a miracle for weight loss. Another useful aspect of Sirt-1 is its ability to improve skeletal muscle.

Skeletal muscle is all the muscles you voluntarily control, such as the muscles in your limbs, back, shoulders and so on. There are two other types, cardiac muscle is what the heart is formed of, whilst smooth muscle is your involuntary muscles – which includes muscles around your blood vessels, face and various parts of organs and other tissues.

Skeletal muscle is separated into two different groups, the blandly named type-1 and type-2. Type 1 muscle is effective at continued, sustained activity whereas type-2 muscle is effective at short, intense periods of activity. So, for example, you would predominantly use type-1 muscles for jogging, but type-2 muscles for sprinting.

Sirt-1 protects the type-1 muscles, but not the type-2 muscle, which is still broken down for energy. Therefore, holistic muscle mass drops when fasting, even though type-1 skeletal muscle mass increases.

Sirt-1 also influences how the muscles actually work. Sirt-1 is produced by the muscle cells, but the ability to produce Sirt-1 decreases as the muscle ages. As a result, muscle is harder to build as you age and doesn't grow as fast in response to exercise. A lack of sirt-1 also causes the muscles to become tired quicker and gradually decline over time.

When you start to consider these effects of Sirt-1, you can start to form a picture about why fasting helps keep the body supple. Fasting releases Sirt-1, which in turn helps skeletal muscle grow and stay in good shape. Sirt-1 is also released by consuming sirtuin activators, giving the sirtfood diet its muscle retaining power.

Who Should Try the Sirtfood Diet?

Anyone who can make the best use out of this diet should try it. There is no one formula of who should try the sirtfood diet and who shouldn't. However, based on the body's needs and the physical problems a person is suffering from, we can decide on a better utility of this diet. Following are the cases in which the sirtfood diet can prove to be most effective.

Obesity

Sirtuin burns fats quickly, and that's what makes this diet a great help for weight loss. When we study all the cases of the successful sirtfood dieters, we can clearly see how well they fought against obesity. Adele is just one example, who has amazed the world with her 30 pounds of weight loss achievement using the sirtfood diet. So, anyone who isn't able to lose some extra pounds for whatever reason, they can switch to sirtfood and then can see the magic happening.

Low or Poor Metabolic Activity

Since sirtuins are mainly responsible for better cell metabolism, lower sirtuin levels in the body can hamper the natural cell activities and hinders the metabolism. Poor metabolic activity results in weakening of physical strength, obesity, hormonal imbalance, low enzymic activity, and several other related problems. The sirtfood diet is therefore suggested to boost the metabolic rates in the body and revitalize the body and the mind with levels of energy.

No workouts

Extraneous workouts are just not for everybody. Sure, working out is a good way to lose some pounds but it is not possible for every other person to invest the required time and energy into the workouts. Therefore, the sirtfood diet can be used by such individuals. Through this diet, they can manage their weight and lose it even while doing some basic physical activities.

Aging

Aging seems like a threat to all when those wrinkles start appearing on the skin, and the person feels weakened inside out! Well, this magic gene sirtuin can also play its part in countering the effects of aging. It helps DNA to prolong its life and also aid in the repair process. Sirtuin is also responsible for apoptosis and leads to the formation of new healthy cells. This is the reason that people who are entering into middle age should consider doing the sirtfood diet so that they could effectively fight the possible signs of aging in the years to come.

Inflammation

What appears to be weight gain or metabolic inactivity is mostly connected to inflammation of both cells and organs in most cases. This inflammation is both the result and cause of several health problems. Sirtfood does not only prevent inflammation at cellular levels but effectively prevents it at the tissue and organ level.

Stress

There is one added advantage that higher sirtuin levels can guarantee and that is the reduction in stress and depression. Research is still being conducted on the relationship between sirtfood and stress, but sirtuin is that element that can enable quick brain cell recovery and boosts brain activity by getting rid of all the unwanted metabolic waste. Efficient brain functioning then leads to a reduction in stress. So, this sirtfood diet can also help with stress relief.

Burn Fat and Skinny Gene

So far, we've taken a look at the impacts of SIRT1 on fat loss on a notable kind of fat called white adipose tissue (WAT). This is the sort of fat-related to weight gain. It spends significant time away and development is appallingly obstinate and secretes a large group of fiery synthetic substances that oppose fat burning and energize further fat collection, making us overweight and stout. This is the reason weight gain regularly begins gradually, however can snowball so rapidly.

However, not exclusively does PGC-1α advance more mitochondria, it likewise urges them to burn fat as the fuel of the decision to make the energy. So, from one viewpoint, fat stockpiling is blocked, and on the other fat burning is expanded.

Ordinarily, accomplishing huge fat loss requires an impressive penance, either seriously decreasing calories or participating in superhuman degrees of activity or both.

It's just when we comprehend what befalls our fat cells when sirtuin movement is expanded that we can start to understand these astounding discoveries.

PPAR-γ (peroxisome proliferator-actuated receptor-γ). PPAR-γ coordinates the fat-gain process by turning on the genes that are expected to begin blending and putting away fat. To stop the multiplication of fat, you should cut the flexibly. Stop PPAR-γ, and you viably stop fat gain.

SIRT1 blocks the procedure of PPAR-γ. With the action of PPAR-γ stopped, SIRT1 washes down the fat in the circulation system. In addition to the fact that this is finished by closing down the creation and ability of fat, as we've seen, however, it really changes our metabolism, so we begin freeing the collection of overabundance fat. A key controller in our cells known as PGC-1α additionally helps with these procedures. This intensely animates the production of what are known as mitochondria. These are the minuscule energy manufacturing parts that exist inside every one of our cells—they power the body. The more efficient the mitochondria work, the more energy we can create.

There is also another captivating edge to the sirtuin procedure, including a lesser-known kind of fat, brown adipose tissue (BAT), which carries on in an unexpected way. In complete complexity to white fat tissue, BAT is useful to us and needs to get spent. Brown adipose tissue really encourages us to consume energy and has advanced in well-evolved creatures to permit them to scatter a lot of energy as heat. Here is the place SIRT1 initiation accomplishes something really astonishing. It turns on genes in our white fat tissue, so it transforms and assumes the properties of brown fat tissue in what is known as a "browning effect." That implies our fat stores begin to carry on in an out and out various way—rather than putting away energy, they begin to assemble it for removal.

As should be obvious, sirtuin activation has intense direct activity on fat cells, urging fat to dissolve away. However, it doesn't end there. Sirtuins additionally emphatically impact the most pertinent hormones engaged with weight control. Sirtuin activation improves insulin movement. This assists with darkinishing insulin resistance—the susceptibility of our cells to react appropriately to insulin—which is intensely involved in weight gain. SIRT1 likewise improves the discharge and movement of our thyroid hormones, which share many covering roles in boosting our metabolism and, at last, the rate at which we copy fat.

How to Hack the Skinny Genes

Genes contain data that determine everything from appearance to intelligence. An individual acquires genes from their parents, and how parents live affects their offspring's genes.

It's a mixed-up supposition that all that you acquired in your genes is changeless. Your way of life and conditions can stir singular genes or potentially smother others. Here are ways you can modify your condition and way of life to improve your body and brain.

1. Your health will depend on the type of food you eat

Food and nutrients are significant - both can impact the body and psyche. On the off chance that you consistently eat solid and nutritious food, your genes will react as needs to be. Sound sustenance stirs basic genes that positively affect your brain and body. It's basic to have a reliably sound diet since you need your great genes to be dynamic.

Keep up a truly thorough food plan consistently. Your food plan might comprise a free form of the paleo diet. In addition to the fact that this keeps will keep the brain sharp, yet it encourages and keeps up an optimal execution when working out. Try not to take alcohol, don't smoke, and don't do any form of drugs. You feel healthier than you will ever be.

2. Stress can initiate changes

Everyone manages pressure, and that can affect our health and genes. In case you're reliably worried, certain valuable genes can progressively get smothered or enacted to enable you to adapt. That can directly affect your efficiency and health.

To battle pressure, you can go on long runs or drive while tuning in to your preferred music. Utilize positive mental quality tricks and breathing activities to help still your mind and slow your pulse down.

3. A functioning way of life will stir the best genes

A functioning way of life impacts changes as well. You don't need to be an activity addict to get great outcomes. You should simply enjoy some physical movement, for example, moving or running all the time. Your body will initiate genes expected to help those exercises after some time. The effect has a net positive on your health, mind, and profitability.

4. Change your condition

Once in a while, changing your condition isn't as simple as affecting different parts of your life; however, you can control it in little manners. Normal introduction to morning daylight, a clean home environment and living close to a lush zone can impact your dynamic genes, mind, body, and even your state of mind.

Keeping the entirety of the workplace clean and mess-free, you should continually change where you work and travel. For me, the result is a substantially more gainful, unique way of life.

The Procedure of the Sirtfood Diet

One step at a time! That's what it takes to incorporate sirtfood into your diet. The diet is simple and easy to follow in a sense that it only calls for a few definite steps to take. Firstly, you will need to increase food consumption that is rich in sirtuin, then you will have to follow the phases of the diet as discussed in the next section of this book, plus you will need to add green juices to your daily diet. Here are a couple of steps that must be followed to achieve your weight loss goals on a sirtfood diet:

Get the right ingredients

Remember that all this diet asks from you is to increase your sirtuins intake. That can be done only through careful and selective grocery shopping. Prepare a list of the ingredients that contain a high amount of sirtuins and check their utility as per your meal plan. There are certain ingredients like coffee, parsley, red wine, and chocolate, that you can have all the time. So, stock up your kitchen cabinets with these ingredients.

Set up the schedule

The sirtfood diet gives you small weight loss targets for each week. In the initial time period, you must prepare a schedule to keep track of your meals, the caloric intake, and the timing of green juices you are consuming in a day. In this way, you will be able to manage the first few days of the diet adoption easily and continue observing body changes and measure your weight to keep track of your pace.

Prepare for the first week

In the first week of the sirtfood diet, the dieter must control his caloric intake. Therefore, to avoid any mistakes or confusion, all the high caloric food items should be removed from sight. Stuff your refrigerator only with the food that is appropriate for the sirtfood diet, and keep the juices, fruits, and vegetables ready to use. Instead of planning your meal every other day, make plans for the entire week according to the caloric limitations.

Caloric intake

Keep in mind that sirtfood is more about weight loss, so mere sirtuins cannot magically work overnight if you keep consuming more calories than your body can actually burn. Do the math and understand your caloric needs, even when the diet does not restrict you from high caloric intake after the first seven days. Still, you must maintain a strict check on the daily caloric intake to keep the weight in control. Otherwise, it does not take much to regain the lost pounds.

Green juices

Green juices are one of the most essential parts of the sirtfood diet. These are your way to detoxification and quick weight loss. Green veggies are full of phytonutrients, minerals, and antioxidants. Having them frequently throughout the day can help boost the metabolism, remove the metabolic waste from the body, and enables the body to metabolize the needed nutrients appropriately. These juices are also great for keeping electrolyte balance in the body.

Maintenance

To harness the benefit of this diet or any other diet for that matter, it is imperative to maintain your new dietary routine. Most people abandon the diet as soon as they are an oven with the first two phases of the diet or when they achieve their weight loss goals. And soon, they regain weight and blame the diet for being ineffective, which is far from true. It all depends on how consistently you follow this diet plan.

Chapter 3: Which Are the Sirtfoods?

1. Birds Eye Chilies

Recently, Bird's eye chilies have become very expensive and sometimes scarce in many countries around the world.

That is because people are becoming increasingly aware of the health benefits of this fruit (yes, it's a fruit not a vegetable), especially for weight loss. And unlike many other chili peppers, this one is grown in very little quantities.

Bird's eye chili has superb Sirtuin-activating properties but its benefits for weight loss don't end there.

Bird's eye chilies also play a key role in enhancing body metabolism. They contain a special compound called Capsaicin that creates a hot and burning sensation when you eat them. This raises your body's temperature and, in order to regulate the temperature, your body will resort to burning more calories to create body heat.

The result of this is a faster weight loss because your body will often have to turn to the unused, stored up fat deposits to make up for the increase in calorie consumption.

Other health benefits of the Bird's eye chili for weight loss include:

Contains Antioxidant Properties: Bird's eye chilies contain at least 4 different antioxidants, among which there are capsaicin, violaxanthin, sinaplic acid, and ferulic acid. Antioxidants also improve the body's natural metabolic processes and lead to increased weight loss.

Reduces Blood Cholesterol: Bird's eye chilies, because they contribute to the burning of old, stored up fats in the body, help to reduce the presence of the bad cholesterol, low-density lipoprotein (LDL) in the body.

Reduces Bloating and Flatulence: If you are looking to reduce the size of your tummy and waistline, you should consider adding more Bird's eye chilies to your diet. They help to stimulate the stomach and intestinal tracts, helping to promote digestion and excretion and the result is reduced bloating and a smaller waistline.

2. Buckwheat

Buckwheat is a crop that originated from Japan. In fact, legend has it that buckwheat was such a favorite amongst Buddhist Monks that sometimes, when they made long trips to the mountains, they would go with bags of buckwheat and cooking utensils so that they could cook some buckwheat whenever they get the chance.

There wasn't so much room for cooking so they often needed foods that could keep them nourished for a very long time after a single consumption and buckwheat was one of their favorites.

Buckwheat contains rutin, a chemical compound that has Sirtuin-activating properties.

But apart from being able to help you activate your skinny genes, buckwheat also has many other benefits for weight loss.

Improves Digestion: Buckwheat helps to speed up weight loss by improving metabolism and digestion.

Its high fiber content helps to increase the rate at which toxins and waste products are expelled from your digestive tracts, leading to a faster metabolism and increased weight loss.

Reduces Blood Cholesterol: With regular consumption, buckwheat can help reduce your bad cholesterol (low-density lipoprotein (LDL) levels.

Reduces Blood Sugar: It is often tagged as a 'diabetic friendly' food because it has a low glycemic rate, which means that its glucose is absorbed much more slowly, which helps keep your blood sugar levels balanced.

A balanced blood sugar level plays a significant role in weight management because reduces food cravings and your overall appetite.

Promotes Gut Flora: Buckwheat also helps to stimulate the growth of healthy bacteria in the gut, which contributes to increased food digestion and absorption, and a reduction in weight gain, especially in the stomach and waist area.

3. Medjool Dates

Medjool dates are sweet, actually extremely sweet, since they have a sugar content of about 66%. So, it's only normal that you'll be wondering what this seemingly abominable food for weight loss is doing in a weight loss diet plan.

But even though Medjool dates have a high sugar content, its high polyphenol properties make it a very great food to include in a weight loss diet because polyphenols are Sirtuin-activating.

Also, the sugar in Medjool dates is different from refined or artificial sugars, which are the ones that are often problematic.

If you have a sweet tooth, and often find it hard to do without sugars on a diet, then Medjool dates are for you. You can even have them dried and grinded, and use the powder to sweeten your teas, smoothies and cereals.

This is way healthier than using table sugar, honey, syrup, or any other sweetener with a high glycemic index.

Medjool dates also have other weight loss properties and benefits:

Prevent and Relieve Constipation: Medjool dates have a high soluble fiber content that helps bulk up your stool and make it move through your intestines faster and more easily.

If you often suffer from constipation, especially when you are on a diet, Medjool dates are good for you.

Boost Energy Levels: One common problem people face during a diet is low energy levels. Because you are not eating as much food as your body is used to, or because your foods now contain less sugars and artificial sweeteners, you may begin to experience lower energy levels or outright body weakness that makes it difficult for you to get through your daily activities.

Medjool dates contain healthy and natural glucose, fructose and sucrose that can easily be processed and utilized by your body for energy.

4. Rocket/Arugula

In some recipes you'll see it written as arugula and some recipes call it rocket – but it's the same thing. It is even called rucola, roquette, or arugula in some countries.

Whatever it is called in your country, the most important thing you need to know about this leafy green is that it is rich in Quercetin and Kaempferol, two Sirtuin-activating compounds.

The Romans and Ancient Greeks used it as a digestive aid in the past. It is also believed to have aphrodisiac properties, which led it to be banned in Monasteries during the Middle Ages.

Arugula is fantastic for helping you activate your skinny genes, but it also helps you lose weight and manage your weight in several other ways:

Has Antioxidant Properties: Arugula contains powerful antioxidant properties that promote the removal of toxins and bad cholesterol from the body.

Restores body pH levels: Arugula is an alkaline food, which means it helps reduce acidity in your body, and helps you maintain a balanced pH level.

What does that have to do with weight loss, right? A balanced pH can help you burn stored up fats faster and keep your body from accumulating fat.

It also helps to promote gut flora, and improve digestion, which contribute to weight loss.

Contains Loads of Nutrients: Arugula supplies your body with a lot of essential vitamins, nutrients and phytonutrients.

This is great for people who are into portion control or calorie counting.

It helps you get all the essential nutrients that your body needs like Vitamin K, Calcium, Magnesium, and a load of others, without eating excessively.

Fights Blood Sugar Fluctuations: Fluctuations in blood sugar levels is one of the biggest culprits of overeating, especially eating of junk or sugary foods.

Increased blood sugar levels make you crave unhealthy foods, the same way abusing drugs make you crave more drugs.

Blood sugar balancing foods like arugula helps to correct this problem by reducing sugar cravings, keeping your appetite in check, and subsequently, helping you lose weight.

5. Capers

You're probably already familiar with capers, especially if you are a pizza lover as they are often used as pizza toppings.

They are also often featured in the Mediterranean diet as they have their origin from the Mediterranean area, that is South Europe and North Africa.

Capers contain several Sirtuin-activating compounds like phenols, quercetin, kaempferol, gingketin, and isoginkgetin.

They also have other properties that contribute to weight loss such as:

Improve Fat Breakdown: Capers help improve the breakdown of fatty cells and contribute to overall weight loss.

Increase Sugar Uptake: Capers can also help slow down blood sugar fluctuations by reducing the sugar uptake in your gut.

Asides their weight loss properties, capers also have antiviral and anti-cancer properties, which make them a must-have in every diet.

6. Celery

Celery has been used to cleanse and detox the body for thousands of years. It was also used to heal liver, kidney, and gut health problems in the ancient times.

Recently, celery has become more popular amongst dieters. In fact, many people swear by the Celery Juice Diet, a detox program that has you drink celery juice every day for several days or weeks.

Celery is one of the top Sirtfoods and consuming it regularly poses a lot of health and weight loss benefits:

Dissolves Fat Cells: Celery helps to dissolve fat cells, especially those ones stored in the liver, leading to improved liver function, metabolism, and overall weight loss.

Helps with Appetite Control: When you consume celery (as veggies not as juice), it fills you up for a very long time, which leads to lesser appetite and cravings, and a reduced overall food intake.

Reduces Cholesterol Levels: Celery can also lead to a significant reduction in overall cholesterol levels.

7. Cocoa

Who doesn't love a diet that allows you to have chocolate? Other diets may require that you stay far away from it, but on the Sirtfood diet you get to have as much as you want because cocoa, the major ingredient in chocolate, has Sirtuin-activating properties.

But you can't have just any chocolate you may find on the supermarket shelf.

You can only have brands that contain 85% cocoa solids or more.

Brands with fewer cocoa solids have diminished Sirtuin-activating properties and cannot be classified as Sirtfoods.

Other benefits of cocoa for weight loss include:

Promotes Sleep and Reduces Stress Levels: Stress contributes to overeating and lack of sleep contributes to weight gain.

Cocoa helps to calm the nerves and reduces stress levels and anxiety, leading to enhanced sleep and healthier eating habits.

Promotes Digestion and Excretion: Cocoa is also rich in fiber and flavonoids that contribute to detoxification and elimination of toxins and waste from the body.

Improves Metabolism: Cocoa is also a thermogenic enhancer. It helps to improve weight loss by increasing the rate at which your body utilizes calories for energy.

8. Coffee

You probably wouldn't have guessed that coffee could make it on the list of foods with 'health benefits' especially since they are often demonized because of their caffeine content.

"Caffeine is bad for you", they say; "Choose decaffeinated beverages", they advise.

While it is true that caffeine is not good for everyone, it is not true that caffeine is dangerous or shouldn't be consumed at all.

Coffee is not just one of the most powerful Sirtfoods, it also contains chlorogenic acid, a chemical compound that helps to slow down the production of glucose in the body.

Other benefits of coffee for weight loss include:

Reduces the Production of New Fat Cells: Coffee reduces the rate at which new fat cells are produced in your body, leading to reduced fat storage and increased fat loss.

Has Antioxidant Properties: If you are a frequent coffee drinker, you probably already know this. Coffee speeds up digestion and excretion and increases the rate at which toxins are expelled from your body.

Suppresses Hunger: Coffee also helps to suppress hunger. It contains chemical compounds that when absorbed in the blood stream, helps to create feelings of fullness in the gut.

Decreases Water Weight: Coffee acts as a diuretic, which means it makes you urinate often, leading to a reduction of excess fluid retention, and water weight in your body.

Of course, like I mentioned earlier, coffee is not for everyone especially if you have underlying health issues that make coffee a health risk for you.

If you can't have caffeine, it's okay to leave coffee out of your diet – you'll still have more than a dozen other Sirtfoods to choose from.

But if you are allowed to have decaffeinated coffee, you can opt for that because decaf coffee contains peptide tyrosine, a chemical compound that reduces hunger, and increases satiety.

9. Extra Virgin Olive Oil

On the Sirtfood diet, you will have to ditch all other cooking oils and start making your food exclusively with Extra Virgin Olive Oil.

Extra Virgin Olive Oil contains Sirtuin-enhancing properties, and has other benefits for weight loss including:

Contains Oleic Acid: Olive oil has oleic acid, which helps it to retain all of its antioxidant properties.

Enriched with Monounsaturated Fatty Acids: Unlike many other cooking oils that contain saturated fats which make them unhealthy for cooking and frying, Extra Virgin Olive oil is a healthier choice as it contains Monounsaturated Fatty Acids, which experts have labeled 'the good fat'.

10. Matcha Green Tea

Another super Sirtfood is Matcha green tea. Green tea, especially Matcha green tea, contains catechins, a group of powerful flavonoids that promote fat loss.

One type of catechins that is primarily found in Matcha green tea, Epigallocatechin Gallate (EGCG), is indeed a Sirtuin activator.

Matcha is processed in a particular way which makes it retain its EGCG properties, unlike other types of green tea.

Green tea also promotes weight loss and weight management due to the fact that:

Improves Breakdown of Fat Cells: Before your body can burn down the excess fat that it has accumulated over time, it must first break down the fat cells.

Some special foods such as green tea however contribute to the breakdown of fat cells by inhibiting norepinephrine, an enzyme that often prevents easy breakdown of fat cells.

Improves Fat Burning During Workout: If you have an active lifestyle or you work out regularly, consuming Matcha green tea will help to increase the rate at which your body burns fat during physical activities.

Reduces Appetite: Just like coffee, Matcha green tea suppresses your appetite and helps you make healthier food choices.

Helps Burn Stubborn Abdominal Fat: We all know how tough it can be to lose belly fat, the type of fat that lodges in your stomach, but Matcha green tea has been proven to be helpful for getting rid of this type of fat.

11. Kale

Everyone loves and eats kale, or don't we all? Well, we all should because kale is another super Sirtfood, thanks to its quercetin and kaempferol contents.

Kale is also great for weight loss because it:

 Acts as a Hunger Suppression: A single cup of kale has around 2.4 g of dietary fiber, and as you already know by now, fiber keeps you filled up for a very long time and prevents hunger.

 Contains Glucosinolate and Sulphur Compounds: Kale is filled with two very strong detoxifiers – sulphur compounds and glucosinolate.

 Both help to rid the body of toxins that make it harder for your body to break down and utilize stored up fats.

 Has Low Energy Density: Researchers have revealed that consuming foods with low energy density like kale can help you lose weight faster.

In one study conducted on a group of 200 obese women, the researchers found that subjects who consumed 2 servings of low energy-dense soup everyday lost 50% more weight compared to people who consumed high energy-dense foods.

In simpler words, it means that if I consume 3 meals of 250 calories each (750 calories in total), but with fewer kilocalories per gram, and you consume the same quantity of meals with similar calorie count but with a higher count of kilocalories per gram, I will most likely lose weight faster than you even though we're pretty much eating the same number of calories daily.

12. Lovage /Sea Parsley

It is important to not confuse lovage with flat-leaf parsley.

If you live in the US, you're probably more familiar with flat-leaf parsley, which is commonly used to garnish and spice up your meals.

But lovage is another member of the parsley family that is also known as sea parsley. Take note of this when you go grocery shopping so you can buy the right 16

Type of parsley.

Lovage contains apigen, another superb Sirtuin-activator. Lovage is also great for people who suffer from insomnia as apigen can bind to the benzodiazepine receptors in the human brain, helping to calm you down and promote sleep.

In addition to be a Sirtfood, lovage also helps with:

Digestion: Lovage promotes digestion and gastrointestinal health. It also reduces stomach bloating and gastrointestinal inflammation.

Kidney Health: A healthy functioning kidney is crucial to weight loss and weight management and lovage helps to promote kidney health by promoting detoxification and urination.

And you know what the best thing about lovage's diuretic effect is? It doesn't cause electrolytes loss like most diuretics do.

13. Red Chicory

Red chicory is a common secret ingredient in many weight loss herbal teas and supplements.

It is a Sirtuin-activator, and it also has many other weight loss benefits.

Contains Inulin: Red chicory is made up of 68% inulin, a type of carbohydrate that acts as a prebiotic.

It feeds the good bacteria in your gut, which is very important because these good bacteria help to fight off the bad bacteria that are often responsible for inflammation and many other digestive issues.

Improves Blood Sugar Control: Inulin also helps to improve blood sugar balance. It promotes carbohydrate absorption and helps to prevent blood sugar fluctuations.

Regulates Appetite: A group of researchers conducted a study where they placed 48 obese adults on 21 g of red chicory-derived oligofructose daily for 12 weeks.

They discovered that that oligofructose helped to reduce ghrelin, the hormone that stimulates hunger.

The participants reported less hunger and cravings and had better control of their appetite.

14. Red Endive

Red endives are rich in luteolin, another Sirtuin-activating compound. It helps to activate your skinny gene, and also helps with:

Helps to Keep Energy Levels Stable: Any successful weight loss program must have this important element. It must be able to keep your energy levels balanced.

If your energy levels keep fluctuating, it is unlikely that you'll be able to follow through with the diet and red chicory really helps with balancing your energy levels.

Slows Down Digestion: Red chicory also helps to slow down digestion, not in the way that you get constipated, but in a way that keeps you satiated for longer periods and keeps your appetite in check.

Rich in Antioxidants: Endives are also rich in powerful chemical compounds that neutralize free radicals and prevent cell damage.

15. Red Onions

The aromatic effect of red onions in your meals is enough reason for anyone to fall in love with them but its benefits surpass food flavoring.

Red onions are a rich source of the Sirtuin-activating compound, quercetin. In fact, of all the foods on this list, red onions have the highest amount of quercetin in them.

Other reasons why red onions are great for weight loss include:

Powerful Probiotic Food: Red onions, just like red chicory, contribute to gut health as they help to feed the good bacteria in your gut. This helps to prevent bloating and reduce abdominal fat.

Good Source of Fiber: Red onions are also a great source of fiber and help to reduce hunger and regulate appetite.

16. Red Wine

A diet that allows you to drink alcohol, who would have thought?

The Sirtfood diet is not one of those diets that won't allow you to have alcohol.

On this diet you can drink a glass of red wine daily as red wine is also Sirtuin-activating.

Women can have one 5-ounce glass of red wine, while men can have up to two 5-ounce glasses of red wine every day. You can also cook with it too.

Recommended red wine brands for the Sirtfood diet include Merlot, Pinot noir, and Cabernet Sauvignon.

17. Soy

Soy is a rich source of the Sirtuin activator, daidzein. It is also rich in another Sirtuin activator, formononetin.

However, you must avoid heavily processed soy products and opt for natural sources like tofu, miso, tempeh, and natto as the natural, unprocessed ones retain the Sirtuin-activating compounds you need.

Soy also promotes:

Satiety: Soy is rich in proteins, and it is a well-known fact that protein is very great for suppressing your appetite.

Appetite Control: Soy has a low glycemic index and can help with hunger prevention and appetite control.

18. Strawberries

Strawberries are great Sirtuin-activators too as they contain the plant compound, fisetin.

Strawberries also promote weight loss by:

Boosting Metabolism: Strawberries are rich in anthocyanins, another chemical compound that promotes the production of adiponectin, a hormone that helps to speed up metabolism and weight loss.

Helping to Reduce Fat: Strawberries are also rich in gallic acid which promotes the normal functioning of weight reducing hormones that are often blocked by chronic inflammation.

19. Turmeric

Turmeric contains curcumin. Curcumin is another Sirtuin-activating compound.

However, for your body to be able to properly and effectively absorb curcumin from turmeric, you have to combine it with black pepper, or cook it in fat or add it to a liquid or teas. This helps to promote the absorption of curcumin in your body.

Turmeric also aids:

Prevention of Metabolic Syndrome: Metabolic syndrome is often characterized by fat accumulation around your abdomen and is caused by insulin resistance.

Turmeric helps to prevent and control metabolic syndrome by controlling blood sugar levels, cholesterol, and triglycerides.

Increases Bile Production: Turmeric increases production of bile in the stomach, which helps to aid food digestion.

20. Walnuts

Walnuts are often listed as one of the top nuts for weight loss and rightly so. Walnuts are Sirtuin-activating, help suppress hunger, and help with appetite control.

Other sirtfoods

There are a lot of other foods out there that produce moderate levels of sirtuin-activating nutrients. The sirtfood is all about inclusion so you are free to incorporate a variety of foods with sirtuin-activators in moderation. The more sirtfoods included in your diet the better. This enables you to include more of your favorite foods to derive the maximum satisfaction and pleasure from your meal.

To maintain and continue your weight loss and wellbeing, you are encouraged to include these foods as you expand the skills of your diet

Vegetables: artichokes, asparagus, bok choy/pakchoi, broccoli, frisée, green beans, shallots, watercress, white onions, yellow endive.

Nuts and seeds: chestnuts, chia seeds, peanuts, pecan nuts, pistachio nuts, sunflower seeds

Grains and pseudo-grain: popcorn, quinoa, whole-wheat flour

Beans: fava beans, white beans (e.g., cannellini or navy)

Beverages: black tea, white tea

Chapter 4: The Benefits of the Sirtfood Diet

Yes, you would lose weight, and you would be able to fit in your skinny jeans, and your friends wouldn't be able to hide their shock and admiration when they see the new you, and maybe you would even make headlines like our dear singer Adele, but that is not where the benefits of this diet ends.

Along with weight loss and weight management, the Sirtfood diet also offers a lot of health benefits.

The Health Benefits of the Sirtfood Diet

These are all the benefits you will enjoy following the Sirtfood diet:

- Muscle Gain: This is everyone's dream - we all want to lose weight without losing muscle tone. We don't want the loose skin and flabby abs, stomachs, and breasts that drastic weight loss often leaves behind.
- The Sirtfood diet will help you achieve this dream because it incorporates a lot of proteins in your daily diet, which help to promote muscle gain during fat loss.
- Diabetes: If you are suffering from diabetes or already showing symptoms of pre-diabetes, this diet can help to reboot your body and stop insulin resistance, which is often a precursor to diabetes.
- Memory Improvement: Some of the meals you'll be having on this diet, such as turmeric, are known to help with cognition problems and help with memory improvement.
- Lowers Blood Pressure and Improves Cardiovascular Health: By helping to rid the body of bad cholesterol and triglycerides that often block the arteries and make it harder for your body to pump blood, leading to high blood pressure.
- Boosts Energy: The Sirtfood diet, unlike many other diets that leave you feeling weak and un-der-motivated, helps to boost your energy levels 29
- Along with improving concentration so that it is easier for you to be productive and be your usual self even though you are on a diet.
- Appetite Control: Inability to control appetite is often a clog in the wheel of progress on any weight loss diet.
- Sirtuins will not only help you control your appetite by reducing blood sugar spikes, but it will also help to improve hormone balance so that your hunger and satiety hormones, ghrelin and leptin can start working normally again.
- Healthy Hair, Skin and Nails: Most of the Sirtfoods contain ingredients that help to boost hair, nail and skin health so get ready to glow and have better hair and nails on this diet.
- Boosts Fertility: This diet is also rich in vegetables, fruits and superfoods that are known to help boost fertility.

- It can also help to reverse the symptoms of Polycystic Ovary Syndrome (PCOS), which is often linked to obesity and excess weight.

Chapter 5: A 21 Days Sirt-food Diet Meal Plan

Experts in psychology have proven repeatedly over the years that it takes 21 days for the average human being to build a habit, and 90 days for that habit to become fully incorporated into his lifestyle. Building a habit can be challenging if you do not have a solid game plan, and that is our ambition for this chapter. In this chapter, we would build a 21-days sirtfood timetable that would help you get through Phases One and Two of the Sirtfood diet. Let's get moving!

DAYS	BREAKFAST	LUNCH	DINNER	SNACKS/DES-SERTS
1	Chocolate Gran-ola	Butternut pump-kin with buck-wheat	Tofu Thai Curry	Chocolate Maple Walnuts
2	Oatmeal Pan-cakes	Roasted Arti-choke Hearts	Beef bourgui-gnon with Mashed potatoes and kale	Matcha and Chocolate Dipped Straw-berries
3	Cinnamon Qui-noa	Beef Broth	Turkish fajitas	Vegan Rice Pud-ding
4	Buckwheat Por-ridge	Salmon and Ca-pers	Sirt Chicken Korma	Plum Oat Bars
5	Chocolate Gran-ola	Pasta Salad	Tomato Chicken Mix	Spinach and Kale Mix
6	Apple Pancakes	Sirtfood Cara-mel Coated Cat-fish	Chicken and Veggies	Kale Dip with Cajun Pita Chips
7	Breakfast Muesli	Lentil Tacos	Japanese Chicken Thighs	Triple Chocolate Chip Deep Dish Cookies
8	Sirtfood Scram-bled Eggs	Lentil and Qui-noa Salad	Air Fried Whole Chicken	Protein Brown-ies

9	Strawberry Buckwheat Pancakes	Sloppy Joes	Perfect Garlic Butter Steak	Protein Pumpkin Spiced Donuts
10	Blackcurrants Pancakes	Lentil Burgers	Crispy Pork Medallions	Wrapped Plums
11	Creamy Coconut Porridge	Potato Salad	Prawns, Pak Choi and broccoli	Cucumber Sandwich Bites
12	Salmon & Kale Omelet	Ginger Brown Rice	Cocoa spaghetti <u>Bolognese</u>	Cocoa and Nuts Bombs
13	Sirtfood Green Onion and Mushroom Omelet	Pasta with kale and Black Olive	Baked salmon with Watercress sauce and <u>Potatoes</u>	Sweet Cinnamon Peaches
14	Buckwheat Granola	Asparagus Soup	Coq au vin with potatoes and green beans	Chocolate strawberry milk
15	Sirtfood Muffins	Kale White Bean Pork chops	Beans & Kale Soup	Green tea and Rocket smoothie
16	Fruity Tofu Smoothie	Tuna Salad	Beef bourguignon with Mashed potatoes and kale	Chocolate strawberry milk
17	Black currants and oat yogurt	Turkey Curry	Barbecued Lime Shrimp	Pineapple Lassi
18	Easy Granola Clusters	Tofu and Curry	Crispy Shrimp	Sirt shot
19	Stovetop Granola	Chicken and Bean Casserole	Spicy Air-Fried Cheese Tilapia	Hot chocolate eggnog
20	No Bake Peanut Butter Granola Bars	Prawn and Coconut Curry	Cheese Salmon	Mint julep
21	Banana Muesli with Dates	Moroccan Chicken Casserole	Herb Salmon Fillet	Gingerbread latte

Chapter 6: Phase 1 of the Sirtfood Diet: Restriction

The first stage of the sirtfood is known as the first phase, or more commonly, 'Phase 1'. Phase 1 is basically the first seven days of the sirtfood diet regimen. Phase 1 is the most intense phase of the sirtfood diet as it is the only phase where you cannot consume above a specified number of calories. In the first three days of phase 1, the maximum permissible number of calories that can be consumed per day is one thousand. In the last four days, the maximum permissible number of consumable calories moves up to 1500. The ambition of the first phase of the sirtfood diet is to help you hit the ground running and activate your sirtuin genes. The restricted number of calories will aid in the activation of your body's stress pathways, which would eventually, together with the action other polyphenols in the sirtfoods, lead to the activation of the sirtuin genes.

At the conclusive end of the first phase, the average mass of fat that would be lost should be between 5 to 7 pounds. However, your body is most likely going to retain all of its muscle or even add up some more, so using a weighing scale to judge the progress of phase 2 might not be such a good idea. So, phase 1 is basically the first seven days of your sirtfood diet.

How do you prepare for phase 1?

When you start out on the sirtfood diet, you are preparing to begin a journey to a new kind of freedom and liberation – freedom from your self-imposed shackles of poor eating habits into a world where you have control over what goes in your body. To get started out for phase 1, you will need to put a couple of things in place. These include:

A juicer: A lot of modern households already use a juicer in one way or the other on a fairly regular basis. The juicer would be used in the preparation of the sirtfood green juice, a natural concoction of herbs that would help detoxify your body and get you started on dissolving those fatty deposits. Since the aim of the juicer is to extract as much liquid as possible from vegetables, be sure to get one that is better equipped for the type of food products you would be putting in it.

Secondly, you would need to get familiar with your sirtfood menu and see where exactly you can get all these foods in your neighborhood. Depending on your city, you may be able to get all the sirtfoods you need in your local grocery store, or you may need to try shopping in the open market to get some of the vegetables and food items on the list. The point, however, is to get familiar with the foods that will be forming your new regimen and to figure out how you'd be sourcing these foods.

Thirdly, you need to figure out a means of preserving the foods you'd be purchasing beforehand. If you have steady access to electricity and a refrigerator, it is advised that you shop for three days' worth of vegetable supplies at once and store the veggies in your fridge for when you need to make your meals. After three days, you'd need another supply of veggies. The three-day limit is set to prevent spoilage of the veggies, which would only affect the quality of your food and the rate of your development.

It is also pertinent for you to learn how to prepare the foods you would prepare beforehand. The sirtfood menu features a variety of food options, so it's okay for you to select a few that you can confidently cook right away. As you progress in your journey in the diet, you will gradually learn how to cook more foods and expand your diet.

Next, it is also critically important for you to plan your eating timetable beforehand. Your sirtfood green juice should be consumed three times per day in the first three days – once when you wake up, thirty minutes to one hour before any meal, and then two other times within the day. Look at your number of calories and plan out when you would be eating and what you would be eating on each day. This will make it an effortless route for you to make these decisions when you finally begin your diet.

Journaling can be very helpful in helping you stay steadfast on your personal journey. Keeping a journal allows you to keep a chronological record of your struggles and your victories as you go through the sirtfood diet. Trying to use the scales to monitor your progress, especially so early into your dieting journey, is a bad idea. As has been repeatedly mentioned, the sirtfood diet helps you to burn fats as well as maintain and even build muscle mass. So, as you gear up to begin phase 1 of your diet, try as much as possible to stay off the scales for the meantime and just focus on sticking to this wonderful dieting system.

Finally, get excited about the journey ahead. To accomplish this, it helps if you can figure out exactly why you are embarking on the sirtfood diet. Are you doing it to reduce your risk of contracting a dangerous life-threatening disease along the line? Are you doing it to enhance your career in the media or modeling industry? Are you doing it to improve your mental health and improve your moods, focus, and concentration? Whatever be your reason for wanting to make the important personal sacrifice of starting up the sirtfood diet, remind yourself that you are finally about to achieve those aims. Be excited that your life is about to experience a positive turn around.

Expectations for Phase 1

You may wonder – what exactly is Phase 1 going to entail, and what results can I expect to achieve after the first week of my diet? With great sacrifice, they say, comes great rewards. Phase 1 is going to be the most tasking phase of your diet, no doubt, but it will also be the phase that provides you with the most pleasantly surprising results. At the end of phase 1, you can expect to lose between 5 to 7 pounds of weight in pure fat, as evidenced by the results of the cohort study carried out in London. You can also expect to experience enhanced mental clarity and focus, and a general feeling of lightness and agility. However, since phase 1 is going to be your stage of making the most important sacrifices for future benefits, it also means you would probably have to deal with some discomfort during this phase. Not everybody would experience these signs, but some participants in the diet have reported feelings of hunger, lethargy, slight irritability, and even strong cravings for junk food and sugary snacks and drinks during the first phase. It is believed that the restriction of the calories consumed by the participant in the first three days to one thousand calories, and to fifteen hundred calories in the last four days of phase one is responsible for these challenges.

So, if you feel really hungry, tired, or extremely desirous of junk food during your first phase, be patient. Remember your reason for starting this and renew your resolve to stay strong and fight for the dazzling life you've dreamed of every single day. Usually, in the final days of phase one, as your body gets used to the diet, you will feel your fatigue and tiredness slipping away, and these feelings would become replaced by feelings of strength, clarity, and agility. As you switch from one thousand calories to fifteen hundred calories per day, you will feel more satiated and energized too, and your moods will generally improve. From this point onwards, your journey becomes progressively easier.

Meal plan for Phase 1

For the first three days of the sirtfood diet, you will be expected to drink three sirtfood juices and eat one mail sirtfood meal per day. This combination helps to keep the number of calories consumed just under one thousand. For the last four days of the first phase, however, you will be required to eat two main sirtfood meals and two sirtfood juices on a daily basis. This combination would sum up to about fifteen hundred calories.

As you can probably already predict, the sirtfood green juice would be an essential part of your sirtfood diet in phase one and beyond. After water, this drink would constitute a major percentage of your total fluid intake as you proceed with the sirtfood diet. Other fluids that you would be permitted to consume would include black coffee (i.e., without milk) and green tea. Milk should be abstained from during the first phase of the sirtfood diet as it contains active substances that may hamper the activation of the sirtuin genes.

Since the sirtfood green juice is so critical to the success of your sirtfood diet, let's examine exactly how to make the sirtfood green juice before delving into what your model meal plan should look like.

To prepare the sirtfood green juice, you'll need:

2.5 oz. kale

1 oz. arugula

0.25 oz. flat-leaf parsley

5.5 oz. celery stalks (with leaves)

0.5 medium green apple

1 in. ginger

Half of a lemon squeezed or juiced.

0.5 tsp. matcha powder

Note that the matcha powder should only be included only in the first two juices of the day during the first three days of phase one. Basically, between day 1 and 3, only the juice you'd be drinking very early in the morning before breakfast, and the drink you'll be having by midmorning should contain matcha. Your third sirtfood juice of the day should not contain matcha powder because the substance has been found to be caffeinated and may alter your sleep pattern if taken too late in the day. So, do not forget – no matcha for the last juice of the day between days 1 and 3.

For the final four days of phase one, however, it is okay to put matcha powder in the two sirtfood juices you'll be drinking daily. This is because you'd have completed your daily required sirtfood juice intake by midday, provided you follow the laid-down guidelines.

So, now that you know the ingredients and you know the sirtfood juice rules let's get into the nitty-gritty of making this wonderfully wholesome drink.

First of all, mix your veggies in the juicer. This means your arugula, kale, and parsley should be loaded into the juicer. Ensure to extract as much fluid as possible from these greens to ensure that you get maximum value for your time, effort, and money. After the juicing process, you should have obtained about a quarter of a cup of veggie juice. Absolutely delicious, yeah?

The next step is to lead your apples, ginger, and celery into the juicer and extract the fluid from those too. Add this new mixture to the one obtained in the first step.

Next, peel your lemon, cut it in half, and squeeze out the juice. If you feel that your squeezing is not efficient enough, you can use the juicer instead. After adding the lemon juice to your mixture, you should have about a cup of juice ready.

Pour out a small portion of your juice and add in your half teaspoon of matcha powder. Ensure that the matcha dissolves properly in the juice, and then pour the matcha-containing juice into the rest of the juice.

Stir your juice properly, and you may add a little water to adjust the taste if you like. Enjoy the immaculate taste of good health!

Now that you have gotten a good grasp of how to make your sirtfood green juice, it's time to design a workable meal plan that would allow you to access a variety of sirtfoods to aid your progress in phase 1. Remember that in each day for your first three days, you must drink a cup of sirtfood green juice thrice and eat a sirtfood main meal once. For the remaining four days of Phase 1, its two sirtfood juices and two main meals to give fifteen hundred calories.

Let's break the meal plan down now.

Day 1: Sirtfood green juice – 3 times Main meal – 1 time

Meal idea: Stir-fried Asian shrimp, buckwheat noodles and dark chocolate (85% cocoa) Vegan option: Sesame glazed tofu, miso, ginger, chili, stir-fried greens, and dark chocolate (85% cocoa).

Day 2: Sirtfood green juice – 3 times Main meal: 1 time

Meal idea: Aromatic chicken breast, kale, red onions, tomato, and chili salsa Vegan option: Kale, red onion dal, and buckwheat.

Day 3: Sirtfood green juice – 3 times Main meal: 1 time

Meal idea: Turkey escalope, capers, sage, parsley, cauliflower, and dark chocolate.

Vegan option: Baked tofu, cauliflower, and dark chocolate.

From day four onwards, you can eat ½ oz. Dark chocolate once a day, preferably alongside one meal.

Day 4: Sirtfood green juice – 2 times Main meal: 2 times

Meal 1: Sirt muesli

Meal 2: Salmon fillet, endive, arugula, and celery salad.

Vegan option 1: Sirt muesli

Vegan option 2: Tuscan bean stew.

Day 5: Sirtfood green juice – 2 times Main meal: 2 times

Meal 1 (Vegan and regular diets): Sirt super salad.

Meal 2 (regular diet): Grilled beef, red wine, onion rings, garlic, kale, and roasted potatoes.

Meal 2 (Vegan diet): Kidney bean mole and baked potatoes.

Day 6: Sirtfood green juice – 2 times Main meal: 2 times

Meal 1: Sirtfood omelet

Meal 2: Baked chicken breast, parsley pesto, red onion salad.

Vegan option 1: Waldorf salad.

Vegan option 2: Roasted eggplants, walnuts, parsley pesto, and tomato salad.

Day 7: Sirtfood green juice – 2 times Main meal: 2 times

Meal 1: Strawberry buckwheat salad

Meal 2: Baked cod marinated in miso, sesame, and stir-fried greens Vegan option 1: Strawberry buckwheat salad.

Vegan option 2: Buckwheat noodles in miso broth, tofu, celery, and kale.

Lara Burns

Breakfasts

Chocolate Granola

Preparation Time: 10 minutes

Cooking Time: 38 minutes

Servings: 8

Ingredients:

- ¼ cup cacao powder
- ¼ cup maple syrup
- 2 tablespoons coconut oil, melted
- ½ teaspoon vanilla extract
- 1/8 teaspoon salt
- 2 cups gluten-free rolled oats
- ¼ cup unsweetened coconut flakes
- 2 tablespoons chia seeds
- 2 tablespoons unsweetened dark chocolate, chopped finely

Directions:

1. Preheat your oven to 300°F.
2. Line a medium baking sheet with parchment paper.
3. In a medium pan, add the cacao powder, maple syrup, coconut oil, vanilla extract and salt and mix well.
4. Now, place pan over medium heat and cook for about 2-3 minutes or until thick and syrupy, stirring continuously.
5. Remove the pan of mixture from the heat and set aside.
6. In a large bowl, add the oats, coconut and chia seeds and mix well.
7. Add the syrup mixture and mix until well combined.
8. Transfer the granola mixture onto a prepared baking sheet and spread in an even layer.
9. Bake for approximately 35 minutes.
10. Remove the baking sheet from oven and set aside for about 1 hour.
11. Add the chocolate pieces and stir to combine.
12. Serve immediately.

Nutrition:

Calories 193

Total Fat 9.1 g

Saturated Fat 5.2 g

Cholesterol 0 mg

Sodium 37 mg

Total Carbs 26.1 g

Fiber 4.6 g

Sugar 5.9 g

Protein 5 g

Oatmeal Pancakes

Preparation Time: 15 minutes

Cooking Time: 5 minutes

Servings: 8

Ingredients:

- 1 cup whole wheat pancake mix
- 1/8 cup chopped walnuts
- ¼ cup old-fashioned oats

Directions:

1. Make the pancake mix according to the directions on the package.
2. Add walnuts, and oats.
3. Coat a skillet with cooking spray.
4. Add about ¼ cup of the batter onto the griddle when hot.
5. Turn pancake over when bubbles form on top.
6. Cook until golden brown.
7. Serve immediately.

Nutrition:

Calories - 155

Fat - 4 g

Carbs – 28 g

Protein – 7 g

Cinnamon Quinoa

Preparation Time: 5 minutes

Cooking Time: 6 minutes

Servings: 4

Ingredients:

- Chopped walnuts
- 1 ½ cup water
- Maple syrup
- 2 cinnamon sticks
- 1 cup quinoa, washed and drained

Directions:

1. Prepare your pressure cooker with a trivet and steaming basket.
2. Place the quinoa, and the cinnamon sticks in the basket and pour the water, then close and lock the lid.
3. Cook at high pressure for 6 minutes. When the cooking time is up, release the pressure using the quick-release method.
4. Fluff the quinoa with a fork and remove the cinnamon sticks.
5. Divide the cooked quinoa among serving bowls and top with maple syrup and chopped walnuts.

Nutrition:

Calories - 160

Fat - 3 g

Carbs – 28 g

Protein – 6 g

Buckwheat Porridge

Preparation Time: 10 minutes

Cooking Time: 15 minutes

Servings: 2

Ingredients:

- 1 cup buckwheat, rinsed
- 1 cup unsweetened almond milk

- 1 cup water
- ½ tsp. Ground cinnamon
- ½ tsp. vanilla extract
- 2 tbsp. raw honey
- ¼ cup fresh blueberries

Directions:

1. In a pan, add all the ingredients (except honey and blueberries) over medium-high heat and bring to a boil.
2. Reduce the heat to low and simmer, covered for about 10 minutes.
3. Stir in the honey and remove from the heat. Set aside, covered, for about 5 minutes.
4. With a fork, fluff the mixture, and transfer into serving bowls.
5. Top with blueberries and serve.

Nutrition:

Calories - 358

Fat - 4.7 g

Carbs – 3.7 g

Protein – 12 g

Chocolate Granola

Preparation Time: 10 minutes

Cooking Time: 38 minutes

Servings: 8

Ingredients:

- ¼ cup cacao powder
- ¼ cup maple syrup
- 2 tbsp. Coconut oil, melted
- ½ tsp. vanilla extract
- 1/8 tsp. salt
- 2 cups gluten-free rolled oats
- ¼ cup unsweetened coconut flakes
- 2 tbsp. chia seeds
- 2 tbsp. unsweetened dark chocolate, chopped finely

Directions:

1. Preheat your oven to 300ºF and line a medium baking sheet with parchment paper.
2. In a medium pan, add the cacao powder, maple syrup, coconut oil, vanilla extract, and salt, and mix well.
3. Place a pan over medium heat and cook for about 2–3 minutes, or until thick and syrupy, stirring continuously.
4. Remove from the heat and set aside. In a large bowl, add the oats, coconut, and chia seeds and mix well.
5. Add the syrup mixture and mix until well combined.
6. Transfer the granola mixture onto a prepared baking sheet and spread it in an even layer—Bake it for about 35 minutes.
7. Remove from the oven and set aside to cool.
8. Add the chocolate pieces and stir to combine.
9. Enjoy.

Nutrition:

Calories - 193

Fat - 9.1 g

Carbs – 26.1 g

Protein – 5 g

Apple Pancakes

Preparation Time: 10 minutes

Cooking Time: 24 minutes

Servings: 6

Ingredients:

- ½ cup buckwheat flour
- 2 tbsp. coconut sugar
- 1 tsp. Baking powder
- ½ tsp. ground cinnamon
- 1/3 cup unsweetened almond milk
- 1 egg, beaten lightly

- 2 granny smith apples, peeled, cored, and grated

Directions:

1. In a bowl, place the flour, coconut sugar, and cinnamon, and mix well.
2. In another bowl, place the almond milk and egg and beat until well combined.
3. Place the flour mixture and mix until well combined.
4. Fold in the grated apples.
5. Add the desired amount of mixture and, with a spoon, spread into an even layer.
6. Cook for 2 minutes on each side.
7. Repeat with the remaining mixture.
8. Serve warm with the drizzling of honey.

Nutrition:

Calories - 93

Fat - 2.1 g

Carbs – 22 g

Protein – 2.5 g

Breakfast Muesli

Preparation Time: 10 minutes

Cooking Time: 0 minutes

Servings: 2

Ingredients:

- ¾ oz. Buckwheat drops
- ⅜ oz. Buckwheat puffs
- ½ oz. coconut drops or dried up coconut
- 1 ½ oz. Medjool dates hollowed and slashed
- ½ oz. Pecans slashed
- ⅜ oz. cocoa nibs
- 3 ½ oz. strawberries, hulled and slashed
- 3 ½ oz. plain Greek yogurt

Directions:

1. In a blender, put all the listed ingredients.
2. Blend until smooth

3. Serve straight away.

Nutrition:

Calories - 334

Fat - 22.58 g

Carbs – 34.35 g

Protein – 4.39 g

Sirtfood Scrambled Eggs

Preparation Time: 15 minutes

Cooking Time: 7 minutes

Servings: 1

Ingredients:

- 1 tsp extra virgin olive oil
- ¾ oz. red onion, finely chopped
- ½ bird's eye chili, finely chopped
- 3 medium eggs
- 1.7 fl. oz. milk
- 1 tsp ground turmeric
- 3/16 oz. parsley, finely chopped

Directions:

1. In a skillet, heat the oil over high heat.
2. Toss in the red onion and chili, frying for 3 minutes.
3. In a large bowl, whisk together the milk, parsley, eggs, and turmeric.
4. Pour into the skillet and lower to medium heat.
5. Cook for 4 minutes, scrambling the mixture as you do with a spoon or spatula.
6. Serve immediately.

Nutrition:

Calories - 224

Fat - 14.63 g

Carbs – 4.79 g

Protein – 17.2 g

Strawberry Buckwheat Pancakes

Preparation Time: 5 minutes

Cooking Time: 6 minutes

Servings: 4

Ingredients:

- 3½ oz. strawberries, chopped
- 3½ oz. buckwheat flour
- 1 egg
- 8 fl oz. milk
- 1 tsp. olive oil
- 1 tsp. olive oil for frying
- Freshly squeezed juice of 1 orange

Directions:

1. Pour the milk into a bowl and mix in the egg and a tsp. of olive oil.
2. Sift in the flour to the liquid mixture until smooth and creamy.
3. Allow it to rest for 15 minutes.
4. Heat a little oil in a pan and pour in a quarter of the mixture or to the size you prefer.
5. Sprinkle in a quarter of the strawberries into the batter.
6. Cook for around 2 minutes on each side.
7. Serve hot with a drizzle of orange juice.

Nutrition:

Calories - 180

Fat - 7.5 g

Carbs – 22.58 g

Protein – 7.46 g

Blackcurrants Pancakes

Preparation Time: 5 minutes

Cooking Time: 50 minutes

Servings: 4

Ingredients:

- 2 apples, cut into small chunks
- 2 cups of quick-cooking oats

- 1 cup flour of your choice
- 1 tsp baking powder
- 2 tbsp. honey
- 2 egg whites
- 1 ¼ cups of milk
- 2 tsp extra virgin olive oil
- A dash of salt
- For the berry topping:
- 1 cup blackcurrants, washed and stalks removed
- 3 tbsp. water
- 2 tbsp. honey

Directions:

1. Place the ingredients for the topping in a small pot simmer, frequently stirring for about 10 minutes until it cooks down and the juices are released.
2. Take the dry ingredients and mix them in a bowl. Afterward, add the apples and the milk a bit at a time you may not use it all) until it is a batter.
3. Stiffly whisk the egg whites and then gently mix them into the pancake batter. Set aside in the refrigerator.
4. Pour a one-quarter of the oil onto a flat pan or flat griddle, and when hot, pour some of the batter into it in a pancake shape.
5. When the pancakes start to have golden brown edges and form air bubbles, they may be ready to be gently flipped.
6. Repeat for the next three pancakes.
7. Top each pancake with the berries.

Nutrition:

Calories - 470

Fat - 16.83 g

Carbs – 79 g

Protein – 11.

71 g

Creamy Coconut Porridge

Preparation Time: 24 hours 20 minutes

Cooking Time: 5 minutes

Servings: 2

Ingredients:

- ¼ cup walnuts
- ½ cup Roasted Buckwheat Kernels
- 2 Medjool dates pitted
- 1 tbsp. chia seeds
- 1 tbsp. pure maple syrup
- 1 cup of coconut milk
- Pinch of salt

Directions:

1. In a large glass jar, soak the kasha and walnuts overnight.
2. Rinse the kasha and walnuts through a fine-mesh strainer under running water. Shaking the strainer several times, ensures thorough rinsing.
3. Place all the ingredients in a blender and blend for about 20 seconds.
4. Scrape down sides and blend again for another 10 seconds.
5. It can be served chilled or gently warmed.
6. Top with favourite toppings, and enjoy!

Nutrition:

Calories – 420

Fat - 28g

Carbs – 57g

Protein – 12g

Salmon & Kale Omelet

Preparation Time: 10 minutes

Cooking Time: 6 minutes

Servings: 4

Ingredients:

- 6 eggs

- 2 tbsp unsweetened almond milk
- Salt and black pepper, to taste
- 2 tbsp olive oil
- 4 oz. smoked salmon, cut into bite-sized chunks
- 2 cups fresh kale, tough ribs removed and chopped finely
- 4 scallions, chopped finely

Directions:

1. In a bowl, place the eggs, coconut milk, salt, and black pepper, and beat well then set aside.
2. In a non-stick wok, heat the oil over medium heat. Place the egg mixture and cook for about 30 seconds, without stirring.
3. Place the salmon kale and scallions on top of egg mixture evenly.
4. Reduce the heat to low.
5. With the lid, cover the wok and cook for about 4 minutes, or until omelet is done completely.
6. Uncover the wok and cook for about 1 minute.
7. Transfer the omelet onto a serving plate and serve.

Nutrition:

Calories 210

Fat 14.9 g

Carbs 5.2 g

Protein 14.8 g

Sirtfood Green Onion and Mushroom Omelet

Preparation Time: 10 minutes

Cooking Time: 5 minutes

Servings: 2

Ingredients:

- 6 oz. crimini mushrooms
- 2 tbsps. Plus 2 tsps. Butter

- 5 tbsps. Chopped green onions
- 1/4 cup dry vermouth
- 6 large eggs
- 1 tbsp. water
- 1/4 tsp. salt
- 1/4 tsp. ground black pepper

Directions:

1. In processor, finely chop mushrooms. Melt 2 tbsp. butter on medium high heat in medium skillet. Add 3 tbsp. onions and mushrooms; sauté for 3 minutes.
2. Add vermouth; boil for 1 1/2 minutes till evaporated. Season with pepper and salt.
3. Whisk pepper, salt, 1 tbsp. water and eggs to blend in medium bowl. Melt 1 tsp. butter on medium heat in small non-stick skillet.
4. Add 1/2 egg mixture; mix with back of a fork till edges start to set. Cook, lifting edges using a spatula so uncooked egg flows underneath, for 2 minutes till omelet is set.
5. Put 1/2 mushroom mixture down the middle of omelet then folds both omelet sides over fillingput onto plate.
6. Repeat using leftover mushroom mixture, egg mixture and butter. Sprinkle leftover onions on omelets.

Nutrition:

Calories per serving: 399

Carbohydrates: 15g

Protein: 1g

Fat: 0g

Sugar: 0.6g

Sodium: 506mg

Fiber: 1g

Lunch

Butternut pumpkin with buckwheat

Preparation Time: 5 Minutes

Cooking time: 50 Minutes

Servings: 4

Ingredients:

- One tablespoon of extra virgin olive oil
- One red onion, finely chopped
- One tablespoon fresh ginger, finely chopped
- Three cloves of garlic, finely chopped
- Two small chilies, finely chopped
- One tablespoon cumin
- One cinnamon stick
- Two tablespoons turmeric
- 800g chopped canned tomatoes
- 300ml vegetable broth
- 100g dates, seeded and chopped
- one 400g tin of chickpeas, drained
- 500g butter squash, peeled, seeded and cut into pieces
- 200g buckwheat
- 5g coriander, chopped
- 10g parsley, chopped

Directions:

1. Preheat the oven to 400 °.
2. Heat the olive oil in a frying pan and sauté the onion, ginger, garlic, and Thai chili. After two minutes, add cumin, cinnamon, and turmeric and cook for another two minutes while stirring.
3. Add the tomatoes, dates, stock, and chickpeas, stir well and cook over low heat for 45 to 60 minutes. Add some water as required. In the meantime, mix the pumpkin pieces with olive oil. Bake in the oven for about 30 minutes until soft.
4. Cook the buckwheat according to the directions and add the remaining turmeric. When everything is cooked, add the pumpkin to the other ingredients in the roaster and serve with the buckwheat. Sprinkle with coriander and parsley.

Nutrition:

Calories per serving 248.1

Total Fat .8.7g

Saturated fat per serving 2.6g

Monounsaturated fat per serving 1.5g

Polyunsaturated fat per serving 4.0g

Protein per serving 8.5g

Roasted Artichoke Hearts

Preparation Time: 5 minutes

Cooking Time: 40 minutes

Servings: 3

Ingredients:

- 2 cans artichoke hearts
- 4 garlic cloves, quartered
- 2 tsp extra virgin olive oil
- 1 tsp dried oregano
- salt and pepper, to taste
- 2-3 tbsp lemon juice, to serve

Directions:

1. Preheat oven to 375F.
2. Drain the artichoke hearts and rinse them very thoroughly.
3. Toss them in garlic, oregano, and olive oil.
4. Arrange the artichoke hearts in a baking dish and bake for about 45 minutes tossing a few times if desired.
5. Season with salt and pepper and serve with lemon juice.

Nutrition:

Calories: 35

Fat: 20 g

Carbohydrates: 3 g

Protein: 1 g

Fiber: 1 g

Beef Broth

Preparation Time: 5 minutes

Cooking Time: 40 minutes

Servings: 3

Ingredients:

- 4-5 pounds beef bones and few veal bones
- 1 pound of stew meat (chuck or flank steak) cut into 2-inch chunks
- Olive oil
- 1-2 medium red onions, peeled and quartered
- 1-2 large carrots, cut into 1-2-inch segments
- 1 celery rib, cut into 1-inch segments
- 2-3 cloves of garlic, unpeeled
- A handful of parsley stems and leaves
- 1-2 bay leaves
- 10 peppercorns

Directions:

1. Heat oven to 375F.
2. Rub olive oil over the stew meat pieces, carrots, and onions.
3. Put stew meat or beef scraps, stock bones, carrots, and onions in a large roasting pan.
4. Roast in the oven for about 45 minutes, turning everything halfway through the cooking.
5. Place everything from the oven in a large stockpot.
6. Pour some boiling water in the oven pan and scrape up all the browned bits and pour all in the stockpot.
7. Add parsley, celery, garlic, bay leaves, and peppercorns to the pot.
8. Fill the pot with cold water, to 1-inch over the top of the bones.

9. Bring the stockpot to a regular simmer and then reduce the heat to low, so it just barely simmers. Cover the pot loosely and let simmer low and slow for 3-4 hours.
10. Scoop away the fat and any scum that rises to the surface occasionally.
11. After cooking, remove the bones and vegetables from the pot.
12. Strain the broth.
13. Let cool to room temperature and then put in the refrigerator.
14. The fat will solidify once the broth has chilled.
15. Discard the fat (or reuse it) and pour the broth into a jar and freeze it.

Nutrition:

Calories: 65

Fat: 1 g

Carbohydrates: 2 g

Protein: 3 g

Fiber: 0 g

Salmon and Capers

Preparation Time: 5 minutes

Cooking Time: 40 minutes

Servings: 3

Ingredients:

- 75g (3oz) Greek yoghurt
- 4 salmon fillets, skin removed
- 4 tsp Dijon mustard
- 1 tbsp capers, chopped
- 2 tsp fresh parsley
- Zest of 1 lemon

Directions:

1. In a bowl, mix the yoghurt, mustard, lemon zest, parsley, and capers.
2. Thoroughly coat the salmon in the mixture.

3. Place the salmon under a hot grill (broiler) and cook for 3-4 minutes on each side, or until the fish is cooked.
4. Serve with mashed potatoes and vegetables or a large green leafy salad.

Nutrition:

Calories: 283

Fat: 25 g

Carbohydrates: 1 g

Protein: 20 g

Fiber: 0 g

Pasta Salad

Preparation Time: 5 minutes

Cooking Time: 40 minutes

Servings: 3

- **Ingredients:**
- A plate of mixed greens ingredients
- 1 box (16 ounces) elbow pasta
- 4 cups of water
- 1 tbsp fit salt
- 2 tbsp olive oil
- ½ cup red onion, diced
- 1 cup simmered red peppers, daintily cut
- ¼ cup dark olives, cut
- ½ pound (8 ounces) crisp mozzarella, diced
- ½ cup slashed basil
- Red wine vinaigrette ingredients
- 1 box (16 ounces) elbow pasta
- 4 cups of water
- 1 tbsp fit salt
- 2 tbsp olive oil
- ½ cup red onion, diced
- 1 cup simmered red peppers, daintily cut
- ¼ cup dark olives, cut
- ½ pound (8 ounces) crisp mozzarella, diced

- ½ cup slashed basil

Directions:

1. Amass pressure top, ensuring the weight discharge valve is in the seal position.
2. Select pressure and set it to high. Set time to 3 minutes.
3. Select start/stop to start.
4. While the pasta is cooking, set up the red wine vinaigrette.
5. In a blending bowl, join all vinaigrette fixings aside from olive oil.
6. Gradually speed in the olive oil until wholly joined.
7. Taste and alter seasonings as wanted.
8. Put in a safe spot.
9. At the point when weight cooking is finished, enable the strain to discharge for 10 minutes regularly.
10. Following 10 minutes, snappy discharge remaining weight by moving the weight discharge valve to the vent position.
11. Cautiously expel top when the unit has completed the process of discharging pressure.
12. Evacuate the pot and strain the pasta in a colander.
13. Move to a bowl and hurl with 2 tbsp of olive oil.
14. Spot bowl in cooler and enable pasta to cool for 20 minutes.
15. When pasta has cooled, mix in red onion, broiled peppers, dark olives, mozzarella, and basil.
16. Delicately crease in the red wine vinaigrette.
17. Serve quickly or cover and refrigerate for serving later.

Nutrition:

Calories: 248

Fat: 6 g

Carbohydrates: 36 g

Protein: 9 g

Fiber: 0 g

Sirtfood Caramel Coated Catfish

Preparation time: 15 minutes

Cooking time: 45 minutes

Serving: 4

Ingredients:

- 1/3 cup water
- 2 tbsps. Fish sauce
- 2 shallots, chopped
- 4 cloves garlic, minced
- 1 1/2 tsps. Ground black pepper
- 1/4 tsp. red pepper flakes
- 1/3 cup water
- 1/3 cup white sugar
- 2 lbs. catfish fillets
- 1/2 tsp. white sugar
- 1 tbsp. fresh lime juice
- 1 green onion, thinly sliced
- 1/2 cup chopped cilantro

Directions:

1. Combine fish sauce and 1/3 cup of water in a small bowl; mix and put aside.
2. Combine together shallots, red pepper flakes, black pepper and garlic in another bowl and put aside.
3. Heat 1/3 cup of sugar and 1/3 cup of water in a big skillet placed over medium heat, stirring from time to time until sugar becomes deep golden brown. Stir in the fish sauce mixture gently and let the mixture boil. Mix and cook the shallot mixture.
4. Once the shallots have softened, add the catfish to the mixture.
5. Cook the catfish with cover for about 5 minutes each side until the fish can be easily flake using a fork. Transfer the catfish to a large plate, place a cover,

and put aside. Adjust the heat to high and mix in a half tsp. of sugar.
6. Stir in any sauce that left on the plate and the lime juice.
7. Let it boil and simmer until the sauce has cooked down.
8. Drizzle the sauce on top of the catfish and sprinkle with cilantro and green onions.

Nutrition:

Calories per serving: 254

Carbohydrates: 4g

Protein: 1g

Fat: 0.5g

Sugar: 3g

Sodium: 96mg

Fiber: 1g

Lentil Tacos

Preparation time: 10 minutes

Cooking time: 12 minutes

Servings: 8

Ingredients:

- 2 cups cooked lentils
- ½ cup chopped green bell pepper
- ½ cup chopped white onion
- ½ cup halved grape tomatoes
- 1 teaspoon minced garlic
- ½ teaspoon garlic powder
- 1 teaspoon red chili powder
- ½ teaspoon smoked paprika
- ½ teaspoon ground cumin
- 8 whole-grain tortillas

Directions:

1. Take a large skillet pan, place it over medium heat, add oil, and let it heat.
2. Add onion, bell pepper, and garlic, stir until mixed, and then cook for 5 minutes until vegetables begin to soften.

3. Add lentils and tomatoes, stir in all the spices and then continue cooking for 5 minutes until hot.
4. Assemble the tacos and for this, heat the tortillas until warmed and then fill each tortilla with ¼ cup of the cooked lentil mixture.
5. Serve straight away.

Nutrition:

Calories: 315

Fat: 7.8 g

Protein: 13 g

Carbs: 49.8 g

Fiber: 16.2 g

Lentil and Quinoa Salad

Preparation time: 5 minutes

Cooking time: 15 minutes

Servings: 4

Ingredients:

- 2 medium green apples, cored, chopped
- 3 cups cooked quinoa
- ½ of a medium red onion, peeled, diced
- 3 cups cooked green lentils
- 1 large carrot, shredded
- 1 ½ teaspoon salt
- 1 teaspoon ground black pepper
- 2 tablespoons olive oil
- ¼ cup balsamic vinegar

Directions:

1. Take a large bowl, place all the ingredients in it and then stir until combined.
2. Let the salad chill in the refrigerator for 1 hour, divide it evenly among six bowls and then serve.

Nutrition:

Calories: 199

Fat: 10.7 g

Protein: 8 g

Carbs: 34.8 g

Fiber: 5.9 g

Sloppy Joes

Preparation time: 5 minutes

Cooking time: 15 minutes

Servings: 4

Ingredients:

- 2 cups cooked lentils
- 2/3 cup diced white onion
- 1 medium sweet potato, peeled, chopped
- 1 medium red bell pepper, cored, diced
- 1 teaspoon minced garlic
- ¾ cup chopped mushrooms
- 1 teaspoon red chili powder
- 1 teaspoon paprika
- 1 teaspoon ground cumin
- 1 tablespoon brown sugar
- 1 tablespoon Worcestershire sauce
- 1 tablespoon olive oil
- ½ cup vegetable broth
- 15 ounces tomato sauce

Directions:

1. Take a large pan, place it over medium-high heat, add oil, and then let it heat.
2. Add onion, bell pepper, garlic, mushroom, and sweet potato, stir until mixed, and then cook for 8 minutes or more until potatoes turn tender.
3. Add lentils, stir in sugar and all the spices, pour in the tomato sauce and then cook for 3 minutes until thoroughly hot.
4. Pour in the broth, bring the mixture to a simmer, and then remove the pan from heat.
5. Ladle the sloppy Joes mixture over the bun and then serve.

Nutrition:

Calories: 125.3

Fat: 3.6 g

Protein: 2.8 g

Carbs: 20.1 g

Fiber: 3 g

Lentil Burgers

Preparation time: 10 minutes

Cooking time: 10 minutes

Servings: 4

Ingredients:

- 2 cups cooked green lentils
- 2 tablespoons chopped white onion
- 4 ounces sliced mushrooms
- 1 teaspoon minced garlic
- 2 teaspoons garlic powder
- 2/3 teaspoon salt
- ½ teaspoon ground black pepper
- 1 tablespoon Worcestershire sauce
- 1 tablespoon yellow mustard
- 2 tablespoons olive oil
- 5 hamburger buns

Directions:

1. Place the cooked lentils in a blender, pulse until blended, and then tip the mixture into a medium bowl, set aside until required.
2. Place 1 tablespoon oil in a medium skillet pan, place it over medium heat, and when hot, add onion, mushrooms, and garlic.
3. Cook for 3 minutes, spoon the mixture to a food processor, add mustard, Worcestershire sauce, and 1 bun, and then pulse until slightly smooth.
4. Tip the mushroom mixture to lentil, and then stir until combined.

5. Add salt, black pepper, and garlic powder, stir until mixed, and then shape the mixture into four patties.
6. Place a skillet pan over medium heat, add remaining oil and when hot, add patties and then cook for 3 minutes per side until golden brown.
7. Arrange the patty on a bun and then serve with favorite condiments.

Nutrition:

Calories: 184

Fat: 4 g

Protein: 11 g

Carbs: 28 g

Fiber: 9 g

Potato Salad

Preparation time: 5 minutes

Cooking time: 25 minutes

Servings: 4

Ingredients:

- 2 medium potatoes
- 2 medium tomatoes, diced
- 2 celery, diced
- 1 green onion, chopped

Directions:

1. Place the potatoes into a pan, cover with water, and then place the pan over medium-high heat.
2. Cook the potatoes for 20 minutes, and when done, drain them and let them cool.
3. Peel the potatoes, cut them into cubes, and then place them into a large bowl.
4. Add tomatoes, celery, and green onion, season with salt and black pepper, drizzle with oil and then toss until coated.
5. Divide the salad between three bowls and then serve.

Lara Burns

Nutrition:

Calories: 268.5

Fat: 15.8 g

Protein: 5 g

Carbs: 21 g

Fiber: 2.5 g

Ginger Brown Rice

Preparation time: 5 minutes

Cooking time: 40 minutes

Servings: 3

Ingredients:

- 1 cup brown rice, rinsed
- 1-inch grated ginger
- ½ of Serrano pepper, chopped
- 1 green onion, chopped
- 2 cups of water

Directions:

1. Take a medium pot, place it over medium-high heat, and then pour in water.
2. Add rice, green onion, Serrano pepper, and ginger, bring to a boil, switch heat to medium and then simmer for 30 minutes.
3. Divide rice among three bowls and then serve.

Nutrition:

Calories: 125

Fat: 1 g

Protein: 3 g

Carbs: 26 g

Fiber: 0 g

Pasta with kale and Black Olive

Preparation time: 10 minutes

Cooking time: 40 minutes

Servings: 3

Ingredients:

- 60 g of buckwheat pasta
- 180 gr of pasta
- Six leaves of washed curly kale
- 20 black olives
- Two tablespoons of oil
- ½ chili pepper

Directions:

1. Cut the curly kale leaves into strips about 4 cm wide; cook them in salted boiling water for 5 minutes. Also, add the pasta to the pan. While the pasta is cooking, in a nonstick pan, towards the oil and olives. Drain the pasta and cabbage (keeping some cooking water aside) and add them to the olives. Mix well, adding, if needed, a little cooking water. Add the chili pepper and keep everything well.

Nutrition:

Calories per serving 372.7

Total Fat .28.0g

Saturated fat per serving 2.7g

Monounsaturated fat per serving 10.0g

Polyunsaturated fat per serving 2.1g

Protein per serving 3.6g

Dinner
Tofu Thai Curry

Preparation Time: 5 Minutes

Cooking time: 65 Minutes

Servings: 2

Ingredients:

- 400g (14oz) tofu, diced
- 200g (7oz) sugar snaps peas
- 5cm (2 inches) chunk fresh ginger root, peeled and finely chopped

- 2 red onions, chopped
- 2 cloves of garlic, crushed
- 2 bird's eye chilies
- 2 tablespoons tomato puree
- 1 stalk of lemongrass, inner stalks only
- 1 tablespoon fresh coriander (cilantro), chopped
- 1 teaspoon cumin
- 300mls (½ pint) coconut milk
- 200mls (7fl oz) vegetable stock (broth)
- 1 tablespoon virgin olive oil
- Juice of 1 lime

Directions:

2. Heat the oil in a frying pan, add the onion and cook for 4 minutes. Add in the chilies, cumin, ginger, and garlic and cook for 2 minutes. Add the tomato puree, lemongrass, sugar-snap peas, lime juice, and tofu and cook for 2 minutes. Pour in the stock (broth), coconut milk and coriander (cilantro) and simmer for 5 minutes. Serve with brown rice or buckwheat and a handful of rockets (arugula) leaves on the side.

Nutrition:

Calories 346.3

Total fat 26.4 g

Saturated fat Trace 2.0 g

Trans fat 0 g

Monounsaturated fat 5.4 g

Cholesterol Trace. 0.0 mg

Beef bourguignon with Mashed potatoes and kale

Preparation time: 15 minutes

Cooking time: 2 - 3 hours

Serving: 4

Ingredients:

- 800 g diced beef

- 2–3 tbsp buckwheat flour
- 1 tbsp extra virgin olive oil
- 150 g red onion, roughly chopped
- 200 g celery, roughly chopped
- 100 g carrots, roughly chopped
- 2–3 cloves of garlic, chopped
- 375 ml of red wine
- 2 tbsp tomato puree
- 750 ml beef broth
- 2 bay leaves
- 1 sprig of fresh thyme or 1 tablespoon of dried thyme
- 75 g diced pancetta or smoked lard
- 250 g mushrooms
- 2 tbsp chopped parsley
- 200 g kale
- 1 tbsp corn flour or arrowroot (optional)
- For the porridge:
- 500g Edward potatoes
- 1 tbsp milk and 1 tbsp olive oil

Directions:

3. Pat the beef dry with kitchen paper. Heat a heavy saucepan over medium-high heat. Add the olive oil, then the beef and saute the meat until it is browned nicely all over. Depending on the size of your pan, it's best to do this in 3-4 small loads.

4. When all of the meat is brown, remove it from the pan with a slotted spoon and set aside. In the same pan, add the onion, celery, carrot and garlic and fry over medium heat for 3 to 4 minutes until tender. Add the wine, tomato paste and broth and bring to a boil. Add the browned beef, bay leaves and thyme and reduce the heat to a simmer. Cover the pan with a lid and cook for 2 hours, stirring from time to time to make sure nothing sticks to the bottom. While the beef is cooking, peel your potatoes and cut them into quarters (or smaller pieces if they're quite large).

5. Put in a pan with cold water and bring to a boil. Reduce the heat to a simmer and cook for 20-25 minutes, covered with a lid. When soft, drain and mash with olive oil and milk. Keep warm. While the potatoes are boiling, heat a pan over high heat. When it's hot but not smoking, add the diced pancetta.

6. The fat content of the bacon means you don't need oil to cook it. When some of the fat has been released and it's starting to brown, add the mushrooms and cook over medium heat until both are nicely browned. Depending on the size of your pan, you may need to do this in multiple loads. Set aside after cooking. Cook or steam the kale for 5–10 minutes until soft. Once the beef is tender enough and the sauce has thickened to your liking, add the pancetta, mushrooms, and parsley. If your sauce is still a little runny, you can mix the corn flour or arrowroot with a little water and then stir the paste into the sauce until you have the consistency you want. Cook for 2-3 minutes and serve with porridge and kale.

Nutrition:

Carbohydrates: 34

Fat: 25

Protein: 31

Kcal: 510

Turkish fajitas

Preparation time: 15 minutes

Cooking time: approx. 1 hour

Serving: 4

Ingredients:

- For the filling
- Cut 500 g turkey breast into strips
- 1 tablespoon of extra virgin olive oil 1-2 chilies, depending on taste, chopped

- 150 g red onion, thinly sliced
- 150 g red pepper, cut into thin strips
- 2–3 cloves of garlic, chopped
- 1 tbsp paprika
- 1 tbsp ground cumin
- 1 teaspoon chili powder
- 1 tbsp chopped coriander
- For the guacamole
- 2 ripe avocados, peeled (reserve one of the stones)
- Juice of 1 lime
- Pinch of chili powder
- Pinch of black pepper
- For the salsa
- 1 × 400 g can of chopped tomatoes
- 20 g red onion, diced
- 20 g red pepper, deseeded and diced
- Juice of ½ - 1 lime, depending on the size
- 1 teaspoon chopped coriander
- 1 teaspoon capers

For the salad

- 100 g rocket
- 3 tomatoes, cut
- 100 g cucumber, thinly sliced
- 1 tbsp extra virgin olive oil juice of ½ lemon
- For serving
- 100 g cheddar cheese
- 8 grated whole grain tortilla wraps

Directions:

1. Mix the filling ingredients together and set them aside while you prepare the other parts.
2. Put all of the guacamole ingredients in a small food processor and flash until a smooth paste is formed. Alternatively, you can mash them all together with the back of a fork or spoon.
3. Place the reserved avocado stone in the guacamole - it will keep it from turning

brown. Mix all the ingredients for the salsa.

4. Put all the salad ingredients in a large bowl. Put your largest pan on high heat until it starts to smoke.
5. Put the turkey filling in the hot pan - you may need to cook it in 2 to 3 loads as overcrowding the pan will create too much moisture and it will start boiling instead of frying.
6. Keep the pan over high heat and keep moving the mixture so the turkey colors nicely but doesn't burn.
7. In a low oven, keep the cooked meat warm. To serve, reheat the tortillas according to the directions in the package, then sprinkle some guacamole over each package.
8. Top with some cheese and some salsa, then stack the turkey mixture in the middle and roll it up like a large cigar. Serve with the salad.

Nutrition:

Carbohydrates: 44

Fat: 21

Protein: 30

Kcal: 450

Sirt Chicken Korma

Preparation time: 10 minutes

Cooking time: 50 minutes

Serving: 4

Ingredients:

- 350 ml chicken stock
- 30 g Medjool date, chopped
- 2 cinnamon sticks
- 4–5 cardamom pods, slightly split
- 250 ml coconut milk
- 8 boneless, skinless chicken thighs
- 1 tbsp ground turmeric
- 200 g buckwheat

- 150 ml of Greek yogurt
- 50 g of ground walnuts
- 2 tbsp chopped coriander

For the curry paste

- 1 large red onion, quartered
- 3 cloves of garlic
- 2 cm piece of fresh ginger
- 1 tbsp mild curry powder
- 1 teaspoon ground cumin
- 1 tbsp ground turmeric
- 1 tbsp coconut oil

Directions:

1. Put the ingredients for the curry paste in a food processor and flash for about a minute until you have a nice paste.
2. Alternatively, you can grind it with a pestle and mortar. Fry the paste in a heavy pan over medium heat for 1-2 minutes then add the broth, date, cinnamon, cardamom pods, and coconut milk.
3. Bring to a boil then add the chicken legs. Reduce the heat, cover the pan with a lid, and simmer for 45 minutes.
4. In the meantime, bring a pan of water to the boil and stir in the turmeric.
5. Add the buckwheat and cook according to the directions on the package. As soon as the chicken is tender, stir in the yogurt and cook the walnuts over low heat for a few more minutes.
6. Add the coriander and serve with the buckwheat

Nutrition:

Carbohydrates: 21

Fat: 16

Protein: 32

Kcal: 330

Tomato Chicken Mix

Preparation Time: 10 minutes

Cooking Time: 20 minutes

Serve: 6

Ingredients:

- 14 ounces tomato sauce
- 1 tablespoon olive oil
- 4 medium chicken breasts, skinless and boneless
- Salt and black pepper to taste
- 1 teaspoon oregano, dried
- 6 ounces mozzarella cheese, grated
- 1 teaspoon garlic powder

Directions:

1. Put the chicken in your air fryer and season with salt, pepper, garlic powder, and the oregano.
2. Cook the chicken at 360 degrees F for 5 minutes; then transfer to a pan that fits your air fryer, greased with the oil.
3. Add the tomato sauce, sprinkle the mozzarella on top, place the pan in the fryer, and cook at 350 degrees F for 15 minutes more.
4. Divide between plates and serve.

Nutrition:

calories 270

fat 10

fiber 16

carbs 16

protein 18

Chicken and Veggies

Preparation Time: 10 minutes

Cooking Time: 25 minutes

Serve: 4

Ingredients:

- 1 red onion, chopped
- 1 carrot, chopped
- 3 garlic cloves, minced
- 4 chicken breasts, boneless and skinless
- 1 celery stalk, chopped
- 1 cup chicken stock
- 2 tablespoons olive oil
- ½ teaspoon rosemary, dried
- 1 teaspoon sage, dried
- Salt and black pepper to taste

Directions:

1. In a pan that fits your air fryer, place all ingredients and toss well.
2. Put the pan in the fryer and cook at 360 degrees F for 25 minutes.
3. Divide everything between plates, serve, and enjoy!

Nutrition:

calories 292

fat 12

fiber 16

carbs 19

protein 15

Japanese Chicken Thighs

Preparation Time: 10 minutes

Cooking Time: 30 minutes

Serve: 5

Ingredients:

- 2 pounds chicken thighs
- Salt and black pepper to taste
- 5 spring onions, chopped
- 2 tablespoons olive oil
- 1 tablespoon sherry wine
- ½ teaspoon white vinegar
- 1 tablespoon soy sauce
- ¼ teaspoon sugar

Directions:

1. Season the chicken with salt and pepper, rub with 1 tablespoon of the oil, and put it in the air fryer's basket.
2. Cook at 360 degrees F for 10 minutes on each side and divide between plates.
3. Heat up a pan with the remaining tablespoon of oil over medium-high heat, and add the spring onions, sherry wine, vinegar, soy sauce, and sugar; whisk.
4. Cook for 10 minutes, drizzle over the chicken, and serve.

Nutrition:

calories 271

fat 8

fiber 12

carbs 26

protein 17

Air Fried Whole Chicken

Preparation Time: 10 minutes

Cooking Time: 20 minutes

Serve: 8

Ingredients:

- 1 whole chicken, cut into medium pieces
- 3 tablespoons white wine
- 2 carrots, chopped
- 1 cup chicken stock
- 1 tablespoon ginger, grated
- Salt and black pepper to taste

Directions:

1. In a pan that fits your air fryer, mix all of the ingredients.
2. Put the pan in the air fryer and cook at 370 degrees F for 20 minutes.
3. Divide between plates and serve.

Nutrition:

calories 220

fat 10

fiber 8

carbs 20

protein 16

Perfect Garlic Butter Steak

Preparation Time: 20 minutes

Cooking Time: 13 minutes

Serve: 4

Ingredients:

- 2 Rib eye steaks
- Salt
- Pepper
- Olive oil
- Garlic butter:
- ½ cup softened butter
- 2 tbsp chopped fresh parsley
- 2 garlic cloves, minced
- 1 tsp Worcestershire sauce
- ½ tsp salt (optional)

Directions:

1. Prepare the garlic butter by mixing all the ingredients together.
2. Place in parchment paper. Roll up and put in the fridge.
3. Let the steaks sit for 20 minutes at room temperature.
4. Brush with a little oil, salt, and pepper.
5. Preheat your hot air fryer to 400°F (200°C).
6. Cook for 12 minutes, turning halfway through cooking. Serve.
7. Place the garlic butter on the steaks and let sit for 5 minutes.
8. Enjoy!

Nutrition:

Calories 250

Fat 10g

Carbohydrates 2g

Sugars 1g

Protein 36g

Cholesterol 100mg

Crispy Pork Medallions

Preparation time: 20 minutes

Cooking time: 5 minutes

Serve: 2

Ingredients:

- 1 pork loin, 330 g, cut into 6 or 7 slices of 4 cm
- 1 tsp Dijon mustard
- 1 tsp oil
- Salt, pepper and paprika
- Asian marinade
- 1 tsp salt reduced tamari sauce
- 1 tsp olive oil
- 1 clementine juice
- 1 pinch cayenne pepper
- 2 cloves garlic, pressed
- Crunchy coating
- 1/3 cup breadcrumbs
- ½ orange zest
- 2g freshly grated Parmesan cheese

Direction:

1. Prepare the marinade first. In a bowl, combine all the ingredients. Lightly salt the medallions, pepper, and sprinkle with paprika. Place these in the marinade and turn them several times to impregnate them completely. Cover with plastic wrap and marinate for 1 hour at room temperature.
2. Prepare the coating by combining the breadcrumbs, the orange zest, and the Parmesan cheese in a deep dish.
3. When the maceration time has elapsed, remove the marinade medallions, and dry them on absorbent paper. Spread with mustard, then move on to the crunchy layer. Brush lightly with oil.

4. Heat the air fryer to 350°F. Place the medallions in the fryer basket. Cook 5 minutes, stir, and then return to the fryer for another minute. Serve immediately.

Nutrition:

Calories 222

Carbohydrates 13g

Fat 6g

Protein 24g

Sugars 0h

Cholesterol 74mg

Prawns, Pak Choi and broccoli

Preparation time: 15 minutes

Cooking time: 20 minutes

Serving: 5

Ingredients:

- 1 tbsp ground turmeric
- 400 g raw shrimp, peeled and deveined
- 1 tbsp coconut oil
- 280 g buckwheat noodles
- 1 teaspoon virgin olive oil
- For the china pan
- 1 tbsp coconut oil
- Cut 250 g broccoli into bite-sized pieces
- 250 g pak choi, roughly chopped
- 1 red onion, thinly sliced
- 2 cm piece of fresh ginger, chopped
- 1–2 chili peppers, chopped
- 3 cloves of garlic, chopped
- 150 ml vegetable broth
- 1 bunch of basil, removed leaves and chopped stems
- 1 tbsp Thai fish sauce or tamari

Directions:

1. Mix the turmeric with the prawns. Place the coconut oil in a wok or pan and cook the shrimp over medium-high heat for 3 to 4 minutes, or until opaque.

2. After cooking, remove from pan and set aside. Wipe the pan for the pan and put it on high heat until it starts to smoke.
3. Add the coconut oil then add the vegetables, ginger, chili peppers, and garlic.
4. Keep moving the vegetables in the pan so they don't burn. Cook for 3–5 minutes - lower the heat a little if the vegetables look charred - until they are fried but crispy.
5. Add the broth, whole basil and fish sauce.
6. Bring to the boil, then add the shrimp and let heat. In the meantime, cook the pasta according to the instructions on the package.
7. Freshen up in cold water and mix with the olive oil to prevent them from sticking together. Serve the pan with the hot noodles.

Nutrition:

Carbohydrates: 13

Fat: 15

Protein: 26

Kcal: 270

Cocoa spaghetti Bolognese

Preparation time: 15 minutes

Cooking time: approx. 1 hour

Serving: 4

Ingredients:

- 1 tbsp virgin olive oil
- 1 red onion, finely diced
- 100 g celery, finely diced
- 100 g carrots, finely diced
- 3 cloves of garlic, chopped
- 400 g of lean ground beef
- 1 tbsp Herbs de Provence
- 1–2 bay leaves
- 150 ml red wine
- 300 ml beef broth

- 1 tbsp cocoa powder
- 1 tbsp tomato paste
- 2 × 400 g cans of chopped tomatoes
- 280 g whole wheat spaghetti
- 1 teaspoon ground black pepper
- 1 bunch of fresh basil
- 20 g parmesan cheese

Directions:

1. Heat the oil in a pan, then cook the onion, celery, carrot and garlic over medium heat for 1–2 minutes until they are a little softer.
2. Add the ground beef and dried herbs and cook over medium-high heat until the ground beef is brown.
3. Add the wine, stock, cocoa powder, tomato paste and canned tomatoes, bring to a boil and simmer for 45 to 60 minutes with the lid closed.
4. When you're almost done, cook the pasta as directed on the package.
5. Finally stir the pepper and basil leaves into the sauce. Serve with the pasta and rub some parmesan on top.

Nutrition:

Carbohydrates: 43

Fat: 21

Protein: 11

Kcal: 450

Baked salmon with Watercress sauce and Potatoes

Preparation time: 10 minutes

Cooking time: 35 minutes

Serving: 4

Ingredients:

- 400 g of new potatoes
- 4 × 125 g skinless salmon fillets
- 1 teaspoon extra virgin olive oil
- 1 piece of broccoli, cut into florets

- 1 bunch of asparagus spears
- For the watercress sauce
- 30 g of watercress
- 5 g parsley
- 1 tbsp capers
- 2 tbsp virgin olive oil
- Extra juice of 1 lemon

Directions:

1. Heat the oven to 200 ° C / gas. 6. Put the potatoes in a pan with cold water.
2. Bring to a boil and simmer for 15-20 minutes or until tender.
3. Brush the salmon fillets with the olive oil, place on a baking sheet and bake in the oven for 10 minutes.
4. Reduce the cooking time by 2 to 3 minutes if you prefer your salmon to be lightly cooked.
5. In the meantime, cook or steam the broccoli and asparagus until tender.
6. Put the ingredients for the sauce in a food processor or blender and stir until smooth. Serve the salmon with the sauce and the vegetables.

Nutrition:

Carbohydrates: 9

Fat: 15

Protein: 31

Kcal: 250

Coq au vin with potatoes and green beans

Preparation time: 10 minutes

Cooking time: 35 minutes

Serving: 4

Ingredients:

- 4 skinless chicken legs
- 4 skinless chicken legs
- 1-2 tbsp buckwheat flour
- 1 tbsp extra virgin olive oil

- 150 g red onion
- 150 g carrot
- 200 g celery
- 3 cloves of garlic, chopped
- 400 ml red wine
- 400 ml of chicken broth
- 1 sprig of fresh thyme
- 2–3 bay leaves
- 100 g pancetta or smoked bacon, diced
- 250 g mushrooms
- 400 g of new potatoes
- 2 tbsp chopped parsley
- 250 g green beans

Directions:

1. Roll the chicken pieces in the flour. Heat a heavy saucepan over medium-high heat. Add the olive oil then the chicken and cook until nicely browned all over.
2. Remove from pan and set aside. In the same pan, add the onion, carrot, celery and garlic and cook gently for 2-3 minutes until they soften.
3. When the pan is dry, you can add some water here. Add the wine and chicken stock and bring to a boil. Add the thyme, bay leaves, and chicken. Cover with a lid and simmer gently for 45 minutes.
4. Check the amount of fluid from time to time and add a little more. Heat a pan over high heat. When it's hot but not smoking, add the diced pancetta.
5. When some of the fat has been released and it starts to brown, add the mush-rooms and cook over medium heat until both it and the pancetta are nicely browned.
6. Depending on the size of your pan, you may need to do this in multiple loads. Set aside after cooking.
7. Put the potatoes in a pan with cold wa-ter. Bring to a boil and simmer for 15-20 minutes or until tender. When you're

done, drain it and return to the pan to keep it warm.

8. Add the pancetta, mushrooms and parsley to the Coq au Vin and cook for another 15 minutes.
9. To cook the green beans, steam them or cook them for 4 to 6 minutes, depending on how crispy you like them.
10. Serve the Coq au Vin with the potatoes and beans.

Nutrition:

Carbohydrates: 13

Fat: 15

Protein: 26

Kcal: 270

Beans & Kale Soup

Preparation Time: 15 minutes

Cooking Time: 30 minutes

Servings: 6

Ingredients:

- 2 tablespoons olive oil
- 2 onions, chopped
- 4 garlic cloves, minced
- 1-pound kale, tough ribs removed and chopped
- 2 (14-ounce) cans cannellini beans, rinsed and drained
- 6 cups of water
- Salt and ground black pepper, as required

Directions:

1. In a large pan, heat the oil over medium heat and sauté the onion and garlic for about 4-5 minutes.
2. Add the kale and cook for about 1-2 minutes.
3. Add beans, water, salt, and black pepper and bring to a boil.

4. Cook partially covered for about 15-20 minutes.
5. Serve hot.

Nutrition:

Calories 270.4.

Total fat 4.7 g.

Saturated fat Trace 0.6 g.

Trans fat 0 g.

Monounsaturated fat 2.6 g.

Cholesterol Trace. 0.0 mg

Salad

Orange & Beet Salad

Preparation Time: 15 minutes

Servings: 4

Ingredients:

- 3 large oranges, peeled, seeded and sectioned
- 2 beets, trimmed, peeled and sliced
- 6 cups fresh rocket
- ¼ cup walnuts, chopped
- 3 tablespoons olive oil
- Pinch of salt

Directions:

1. In a salad bowl, place all ingredients and gently, toss to coat.
2. Serve immediately.

Nutrition:

Calories 233

Total Fat 15.6 g

Saturated Fat 1.8 g

Cholesterol 0 mg

Sodium 86 mg

Total Carbs 23.1 g

Fiber 5.3 g

Sugar 17.6 g

Protein 4.8 g

Faro Salad with White Beans

Preparation time: 30 minutes

Cooking time: 32 minutes

Servings: 4

Ingredients:

- 12 ounces (340 g) sugar snap peas, strings removed and cut into 1-inch lengths
- 3¼ teaspoon sea salt, plus more to taste, divided (optional)
- 1½ cups whole faro
- 3 tablespoons extra-virgin olive oil (optional)
- 2 tablespoons lemon juice
- 2 tablespoons minced shallot
- 1 teaspoon Dijon mustard
- ¼ teaspoon black pepper, plus more to taste, divided
- 1 (15-ounce / 425-g) can cannellini beans, rinsed
- 6 ounces (170 g) cherry tomatoes, halved
- ⅓ cup chopped pitted calamite olives 2 tablespoons chopped fresh dill

Directions:

1. Pour the water in a pot over medium heat and bring to a boil. Add the snap peas and 3 teaspoon sea salt (if desired) to the pot and cook for 2 minutes, or until tender crisp. Drain the snap peas and transfer to a bowl. Let rest for 15 minutes to cool completely.
2. Pour the water in the pot over medium heat. Add the faro to the pot and bring to a boil. Cover and cook for 15 to 30 minutes, or until tender. Drain the faro and spread evenly on a baking pan. Let rest for 15 minutes to cool completely.

3. In a large bowl, stir together the olive oil (if desired), lemon juice, shallot, Dijon mustard ¼ teaspoon sea salt (if desired) and ¼ teaspoon black pepper. Add the cooled snap peas, cooled faro, cannellini beans, tomatoes, olives, and dill to the bowl. Toss until well blended. Sprinkle with sea salt (if desired) and pepper to taste.
4. Transfer the salad to 4 to 6 bowls and serve immediately.

Nutrition:

Calories: 501

Fat: 14.9g

Carbs: 81.6g

Protein: 16.6g

Fiber: 7.3g

Wheat Berry Salad with Chickpeas

Preparation time: 25 minutes

Cooking time: 60 minutes

Servings: 4

Ingredients:

- 1½ cups wheat berries
- 16 cups water
- 2 teaspoons sea salt (optional)
- ¼ teaspoon ground black pepper
- 4 teaspoons sherry vinegar
- 2 teaspoons Dijon mustard
- 1 garlic clove, minced
- ¾ teaspoon smoked paprika
- 3 tablespoons extra-virgin olive oil (optional)
- 1 (15-ounce / 425-g) can chickpeas, rinsed
- 3 ounces (85 g) baby spinach, chopped
- 1 small red onion, thinly sliced
- 3 oranges, peeled, pitted and thinly sliced
- ¼ cup minced fresh mint

Directions:

1. Pour the water in a pot over medium heat and bring to a boil. Add the wheat berries and 1½ teaspoons salt (if desired) to the pot and bring to a boil. Reduce the heat to low and simmer for 1 hour to 1 hour 10 minutes, or until the wheat berries become just tender and still chewy. Drain the wheat berries and place on a baking pan to let rest for 15 minutes until completely cool.
2. In a large bowl, stir together the sherry vinegar, Dijon mustard, garlic, smoked paprika, ½ teaspoon salt (if desired), ¼ teaspoon pepper and the olive oil (if desired).
3. Combine the cooled wheat berries, chickpeas, spinach, onion, oranges and mint to the bowl. Toss to blend well.
4. Transfer to bowls and serve immediately.

Nutrition:

Calories: 327

Fat: 9.3g

Carbs: 54.7g

Protein: 10.7g

Fiber: 4.9g

Chickpea and Heart of Palm Salad

Preparation time: 10 minutes

Cooking time: 0 minutes

Servings: 4

Ingredients:

- 1 (15.5-ounce / 439-g) can chickpeas, drained and rinsed
- 1 (14-ounce / 397-g) can hearts of palm, drained and chopped
- ½ cup diced celery
- ½ cup chopped white onion
- ¼ cup almond butter

- ½ teaspoon sea salt (optional)
- ¼ teaspoon freshly ground black pepper

Directions:

1. Place the chickpeas in a large bowl and mash them into a chunky paste with a hand masher.
2. Make the salad: Add the remaining ingredients to the bowl and toss to combine well.
3. Divide the salad among 4 bowls and serve immediately.

Nutrition:

Calories: 212

Fat: 5.7g

Carbs: 34.8g

Protein: 8.8g

Fiber: 8.1g

Citrus Fruit Salad

Preparation Time: 15 minutes

Servings: 2

Ingredients: For Salad:

- 3 cups fresh kale, tough ribs removed and torn
- 1 orange, peeled and segmented
- 1 grapefruit, peeled and segmented
- 2 tablespoons unsweetened dried cranberries

For Dressing:

- 2 tablespoons extra-virgin olive oil
- 2 tablespoons fresh orange juice
- 1 teaspoon Dijon mustard
- ½ teaspoon raw honey
- Salt and ground black pepper, as required

Directions:

1. For salad: in a salad bowl, place all ingredients and mix.

---

2. For dressing: place all ingredients in another bowl and beat until well combined.
3. Place dressing on top of salad and toss to coat well.
4. Serve immediately.

Nutrition:

Calories 256

Total Fat 14.5g

Saturated Fat 2.1 g

Cholesterol 0 mg

Sodium 150 mg

Total Carbs 31.3 g

Fiber 4.8 g

Sugar 16.6 g

Protein 4.6 g

Soup

Shrimp & arugula soup

Preparation time: 8 minutes

Cooking time: 32 minutes

Serving: 2

Ingredients:

- 5 large prawns, cleaned deveined and chopped into bite-sized pieces
- 1 red onion, sliced very thinly
- 1 cup arugula
- 1 cup baby kale
- 2 large celery stalks, sliced very thinly
- 5 sprigs of parsley, chopped
- 5 cloves of garlic, minced
- 5 cups of chicken or fish or vegetable stock
- 1 tbsp extra virgin olive oil
- Dash of sea salt
- Dash of black pepper

Directions:

1. Sauté the vegetables (not the kale or arugula), in a stock pot, on low heat for about 2 minutes so that they are still tender and still crunchy, but not cooked quite yet
2. Add the salt and pepper.
3. Add the shrimp to the pot, and sauté for 10 more minutes on medium-low heat (Make sure the shrimp is cooked thoroughly and is not translucent).
4. When the shrimp seems to be cooked through, add the stock to the pot and cook on medium for about 20 more minutes.
5. Remove from heat and cool before serving.

Nutrition:

Calories - 450

Fat - 27g

Carbs – 32g

Protein – 23g

Curry Lentil Soup

Preparation time: 5 minutes

Cooking time: 40 minutes

Servings: 6

Ingredients:

- 1 cup brown lentils
- 1 medium white onion, peeled, chopped
- 28 ounces diced tomatoes
- 1 ½ teaspoon minced garlic
- 1 inch of ginger, grated
- 3 cups vegetable broth
- 1/2 teaspoon salt
- 2 tablespoons curry powder
- 1 teaspoon cumin
- 1/2 teaspoon cayenne
- 1 tablespoon olive oil
- 1 1/2 cups coconut milk, unsweetened
- ¼ cup chopped cilantro

Directions:

1. Take a soup pot, place it over medium-high heat, add oil and when hot, add onion, stir in garlic and ginger and cook for 5 minutes until golden brown.
2. Then add all the ingredients except for milk and cilantro, stir until mixed and simmer for 25 minutes until lentils have cooked.
3. When done, stir in milk, cook for 5 minutes until thoroughly heated and then garnish the soup with cilantro.
4. Serve straight away

Nutrition:

Calories: 269 Cal

Fat: 15 g

Carbs: 26 g

Protein: 10 g

Fiber: 10 g

Chickpea Noodle Soup

Preparation time: 5 minutes

Cooking time: 18 minutes

Servings: 6

Ingredients:

- 1 cup cooked chickpeas
- 8 ounces rotini noodles, whole-wheat
- 4 celery stalks, sliced
- 2 medium white onions, peeled, chopped
- 4 medium carrots, peeled, sliced
- 2 teaspoons minced garlic
- 8 sprigs of thyme
- 1 teaspoon salt
- 1/3 teaspoon ground black pepper
- 1 bay leaf
- 2 tablespoons olive oil
- 2 quarts of vegetable broth
- ¼ cup chopped fresh parsley

Directions:

1. Take a large pot, place it over medium heat, add oil and when hot, add all the vegetables, stir in garlic, thyme and bay leaf and cook for 5 minutes until vegetables are golden and sauté.
2. Then pour in broth stir and bring the mixture to boil.
3. Add chickpeas and noodles into boiling soup, continue cooking for 8 minutes until noodles are tender, and then season soup with salt and black pepper.
4. Garnish with parsley and serve straight away

Nutrition:

Calories: 260 Cal

Fat: 5 g

Carbs: 44 g

Protein: 7 g

Fiber: 4 g

Mexican Lentil Soup

Preparation time: 5 minutes

Cooking time: 45 minutes

Servings: 6

Ingredients:

- 2 cups green lentils
- 1 medium red bell pepper, cored, diced
- 1 medium white onion, peeled, diced
- 2 cups diced tomatoes
- 8 ounces diced green chilies
- 2 celery stalks, diced
- 2 medium carrots, peeled, diced
- 1 ½ teaspoon minced garlic
- 1/2 teaspoon salt
- 1 tablespoon cumin
- 1/4 teaspoon smoked paprika
- 1 teaspoon oregano
- 1/8 teaspoon hot sauce
- 2 tablespoons olive oil

- 8 cups vegetable broth
- ¼ cup cilantro, for garnish
- 1 avocado, peeled, pitted, diced, for garnish

Directions:

1. Take a large pot over medium heat, add oil and when hot, add all the vegetables, reserving tomatoes and chilies, and cook for 5 minutes until softened.
2. Then add garlic, stir in oregano, cumin, and paprika, and continue cooking for 1 minute.
3. Add lentils, tomatoes and green chilies, season with salt, pour in the broth and simmer the soup for 40 minutes until cooked.
4. When done, ladle soup into bowls, top with avocado and cilantro and serve straight away

Nutrition:

Calories: 235 Cal

Fat: 9 g

Carbs: 32 g

Protein: 9 g

Cauliflower Soup

Preparation time: 10 minutes

Cooking time: 40 minutes

Servings: 2

Ingredients:

- 1 small head of cauliflower, cut into florets
- 4 tablespoons pomegranate seeds
- 2 sprigs of thyme and more for garnishing
- 1 teaspoon minced garlic
- 2/3 teaspoon salt
- 1/3 teaspoon ground black pepper
- 1 tablespoon olive oil
- 1 1/2 cups vegetable stock

- 1/2 cup coconut milk, unsweetened

Directions:

1. Take a pot, place it over medium heat, add oil and when hot, add garlic and cook for 1 minute until fragrant.
2. Add florets, thyme, pour in the stock and bring the mixture to boil.
3. Switch heat to the medium low level, simmer the soup for 30 minutes until florets are tender, then remove the pot from heat, discard the thyme and puree using an immersion blender until smooth.
4. Stir milk into the soup, season with salt and black pepper, then garnish with pomegranate seeds and thyme sprigs and serve.

Nutrition:

Calories: 184 Cal

Fat: 11 g

Carbs: 17 g

Protein: 3 g

Vegan

Spinach and Kale Stir Fry

Preparation Time: 15 Minutes

Cooking Time: 15 Minutes

Servings: 4

Ingredients:

- 2 chopped shallots
- 1 cup no-salt-added and chopped canned tomatoes
- 2 cup baby spinach
- 2 minced garlic cloves
- 5 cup torn kale
- 1 tbsp. extra virgin olive oil

Directions:

1. Heat up a pan with the oil over medium-high heat
2. Add the shallots, stir and sauté for 5 minutes.
3. Add the spinach, kale, and the other ingredients, toss, cook for 10 minutes more.
4. Divide between plates and serve.

Nutrition:

Calories: 141 Cal

Fat: 28 g

Aromatic Red Endives

Preparation Time: 30 Minutes

Cooking Time: 30 Minutes

Servings: 4

Ingredients:

- 2 tbsp. extra virgin olive oil
- 1 tsp. dried rosemary
- 2 halved endives
- ¼ tsp. black pepper
- ½ tsp. turmeric powder

Directions:

1. In a baking pan, combine the endives with the oil and the other ingredients, toss gently.
2. Insert in the oven and bake at 400 0F for 20 minutes.
3. Divide between plates and serve.

Nutrition:

Calories: 102 Cal

Fat: 38 g

Kale & Chicken Stew

Preparation time: 5 Minutes

Cooking Time: 55 Minutes

Servings 4

Ingredients:

- 1 cup sliced leeks
- 1 sliced carrot
- 1 cup chopped onions
- Salt & 1 Tsp. ground pepper to taste
- 2 cups chicken broth
- 3 cups kale
- 4 pounds chicken

Directions:

1. Put ingredients in the slow cooker. Cover, & cook on low for 7 to 9 hours.

Nutrition:

Calories 273

Fat 15

Fiber 11.6

Carbs 16.9

Protein 18.8

Lemony Wax Beans

Preparation time: 5 minutes

Cooking time: 12 minutes

Servings: 4

Ingredients:

- 2 pounds (907 g) wax beans
- 2 tablespoons extra-virgin olive oil
- Salt
- ground black pepper
- Juice of ½ lemon, for serving

Directions:

2. Line a baking sheet with aluminum foil.
3. Toss the wax beans with the olive oil in a large bowl. Lightly season with salt and pepper.
4. Spread out the wax beans on the sheet pan.
5. Select Roast, set temperature to 400°F (205°C), and set time to 12 minutes.
6. Once preheated, place the baking sheet into the oven.

7. When done, the beans will be caramelized and tender. Serve sprinkled with the lemon juice.

Nutrition:

Calories: 44

Carbs: 6g

Fat: 0g

Protein: 2g

Maple and Pecan Granola

Preparation time: 5 minutes

Cooking time: 20 minutes

Servings: 4

Ingredients:

- 1½ cups rolled oats
- ¼ cup maple syrup
- ¼ cup pecan pieces
- 1 teaspoon vanilla extract
- ½ teaspoon ground cinnamon

Directions:

1. Line a baking sheet with parchment paper.
2. Mix the oats, maple syrup, pecan pieces, vanilla, and cinnamon in a large bowl and stir until the oats and pecan pieces are completely coated. Spread the batter on the baking sheet.
3. Set temperature to 300ºF (150ºC), and set time to 20 minutes.
4. Once preheated, place the baking sheet into the oven. Stir once halfway through the cooking time.
5. When done, cool it for 30 minutes before serving. The granola may still be a bit soft right after removing, but it will gradually firm up as it cools.

Nutrition:

Calories: 137

Carbs: 18g

Fat: 6g

Protein: 3g

Sweet and Spicy Broccoli

Preparation time: 10 minutes

Cooking time: 20 minutes

Servings: 4

Ingredients:

- ½ teaspoon olive oil,
- 1 pound (454 g) f broccoli, cut into florets
- ½ tablespoon garlic
- Salt, to taste
- Sauce:
- 1½ tablespoons soy sauce
- 2 teaspoons hot sauce or sriracha
- 1½ teaspoons honey
- 1 teaspoon white vinegar
- Freshly ground black pepper, to taste

Directions:

1. Grease a perforated pan with olive oil.
2. Add the broccoli florets, ½ teaspoon of olive oil, and garlic to a large bowl and toss well—season with salt to taste.
3. Put the broccoli in the perforated pan in a single layer.
4. Select Air Fry, set temperature to 400ºF (205ºC), and set time to 15 minutes.
5. Once preheated, place the pan into the oven. Stir the broccoli florets three times during cooking.
6. Meanwhile, whisk all the ingredients for the sauce in a small bowl until well incorporated.
7. The broccoli should be lightly browned and crispy. Continue cooking for 5 minutes, if desired. Transfer and pour over the sauce and toss to combine. Add more salt and pepper if needed. Serve warm.

Nutrition:

Calories: 68

Carbs: 4g

Fat: 4g

Protein: 3g

Beverages

Chocolate strawberry milk

Preparation time: 5 minutes

Cooking time: 0 minutes

Serving: 1

Ingredients:

- 200 ml milk or dairy-free alternative 150 g strawberries, peeled and halved
- 1 tbsp cocoa powder (100 percent cocoa)
- 10 g pitted Medjool dates
- 10 g walnuts

Directions:

1. Put all ingredients in a powerful mixer and stir until smooth.
2. Once the matcha has dissolved, add the rest of the juice.

Nutrition:

Carbohydrates: 16

Fat: 6

Protein: 3

Kcal: 130

Green tea and Rocket smoothie

Preparation time: 5 minutes

Cooking time: -0 minutes

Serving: 1

Ingredients:

- 200 ml of water
- 50 g banana, sliced
- 25 g pitted Medjool dates

- 15 g rocket
- 1 teaspoon matcha
- 5 g parsley

Directions:

1. Put all ingredients in a powerful mixer and stir until smooth.
2. Once the matcha has dissolved, add the rest of the juice

Nutrition:

Carbohydrates: 8

Fat: 3

Protein: 1

Kcal: 100

Chocolate strawberry milk

Preparation time: 5 minutes

Cooking time: 0 minutes

Serving: 1

Ingredients:

- 150 g strawberries, peeled and halved
- 1 tbsp cocoa powder (100 percent cocoa)
- 10 g pitted Medjool dates
- 10 g walnuts
- 200 ml milk or dairy-free alternative

Directions:

1. Put all ingredients in a powerful mixer and stir until smooth.
2. Once the matcha has dissolved, add the rest of the juice.

Nutrition:

Carbohydrates: 16

Fat: 6

Protein: 3

Kcal: 130

Pineapple Lassi

Preparation time: 5 minutes

Cooking time: 0 minutes

Serving: 1

Ingredients:

- 200 g pineapple, cut into pieces
- 150 g Greek yogurt
- 4–5 ice cubes
- 1 teaspoon ground turmeric

Directions:

1. Put all ingredients in a powerful mixer and stir until smooth.
2. Once the matcha has dissolved, add the rest of the juice. If the mixture is too thick, just add some water and mix until you get the consistency you want.

Nutrition:

Carbohydrates: 13

Fat: 3

Protein: 2

Kcal: 90

Snacks and Desserts

Triple Chocolate Chip Deep Dish Cookies

Preparation Time: 10 minutes

Cooking Time: 30 minutes

Servings: 1

Ingredients:

- 3/4 cup canned pumpkin
- 3/4 cup chocolate peanut butter
- 1/2 cup powdered chocolate protein
- 1/4 cup honey
- 1 beaten egg
- 1 teaspoon pure vanilla
- 1/2 teaspoon baking soda

- 1/2 cup sugar-free chocolate chips
- Vanilla ice cream or serving

Directions:

1. Add all the ingredients except ice cream and chocolate chips in a bowl
2. Use a mixer (electric) beat until mixed evenly.
3. Heat your oven to 350 degrees Fahrenheit.
4. Gradually add the chocolate chips and gently fold to incorporate.
5. Pour batter into a skillet (medium).
6. Place skillet into a preheated oven to bake for approximately 20 minutes until golden brown.
7. Remove from heat and set aside for roughly 7–10 minutes.
8. Serve using the vanilla ice cream.

Nutrition:

Calories: 502

Protein: 6g

Carbohydrates: 65g

Fats: 24g

Protein Brownies

Preparation Time: 10 minutes

Cooking Time: 30–35 minutes

Servings: 1

Ingredients:

- 1/2 cup almond milk
- 1/2 cup, chocolate flavored egg whites
- 1/2 cup, unsweetened apple sauce
- 1/2 cup+1 tablespoon Greek yogurt
- 1 cup, oat flour
- 2–3 scoops, powdered chocolate protein
- 3 tablespoons, powdered unsweetened cocoa
- 1 teaspoon, baker style baking powder
- 1/2 teaspoon salt

Ingredients for the frosting:

- 1/2 cup, nonfat Greek yogurt
- 1/4 cup cherries
- Sweetener (optional)

Directions:

1. The first step is to heat an oven to 350 degrees Fahrenheit then lightly spray a baking dish using cooking spray.
2. Add the egg whites and whisk well until beaten lightly.
3. Add the protein powder, oat flour, sweetener, powdered cocoa, and the baking powder separately.
4. Stir well until mixed evenly, then pour milk mixture (almond) into the flour mixture.
5. Stir well until thoroughly mixed and set batter aside for approximately 5 minutes.
6. Pour batter into the dish and place into the oven to bake for approximately 25 minutes until thoroughly cooked.
7. Remove brownie from heat then set aside to cool.
8. Add all the frosting ingredients in a food processor then process on the highest setting until it becomes smooth.
9. Spread frosting over the top of brownies. Serve.

Nutrition:

Calories: 466

Protein: 6g

Carbohydrates: 50g

Fats: 29g

Protein Pumpkin Spiced Donuts

Preparation Time: 10 minutes

Cooking Time: 15 minutes

Servings: 1

Ingredients:

- 1 cup oat flour
- 3/4 cup xylitol
- 1 scoop, powdered vanilla protein
- 1 tablespoon, ground flaxseed
- 1 tablespoon, ground cinnamon
- 2 teaspoon baking powder
- 1 teaspoon sea salt
- 3 beaten eggs
- 1/2 cup canned pumpkin
- 1 tablespoon melted coconut oil
- 2 teaspoon pure vanilla
- 1 teaspoon apple cider vinegar

Ingredients for the frosting:

- 1/2 cup whipped cream cheese
- 1/2 teaspoon liquid stevia

Directions:

1. Place the xylitol, oat flour, ground flaxseed, powdered protein, baking powder, ground cinnamon, and a dash of sea salt in a large bowl. Preheat your oven to 350°F.
2. Add the egg (beaten) into another bowl (large) along with the pumpkin (canned), pure vanilla, and vinegar and coconut oil (melted).
3. Whisk until mixed (evenly), then pour the mixture into the flour. Stir until thoroughly mixed.
4. Use cooking spray grease a large donut pan.
5. Pour batter into the donut pan (greased).
6. Place batter into the oven and bake for approximately 10 minutes until thoroughly baked.
7. Remove from heat and set donuts onto a wire rack to cool.
8. Add in the cream cheese (whipped) and liquid stevia in a small bowl, whisk until it becomes smooth.
9. Frost donuts using the frosting and serve with a sprinkle of cinnamon (ground) over the top.

Nutrition:

Calories: 452

Protein: 4.9g

Carbohydrates: 51g

Fats: 25g

Wrapped Plums

Preparation Time: 5 Minutes

Cooking Time: 5 Minutes

Servings: 5

Ingredients:

- 2 ounces prosciutto, cut into 16 pieces
- 4 plums, quartered
- 1 tablespoon chives, chopped
- A pinch of red pepper flakes, crushed

Directions:

1. Wrap each plum quarter in a prosciutto slice, arrange them all on a platter, sprinkle the chives and pepper flakes all over and serve.

Nutrition:

Calories 30

Fat 1 g

Fiber 0 g

Carbs 4 g

Protein 2 g

Cucumber Sandwich Bites

Preparation Time: 5 Minutes

Cooking Time: 0 Minutes

Servings: 5

Ingredients:

- 1 cucumber, sliced
- 8 slices whole wheat bread
- 2 tablespoons cream cheese, soft
- 1 tablespoon chives, chopped

- ¼ cup avocado, peeled, pitted and mashed
- 1 teaspoon mustard
- Salt and black pepper to the taste

Directions:

2. Spread the mashed avocado on each bread slice, also spread the rest of the ingredients except the cucumber slices.
3. Divide the cucumber slices on the bread slices, cut each slice in thirds, arrange on a platter and serve as an appetizer.

Nutrition:

Calories 187

Fat 12.4 g

Fiber 2.1 g

Carbs 4.5 g

Protein 8.2 g

Cocoa and Nuts Bombs

Preparation Time: 13 minutes

Cooking time: 8 minutes

Servings: 12

Ingredients:

- 2 cups macadamia nuts; chopped.
- ¼ cup cocoa powder
- 1/3 cup swerve
- 4 tbsp. coconut oil; melted
- 1 tsp. vanilla extract

Directions:

Take a bowl and mix all the ingredients and whisk well.

Shape medium balls out of this mix, place them in your air fryer and cook at 300°F for 8 minutes. Serve cold

Nutrition:

Calories: 120

Fat: 12g

Fiber: 1g

Carbs: 2g

Protein: 1g

Sweet Cinnamon Peaches

Preparation time: 5 minutes

Cooking time: 10 minutes

Servings: 4

Ingredients:

- 2 tablespoons sugar
- ¼ teaspoon ground cinnamon
- 4 peaches, cut into wedges
- Cooking spray

Directions:

1. Grease your air fryer basket using a cooking spray.

2. In a large bowl, stir the sugar and cinnamon. Add the peaches to the bowl and toss to coat evenly.
3. Spread the coated peaches in a single layer on the basket.
4. Select Air Fry, set the temperature to 350°F (180°C), and set time to 10 minutes.
5. After 5 minutes, remove and flip the peaches over. Lightly mist them with cooking spray. Return until done.
6. Let rest for 5 minutes before serving.

Nutrition:

Calories: 80

Carbs: 20g

Fat: 0g

Protein: 0g

Chapter 7: Phase 2 of Sirt-food Diet: Maintenance

In phase 2 of the sirtfood diet, it is expected that you would progress with your fat loss. As phase 2 progresses, if you stick religiously with your diet, you are likely to find yourself getting slimmer and feeling even more energized and pumped to tackle your daily tasks. In phase 2 of the sirtfood diet, you would be eating three times a day, meaning that issues of hunger, fatigue, and irritability due to restriction of calories should not be a problem here. Even though it is advised that you eat thrice, it is still recommended that you do not over-eat. Eat till you feel reasonably full and satisfied, and then stop. Satisfaction and sustainability are the hallmarks of phase 2, and this phase, if handled well, will help you integrate the sirtfood diet into your lifestyle.

How to Prepare for Phase 2

To help you coast through the second phase of the sirtfood diet successfully, there are trifling pointers that you harmonize and probably start implementing right from your first phase. These tips include:

To ensure that you maximize the benefits of this power drink, it is important that you drink it thirty minutes to one hour before having your main breakfast. Waking up early will help you ensure that you drink your sirtfood green juice, get a little workout done, and get ready for work before finally eating your healthy sirtfood breakfast. The combination of the sirtfood meal and the sirtfood green juice will help fill you up and get you energized to maximize your day, while of course, helping you to melt away those fat deposits along the way.

Eat dinner early: Whether you are on a diet or not, medical experts generally advise against late-might eating. It is healthier to eat your dinner early, between 6 PM and 7 PM, and then get a little rest before retiring to bed. So, instead of working late and wolfing down a heavy dinner in bed at 11 PM, try to take a break, eat your healthy dinner, and then get back to handling the rest of your work. It helps if you are done with your work at least one hour before bed so that you can give your body the opportunity to gradually calm down before you sleep. To ensure the optimal success of the sirtfood diet, you should get an average of 7 -8 hours of sleep per night. If you are extremely busy, try to get at least 6 hours of sleep every night. That will help the nutrients in the food repair and rejuvenate your body cells, which will make you healthier, stronger, and well-built. Sleeping early also generally makes you focused and energized when you wake up to tackle the challenges of the next day.

Eat balanced, measured potions: It is important to strike a balance in the quantity of food you would be eating. Eat too much, and you would be overloading your body with calories. You may think: "But the aim is to get as much of the important chemicals as possible!". Yes, you want to have as many polyphenols as healthily possible into your system, but over-eating can cause constipation and affect the action of the sirtuins in your body. So, eat till you are satiated, and then stop. Since you will be eating three meals per day in the second phase, there is no need for you to overload yourself at any time. Eat till you feel reasonably satisfied, get to work, and then eat another meal later. You don't have to go hungry, but you don't have to overload yourself to the point of lethargy either. Let your appetite guide you and stay energized and focused.

Drink your sirtfood juice once: The sirtfood juice is an excellent source of nutrients and polyphenols for activating your sirtuin genes. However, as you progress with the diet and eat more food on a daily basis, you are required to gradually begin to slow down your consumption of the sirtfood green juice., You will recall that in Phase 1, the sirtfood green juice was recommended to be consumed thrice per day alongside one mail for the first three days. In the last four days of phase 1, the recommended daily intake of the sirtfood green juice reduces to two cups, and you become required to eat two meals per day. Once you transition into phase 2 of your diet, however, things change. You can now eat three meals per day, meaning you can get an optimum supply of your nutrients from your food, and intense calorie restriction is no longer necessary. For this reason, once phase 2 begins, you should only consume your sirtfood green juice only once a day – and that's very early in the morning, thirty minutes to one hour before your main breakfast.

Apart from the sirtfood green juice, you can still drink a couple of liquids in phase 2 of the diet. These liquids include water, flavored water, black coffee, and green tea. You may also consume red wine up to three times a week as soon as you commence phase 2.

Expectations for Phase 2

In phase 2, your weight loss journey will continue. The amount of fat that would be eradicated in this phase would vary from one individual to another. However, it is not unconventional for people to lose up to 10 more pounds in pure fat in this phase. As we constantly advise, do not try to judge the success of your dieting efforts by checking a weighing scale every morning. The diet is aimed to help you burn fat and improve your muscle mass, so while losing fat, your muscle cells may be actively dividing, thereby helping you to increase your muscle mass. To help you track your fat loss rate, you can look at your body periodically in the mirror, check the fit of your clothes, or ask for a few trusted opinions.

Phase 2 will also come with enhanced focus and vitality. The active components of the sirtfoods will continue to keep your sirtuin genes activated, leading to feelings of enhanced mental clarity and boosted concentration. The consumption of the foods contained in the sirtfood diet helps to rejuvenate your brain cells, thereby helping to improve brainpower.

If you were addicted to junk food and sugary products prior to staring the sirtfood diet, phase 2 is the stage where your cravings begin to lessen considerably. This is because you would be having three healthy meals per day, and a nutrient-packed cup of green juice to start your day with. Your body would constantly feel satiated, and that urge to dash across the street to grab a burger and a soda just won't be there since you would not be feeling hungry in the first place.

In the long-term, completing phase 2 of the sirtfood diet and moving on to integrate the sirtfood diet system into your lifestyle would help reduce your susceptibility to debilitating diseases. The consumption of unhealthy food leads to the accumulation of fat deposits in the body, as has been described earlier in this book. When you consume a lot of sugar processed regularly, the sugar will gain easy access to your bloodstream, increasing your blood sugar levels, and by extension, your insulin levels. Once your insulin levels pass a certain safe threshold, the natural burning of fats in the body is suppressed, and you begin to trend towards obesity. With obesity comes a high likelihood of heart disease since the fats would make it compulsory for the heart to pump blood at unhealthily high pressure. In some cases, the fat deposits may even block key blood vessels within the body, which can lead to falling unconscious and even death.

Meal Plan for Phase 2

Throughout the fourteen days of phase 2, you will be drinking one serving of sirtfood juice very early in the morning at least thirty minutes to one hour before food. You will also be consuming three standard meals a day – breakfast, lunch, and dinner. These meals will provide your body with the necessary calories and nutrients it needs to stay energized and satiated while eradicating unhealthy fat deposits and repairing your body's cells. In phase 2, carefully selected sirtfood snacks may also be introduced, and they may be consumed once or twice per day. The sirtfood snacks can particularly come in handy when you are in a position where you cannot have a standard meal right away. So instead of violating your diet's rules and eating unhealthy junk, you can simply have a healthy sirtfood snack, pending the time you can eat a standard meal. Sirtfood snacks can be particularly great for long meetings, flights, and long road travels, shopping, and other related circumstances.

Also, one final reminder, the sirtfood diet works best when the foods digest and get the chance to start working before you go to bed, so your dinner should not exceed 7 PM.

Breakfast Options

The foods in this section may be eaten at 7-day intervals. Depending on your preferences and your schedule, however, you can modify this suggestion to fit your lifestyle. Meal option one may be eaten on the eighth day of your diet and the 15th day, for instance. Meal 2 may be eaten on day 9 of the diet and day 16. The point is to make the food as varied as possible and to eat as many meals as possible before consuming the same food again.

The breakfast options include:

Sirtfood smoothie

Sirt muesli

Yogurt, berries, walnut and dark chocolate

Spicy scrambled eggs

Mushroom/ tofu scramble

Buckwheat pancakes, walnuts, strawberries and chocolate

Sirtfood omelet.

Lunch options

Just as instructed for the breakfast options, the lunch options may also be eaten once a week, preferably on a specific day of the week to help you vary your diet and find your new feeding regimen interesting.

Lunch options include:

Sirt chicken salad.

Waldorf salad – apples, walnuts, celery, and mayonnaise.

Sirt tuna salad.

Strawberry buckwheat salad.

Buckwheat pasta salad.

Tofu and shiitake mushroom soup

Whole wheat leavened bread.

Dinner options

Foods that may be eaten for dinner during phase 2 of the sirtfood diet include:

Stir-fry shrimp and buckwheat noodles.

Tuscan bean stew.

Potatoes, kale, curry, and chicken.

Kale, red onions and buckwheat

Sirt chili con carne

Kidney bean mole and baked potatoes

Sirtfood pizza.

Breakfast Recipes

Buckwheat Granola

Preparation Time: 15 minutes

Cooking Time: 30 minutes

Servings: 10

Ingredients:

- 2 cups raw buckwheat groats
- ¾ cup pumpkin seeds
- ¾ cup almonds, chopped
- 1 cup unsweetened coconut flakes
- 1 teaspoon ground cinnamon
- 1 teaspoon ground ginger
- 1 ripe banana, peeled
- 2 tablespoons maple syrup
- 2 tablespoons olive oil

Directions:

1. Preheat your oven to 350 °F.
2. In a bowl, place the buckwheat groats, coconut flakes pumpkin seeds, almonds and spices and mix well.
3. In another bowl, add the banana and with a fork, mash well.
4. Add to the buckwheat mixture, maple syrup and oil and mix until well combined.
5. Transfer the mixture onto the prepared baking sheet and spread in an even layer.
6. Bake for approximately 25-30 minutes, stirring once halfway through.
7. Remove the baking sheet from oven and set aside to cool.

Nutrition:

Calories 252

Total Fat 14.3 g

Saturated Fat 3.7 g

Cholesterol 0 mg

Sodium 5 mg

Total Carbs 27.6 g

Fiber 4.9 g

Sugar 4.9 g

Protein 7.6 g

Lara Burns

Sirtfood Muffins

Preparation Time: 25 minutes

Cooking Time: 2 hours 16 minutes

Servings: 18

Ingredients:

- 1 cup milk
- 2 tbsps. White sugar
- 1 (.25 oz.) package active dry yeast
- 1 cup warm water (110 degrees F/45 degrees C)
- 1/4 cup melted shortening
- 6 cups all-purpose flour
- 1 tsp. salt

Directions:

1. In a small saucepan, warm milk until it is bubbling. Take away from the heat. Add sugar while stirring until it is dissolved. Allow cooling to lukewarm. Dissolve the yeast in warm water in a small bowl and leave to sit for about 10 minutes until creamy.
2. Combine 3 cups flour, shortening, yeast mixture, and milk in a large bowl. Then beat until the mix is smooth. Pour in salt and remaining flour or enough of it to form a soft dough. Knead and transfer into a greased bowl. Cover the dough and leave it to rise.
3. Press down and then roll out into about half inch thick. Use empty tuna can, drinking glass or a biscuit cutter to cut the rounds. Drizzle cornmeal onto waxed paper and leave the rounds to rise on this. Dust cornmeal onto the tops of muffins. Cover them and allow rising for 1/2 hour.
4. Heat griddle that is greased and then cook the muffins for about 10 minutes per side in the griddle over medium heat. Keep the baked muffins in a warm oven until all are cooked. Cool, transfer into plastic bags and store.
5. To use, cut and then toast. Good together with jam, cream cheese or orange butter.

Nutrition:

Calories per serving: 163

Carbohydrates: 45.6 g

Protein: 3 g

Fat: 0.6g

Sugar: 1g

Sodium: 87mg

Fiber: .7 g

Fruity Tofu Smoothie

Preparation Time: 5 Minutes

Cooking Time: 0 Minutes

Servings: 2

Ingredients:

- 1 c. ice cold water
- 1 c. packed spinach
- ¼ c. frozen mango chunks
- ½ c. frozen pineapple chunks
- 1 tbsp. chia seeds
- 1 container silken tofu
- 1 frozen medium banana

Directions:

1. Add all ingredients in a blender until smooth and creamy.
2. Evenly divide into two glasses, serve and enjoy.

Nutrition:

Calories: 175

Fat: 3.7 g

Carbs: 33.3 g

Protein: 6.0 g

Black currants and oat yogurt

Preparation time: 10 minutes

Cooking time: 0 minutes

Serving: 2

Ingredients:

- 100 g black currants, washed and stems removed
- 2 tbsp powdered sugar + 100 ml water
- 200 g natural yogurt
- 40 g jumbo oats

Directions:

1. Put the black currants, sugar and water in a small pan and bring to a boil. Reduce the heat slightly, simmer vigorously, and continue cooking for 5 minutes.
2. Turn off the stove and let it cool down. The blackcurrant compote can now be refrigerated until it is used. Place the yogurt and oats in a large bowl and stir together. Divide the blackcurrant compote between two bowls and top with yogurt and oats. Use a cocktail stick to toss the compote through the yogurt.

Nutrition:

241 calories

Easy Granola Clusters

Preparation time: 5 minutes

Cooking time: 1 minutes

Servings: 2 cups

Ingredients:

- 1½ cups peanut butter
- ¼ cup maple syrup (optional)
- 1½ cups old-fashioned rolled oats
- ½ cup raisins
- ¾ cup flaxseed meal
- ¾ cup raw sunflower seeds (no shells)

Direction:

1. Place the peanut butter and maple syrup (if desired) in a medium microwave-

safe bowl. Microwave them on high for 30-second intervals, stirring between intervals, or until the mixture is well incorporated and smooth. Allow to cool for a few minutes.
2. Fold in the oats, raisins, flaxseed meal, and sunflower seeds and stir the ingredients until they are completely combined.
3. Spread the mixture evenly on a baking sheet and freeze for at least 25 minutes until firm.
4. Break it into clusters before serving.

Nutrition:

Calories: 493

Fat: 31.0g

Carbs: 49.8g

Protein: 16.0g

Fiber: 12.2g

Stovetop Granola

Preparation time: 5 minutes

Cooking time: 10 minutes

Servings: 6 cups

Ingredients:

- 5 cups rolled oats
- ¾ cup date molasses or brown rice syrup (optional)
- 1 tablespoon ground cinnamon
- ½ teaspoon salt (optional)
- 1 cup chopped dried fruit

Directions:

1. Place the oats in a saucepan over medium-low heat and toast for 4 to 5 minutes, stirring constantly to prevent burning, or until the oats are lightly toasted. Transfer the toasted oats to a medium bowl.
2. Add the date molasses (if desired) to the saucepan and cook over medium-low

heat for 1 minute. Stir in the toasted oats, cinnamon, and salt (if desired). Transfer the mixture to a nonstick baking sheet and allow to cool to room temperature.

3. When cooled, transfer the mixture to a large bowl and add the dried fruit and mix well. Serve immediately.

Nutrition:

Calories: 327

Fat: 5.7g

Carbs: 69.2g

Protein: 14.5g

Fiber: 14.9g

No Bake Peanut Butter Granola Bars

Preparation time: 10 minutes

Cooking time: 0 minutes

Servings: 12 bars

Ingredients:

- 1 cup packed pitted dates
- ¼ cup creamy natural peanut butter or almond butter
- ¼ cup pure maple syrup (optional)
- 1½ cups old-fashioned oats
- 1 cup coarsely chopped roasted unsalted almonds

Directions:

1. Pulse the dates, peanut butter, and maple syrup (if desired) in a food processor until the mixture starts to come together and feels slightly sticky. Stop right before or as it starts to turn into a ball of loose dough.
2. Add the oats and almonds and pulse for 1 minute. Transfer the dough to a baking dish and cover with plastic wrap. Place in the refrigerator for 20 minutes until chilled.
3. Cut into 12 bars and serve immediately.

Nutrition:

Calories: 182

Fat: 8.8g

Carbs: 24.3g

Protein: 5.1g

Fiber: 4.2g

Banana Muesli with Dates

Preparation time: 5 minutes

Cooking time: 0 minutes

Servings: 2

Ingredients:

- 1 banana, peeled and sliced
- 1 cup rolled oats
- ½ cup pitted and chopped dates
- ¾ cup unsweetened almond milk
- ¼ cup unsweetened coconut, toasted

Directions:

1. Mix together all the ingredients in a large bowl until well combined and let soak 15 minutes, or until all the milk is absorbed.
2. Give it a good stir and serve immediately.

Nutrition:

Calories: 391

Fat: 8.1g

Carbs: 82.1g

Protein: 10.5g

Fiber: 13.0g

Apple Muesli

Preparation time: 5 minutes

Cooking time: 0 minutes

Servings: 2

Ingredients:

- 1 cup rolled oats

- ½ cup raisins
- ¾ cup unsweetened almond milk
- 2 tablespoons date molasses or brown rice syrup (optional)
- ¼ teaspoon ground cinnamon
- 1 Granny Smith apple, cored and chopped

Directions:

1. Stir together the oats, raisins, almond milk, date molasses (if desired), and cinnamon in a large bowl and let soak 15 minutes.
2. When ready, add the chopped apple and stir to combine. Serve immediately.

Nutrition:

Calories: 356

Fat: 4.7g

Carbs: 79.9g

Protein: 10.1g

Fiber: 11.5g

Blueberry Oatmeal

Preparation time: 5 minutes

Cooking time: 5 minutes

Servings: 2

Ingredients:

- 1½ cups unsweetened coconut milk
- 1 cup old-fashioned rolled oats
- ½ cup fresh or frozen blueberries, thawed if frozen
- Optional Toppings:
- 2 tablespoons chopped nuts
- 2 to 3 tablespoons granola
- 1 tablespoon maple syrup (optional)
- 2 tablespoons raw sunflower seeds (no shells)
- 1 tablespoon coconut shreds
- 1 teaspoon spices of your choice (like cinnamon or pumpkin pie spice)

Directions:

1. Heat the milk in a medium saucepan over medium-high heat until boiling.
2. Fold in the oats and blueberries and stir well.
3. Reduce the heat to low and let simmer uncovered for 5 minutes, or until the water is absorbed, stirring occasionally.
4. Remove from the heat and top with toppings of choice.

Nutrition:

Calories: 273

Fat: 7.5g

Carbs: 45.4g

Protein: 14.4g

Fiber: 8.5g

Vanilla Steel-Cut Oatmeal

Preparation time: 5 minutes

Cooking time: 40 minutes

Servings: 4

Ingredients:

- 4 cups water
- Pinch sea salt (optional)
- 1 cup steel-cut oats
- ¾ cup unsweetened almond milk
- 2 teaspoons pure vanilla extract

Directions:

1. Place the water and salt (if desired) into a large pot over high heat and bring to a boil.
2. Reduce the heat to low and stir in the oats. Cook for about 30 minutes until the oats are soften, stirring occasionally.
3. Add the milk and vanilla and stir well. Cook for about 10 minutes more until your desired consistency is reached.
4. Remove the cereal from the heat and serve warm.

Nutrition:

Calories: 187

Fat: 0g

Carbs: 28.8g

Protein: 9.2g

Fiber: 5.0g

Easy and Healthy Oatmeal

Preparation time: 5 minutes

Cooking time: 5 minutes

Servings: 2

Ingredients:

- 1 cup rolled oats
- Sea salt, to taste (optional)
- 2 cups unsweetened coconut milk or water

Directions:

1. Cook the oats, salt (if desired), and milk in a small saucepan over medium-high heat. Bring to a boil.
2. Reduce the heat to medium and continue to cook for about 5 minutes, or until the oats have soaked up most of the liquid and are creamy, stirring occasionally.
3. Ladle into bowls and serve hot.

Nutrition:

Calories: 300

Fat: 11.2g

Carbs: 42.7g

Protein: 15.8g

Fiber: 7.2g

Slow Cooker Butternut Squash Oatmeal

Preparation time: 15 minutes

Cooking time: 6 hours

Servings: 4

Ingredients:

- 1 cup steel-cut oats
- 3 cups water
- 2 cups cubed (½-inch pieces) peeled butternut squash
- ¼ cup unsweetened coconut milk
- 1 tablespoon chia seeds
- 1½ teaspoons ground ginger
- 2 teaspoons yellow (mellow) miso paste
- 1 tablespoon sesame seeds, toasted
- 1 tablespoon chopped scallion, green parts only

Directions:

1. Mix together the oats, water, and butternut squash in a slow cooker.
2. Cover and cook on Low for 6 to 8 hours, or until the squash is tender when tested with a fork. Mash the cooked butternut squash with a potato masher or heavy spoon. Stir together the butternut squash and oats until well mixed.
3. Mix together the milk, chia seeds, ginger, and miso paste in a small bowl and stir to combine. Add this mixture to the squash mixture and stir well.
4. Ladle the oatmeal into bowls and serve hot topped with sesame seeds and scallion.

Nutrition:

Calories: 229

Fat: 4.9g

Carbs: 39.7g

Protein: 7.1g

Fiber: 9.0g

Multigrain Hot Cereal with Apricots

Preparation time: 30 minutes

Cooking time: 30 minutes

Servings: 2

Ingredients:

- ¼ cup long-grain brown rice
- 2 tablespoons rye
- 2 tablespoons millet
- 2 tablespoons wheat berries
- 2 tablespoons barley
- 6 dried apricots, chopped

2 cups water

Directions:

1. Rinse the grains and soak them in water for 30 minutes until softened and drain.
2. In a saucepan, add the soaked grains, apricots, and 2 cups of water and stir to combine.
3. Cook for about 17 minutes over low heat, or until the liquid is absorbed, stirring periodically.
4. Allow to cool for 15 minutes before serving.

Nutrition:

Calories: 242

Fat: 1.6g

Carbs: 50.5g

Protein: 6.5g

Fiber: 6.1g

Hot Breakfast Couscous Cereal

Preparation time: 10 minutes

Cooking time: 6 minutes

Servings: 4

Ingredients:

- ¾ cup water
- ½ cup couscous
- ¼ cup squeezed orange juice
- 1 tablespoon maple syrup (optional)
- 1 tablespoon frozen apple juice
- 1 teaspoon finely grated orange zest
- Dash ground cinnamon

Directions:

1. In a large casserole dish, add all the ingredients and stir well. Cover in aluminum foil.
2. Transfer the dish to a microwave oven and cook for 5 to 6 minutes on high heat, stirring occasionally to prevent sticking.
3. Let sit for another 1 minute, covered.
4. Divide the cereal among bowls and serve hot.

Nutrition:

Calories: 47

Fat: 0.3g

Carbs: 10.3g

Protein: 0.9g

Fiber: 0.5g

Apple Pancakes

Preparation Time: 15 minutes

Cooking Time: 24 minutes

Servings: 6

Ingredients:

- ½ cup buckwheat flour
- 2 tablespoons coconut sugar
- 1 teaspoon baking powder
- ½ teaspoon ground cinnamon
- 1/3 cup unsweetened almond milk
- 1 egg, beaten lightly
- 2 granny smith apples, peeled, cored and grated

Directions:

1. In a bowl, place the flour, coconut sugar and cinnamon and mix well.
2. In another bowl, place the almond milk and egg and beat until well combined.
3. Now, place the flour mixture and mix until well combined.
4. Fold in the grated apples.
5. Heat a lightly greased nonstick wok over medium-high heat.

6. Add desired amount of mixture and with a spoon, spread into an even layer.
7. Cook for 1-2 minutes on each side.
8. Repeat with the remaining mixture.
9. Serve warm with the drizzling of honey.

Nutrition:

Calories 93

Total Fat 2.1 g

Saturated Fat 1 g

Cholesterol 27 mg

Sodium 23 mg

Total Carbs 22 g

Fiber 3 g

Sugar 12.1 g

Protein 2.5 g

Lunch

Asparagus Soup

Preparation time: 5 minutes

Cooking time: 28 minutes

Servings: 6

Ingredients:

- 4 pounds potatoes, peeled, chopped
- 1 bunch of asparagus
- 15 ounces cooked cannellini beans
- 1 small white onion, peeled, diced
- 3 teaspoons minced garlic
- 1 teaspoon grated ginger
- ½ teaspoon salt
- ¼ teaspoon ground black pepper
- 1 lemon, juiced
- 1 tablespoon olive oil
- 8 cups vegetable broth

Directions:

1. Place oil in a large pot, place it over medium heat and let it heat until hot.

2. Add onion into the pot, stir in garlic and ginger and then cook for 5 minutes until onion turns tender.
3. Add potatoes, asparagus, and beans, pour in the broth, stir until mixed, and then bring the mixture to a boil.
4. Cook the potatoes for 20 minutes until tender, remove the pot from heat and then puree half of the soup until smooth.
5. Add salt, black pepper, and lemon juice, stir until mixed, ladle soup into bowls and then serve.

Nutrition:

Calories: 123.3

Fat: 4.4 g

Protein: 4.7 g

Carbs: 16.3 g

Fiber: 4.1 g

Kale White Bean Pork chops

Preparation Time: 5 minutes

Cooking Time: 45 minutes

Servings: 4-6

Ingredients:

- 3 tbsp extra-virgin olive oil
- 3 tbsp chili powder
- 1 tbsp jalapeno hot sauce
- 2 pounds bone-in pork chops
- Salt
- 4 stalks celery, chopped
- 1 large white onion, chopped
- 3 cloves garlic, chopped
- 2 cups chicken broth
- 2 cups diced tomatoes
- 2 cups cooked white beans
- 6 cups packed kale

Directions:

1. Preheat the broiler.

2. Whisk hot sauce, 1 tbsp olive oil and chili powder in a bowl.
3. Season the pork chops with ½ tsp salt.
4. Rub chops with the spice mixture on both sides and place them on a rack set over a baking sheet.
5. Set aside.
6. Heat 1 tbsp olive oil in a pot over medium heat.
7. Add the celery, garlic, onion, and the remaining 2 tbsp chili powder.
8. Cook until onions are translucent, stirring (approx. 8 minutes).

Nutrition:

Calories: 140

Fat: 6 g

Carbohydrates: 14 g

Protein: 7 g

Fiber: 3 g

Tuna Salad

Preparation Time: 5 minutes

Cooking Time: 40 minutes

Servings: 3

Ingredients:

- 100g red chicory
- 150g tuna flakes in brine, drained
- 100g cucumber
- 25g rocket
- 6 kalamata olives, pitted
- 2 hard-boiled eggs, peeled and quartered
- 2 tomatoes, chopped
- 2 tbsp fresh parsley, chopped
- 1 red onion, chopped
- 1 celery stalk
- 1 tbsp capers
- 2 tbsp garlic vinaigrette

Directions:

1. Combine all ingredients in a bowl and serve.

Nutrition:

Calories: 240 Cal

Fat: 15 g

Carbohydrates: 7 g

Protein: 23 g

Fiber: 0 g

Turkey Curry

Preparation Time: 5 minutes

Cooking Time: 40 minutes

Servings: 3

Ingredients:

- 450g (1lb), turkey breasts, chopped
- 100g (3½ oz) fresh rocket (arugula) leaves
- 5 cloves garlic, chopped
- 3 tsp medium curry powder
- 2 tsp turmeric powder
- 2 tbsp fresh coriander (cilantro), finely chopped
- 2 bird's eye chilies, chopped
- 2 red onions, chopped
- 400ml (14fl oz) full-fat coconut milk
- 2 tbsp olive oil

Directions:

2. Heat the olive oil in a saucepan, add the chopped red onions and cook them for around 5 minutes or until soft.
3. Stir in the garlic and the turkey and cook it for 7-8 minutes.
4. Stir in the turmeric, chilies and curry powder then add the coconut milk and coriander cilantro).
5. Bring it to the boil, reduce the heat and simmer for around 10 minutes.
6. Scatter the rocket (arugula) onto plates and spoon the curry on top.
7. Serve alongside brown rice.

Lara Burns

Nutrition:

Calories: 400

Fat:6 g

Carbohydrates: 3 g

Protein: 14 g

Fiber: 0 g

Tofu and Curry

Preparation Time: 5 minutes

Cooking Time: 36 minutes

Servings: 4

Ingredients:

- 8 oz dried lentils (red preferably)
- 1 cup boiling water
- 1 cup frozen edamame (soy) beans
- 7 oz (½ of most packages) firm tofu, chopped into cubes
- 2 tomatoes, chopped
- 1 lime juices
- 5-6 kale leaves, stalks removed and torn
- 1 large onion, chopped
- 4 cloves garlic, peeled and grated
- 1 large chunk of ginger, grated
- ½ red chili pepper, deseeded (use less if too much)
- ½ tsp ground turmeric
- ¼ tsp cayenne pepper
- 1 tsp paprika
- ½ tsp ground cumin
- 1 tsp salt
- 1 tbsp olive oil

Directions:

1. Add the onion, sauté in the oil for few minutes then add the chili, garlic, and ginger for a bit longer until wilted but not burned.
2. Add the seasonings, then the lentils and stir

Nutrition:

Calories: 250

Fat: 5 g

Carbohydrates: 15 g

Protein: 28 g

Fiber: 1 g

Chicken and Bean Casserole

Preparation Time: 5 minutes

Cooking Time: 40 minutes

Servings: 3

Ingredients:

- 400g (14oz) chopped tomatoes
- 400g (14oz) tinned cannellini beans or haricot beans
- 8 chicken thighs, skin removed
- 2 carrots, peeled and finely chopped
- 2 red onions, chopped
- 4 sticks of celery
- 4 large mushrooms
- 2 red peppers (bell peppers), deseeded and chopped
- 1 clove of garlic
- 2 tbsp soy sauce
- 1 tbsp olive oil
- 1.75 liters (3 pints) chicken stock (broth)

Directions:

1. Heat the olive oil in a saucepan, put in garlic and onions and cook for 5 minutes.
2. Add in the chicken and cook for 5 minutes then add the carrots, cannellini beans, celery, red peppers (bell peppers) and mushrooms.
3. Pour in the stock (broth) soy sauce and tomatoes.
4. Bring it to the boil, reduce the heat and simmer for 45 minutes.
5. Serve with rice or new potatoes.

Nutrition:

Calories: 324

Fat: 11 g

Carbohydrates: 27 g

Protein: 28 g

Fiber: 7 g

Prawn and Coconut Curry

Preparation Time: 5 minutes

Cooking Time: 35 minutes

Servings: 3

Ingredients:

- 400g (14oz) tinned chopped tomatoes
- 400g (14oz) large prawns (shrimps), shelled and raw
- 25g (1oz) fresh coriander (cilantro) chopped
- 3 red onions, finely chopped
- 3 cloves of garlic, crushed
- 2 bird's eye chilies
- ½ tsp ground coriander (cilantro)
- ½ tsp turmeric
- 400ml (14fl oz) coconut milk
- 1 tbsp olive oil
- Juice of 1 lime

Directions:

1. Place the onions, garlic, tomatoes, chilies, lime juice, turmeric, ground coriander (cilantro), chilies and half of the fresh coriander (cilantro) into a blender and blitz until you have a smooth curry paste.
2. Heat the olive oil in a frying pan, add the paste and cook for 2 minutes.
3. Stir in the coconut milk and warm it thoroughly.
4. Add the prawns (shrimps) to the paste and cook them until they have turned pink and are thoroughly cooked.
5. Stir in the fresh coriander (cilantro).
6. Serve with rice.

Nutrition:

Calories: 163

Fat: 8 g

Carbohydrates: 8 g

Protein: 0 g

Fiber: 1 g

Moroccan Chicken Casserole

Preparation Time: 5 minutes

Cooking Time: 20 minutes

Servings: 3

Ingredients:

- 250g (9oz) tinned chickpeas (garbanzo beans) drained
- 4 chicken breasts, cubed
- 4 Medjool dates halved
- 6 dried apricots, halved
- 1 red onion, sliced
- 1 carrot, chopped
- 1 tsp ground cumin
- 1 tsp ground cinnamon
- 1 tsp ground turmeric
- 1 bird's eye chili, chopped
- 600ml (1 pint) chicken stock (broth)
- 25g (1oz) corn flour
- 60ml (2fl oz) water
- 2 tbsp fresh coriander

Directions:

1. Place the chicken, chickpeas (garbanzo beans), onion, carrot, chili, cumin, turmeric, cinnamon, and stock (broth) into a large saucepan.
2. Bring it to the boil, reduce the heat and simmer for 25 minutes.
3. Add in the dates and apricots and simmer for 10 minutes.
4. In a cup, mix the corn flour with the water until it becomes a smooth paste.
5. Pour the mixture into the saucepan and stir until it thickens.

6. Add in the coriander (cilantro) and mix well.

Nutrition:

Calories: 423

Fat: 12 g

Carbohydrates: 0 g

Protein: 39 g

Fiber: 0 g

Chili con Carne

Preparation Time: 5 minutes

Cooking Time: 30 minutes

Servings: 3

Ingredients:

- 450g (1lb) lean minced beef
- 400g (14oz) chopped tomatoes
- 200g (7oz) red kidney beans
- 2 tbsp tomato purée
- 2 cloves of garlic, crushed
- 2 red onions, chopped
- 2 bird's eye chilies, finely chopped
- 1 red pepper (bell pepper), chopped
- 1 stick of celery, finely chopped
- 1 tbsp cumin
- 1 tbsp turmeric
- 1 tbsp cocoa powder
- 400ml (14 oz) beef stock (broth)
- 175ml (6fl oz) red wine
- 1 tbsp olive oil

Directions:

1. Heat the oil in a large saucepan, add the onion and cook for 5 minutes.
2. Add in the garlic, celery, chili, turmeric, and cumin and cook for 2 minutes before adding then meat then cook for another 5 minutes.
3. Pour in the stock (broth), red wine, tomatoes, tomato purée, red pepper (bell pepper), kidney beans and cocoa powder.

Nutrition:

Calories: 320

Fat: 21 g

Carbohydrates: 8 g

Protein: 24 g

Fiber: 4 g

Tofu Thai Curry

Preparation Time: 5 minutes

Cooking Time: 30 minutes

Servings: 3

Ingredients:

- 400g (14oz) tofu, diced
- 200g (7oz) sugar snap peas
- 5cm (2-inch) chunk fresh ginger root, peeled and finely chopped
- 2 red onions, chopped
- 2 cloves of garlic, crushed
- 2 bird's eye chilies
- 2 tbsp tomato puree
- 1 stalk of lemongrass, inner stalks only
- 1 tbsp fresh coriander (cilantro), chopped
- 1 tsp cumin
- 300ml (½ pint) coconut milk
- 200ml (7fl oz) vegetable stock (broth)
- 1 tbsp virgin olive oil
- juice of 1 lime

Directions:

1. Heat the oil in a frying pan, add the onion and cook for 4 minutes.
2. Add in the chilies, cumin, ginger, and garlic and cook for 2 minutes.
3. Add the tomato puree, lemongrass, sugar-snap peas, lime juice and tofu and cook for 2 minutes.

4. Pour in the stock (broth), coconut milk and coriander (cilantro) and simmer for 5 minutes.
5. Serve with brown rice or buckwheat and a handful of rockets (arugula) leaves on the side.

Nutrition:

Calories: 412

Fat: 30 g

Carbohydrates: 27 g

Protein: 14 g

Fiber: 5 g

Roast Balsamic Vegetables

Ingredients:

- 4 tomatoes, chopped
- 2 red onions, chopped
- 3 sweet potatoes, peeled and chopped
- 100g (3½ oz) red chicory (or if unavailable, use yellow)
- 100g (3½ oz) kale, finely chopped
- 300g (11oz) potatoes, peeled and chopped
- 5 stalks of celery, chopped
- 1 bird's eye chili, deseeded and finely chopped
- 2 tbsp fresh parsley, chopped
- 2 tbsp fresh coriander (cilantro) chopped
- 3 tbsp olive oil
- 2 tbsp balsamic vinegar
- 1 tsp mustard
- Sea salt
- Freshly ground black pepper

Directions:

1. Place the olive oil, balsamic, mustard, parsley, and coriander (cilantro) into a bowl and mix well.

2. Toss all the remaining ingredients into the dressing and season with salt and pepper.
3. Transfer the vegetables to an ovenproof dish and cook in the oven at 200C/400F for 45 minutes.

Nutrition:

Calories: 70

Fat: 0 g

Carbohydrates: 8 g

Protein: 2 g

Fiber: 2 g

Chickpea Salad

Preparation time: 5 minutes

Cooking time: 0 minutes

Servings: 2

Ingredients:

- 1 cup cooked chickpeas
- 16 leaves of butter lettuce
- 1 cup chopped zucchini
- ½ spring onion, chopped
- 1 cup chopped celery
- 1 cup grated carrot
- 1 tablespoon chopped cilantro
- ½ teaspoon salt
- ½ tablespoon lemon juice

Directions:

1. Take a large bowl, place all the ingredients in it, toss until mixed, and let it sit for 15 minutes.
2. Divide the lettuce leaves between two portions, top with the salad evenly and then serve.

Nutrition:

Calories: 166.6

Fat: 7.7 g

Protein: 4.4 g

Carbs: 20.8 g

Fiber: 4.3 g

Tofu and Pesto Sandwich

Preparation time: 5 minutes

Cooking time: 15 minutes

Servings: 4

Ingredients:

- 12 ounces of tofu, pressed, drained
- 4 leaves of butter lettuce
- 4 slices of tomato
- 4 tablespoons basil pesto
- 1 tablespoon olive oil
- 4 slices of whole-wheat sandwich bread

Directions:

1. Switch on the oven, then set it to 375 degrees F and let it preheat.
2. Cut tofu into slices, place them in a bowl, and drizzle with oil and then sprinkle with oregano.
3. Spread tofu pieces on a baking sheet and then roast for 15 minutes.
4. Assemble the sandwich and for this, spread 1 tablespoon of basil pesto on one side of each sandwich slice, top with a lettuce leaf, tomato slice, and tofu.
5. Serve straight away.

Nutrition:

Calories: 219

Fat: 13.5 g

Protein: 8 g

Carbs: 18.5 g

Fiber: 4 g

Dinner

Beef bourguignon with Mashed potatoes and kale

Preparation time: 15 minutes

Cooking time: 2 - 3 hours

Serving: 4

Ingredients:

- 800 g diced beef
- 2–3 tbsp buckwheat flour
- 1 tbsp extra virgin olive oil
- 150 g red onion, roughly chopped
- 200 g celery, roughly chopped
- 100 g carrots, roughly chopped
- 2–3 cloves of garlic, chopped
- 375 ml of red wine
- 2 tbsp tomato puree
- 750 ml beef broth
- 2 bay leaves
- 1 sprig of fresh thyme or 1 tablespoon of dried thyme
- 75 g diced pancetta or smoked lard
- 250 g mushrooms
- 2 tbsp chopped parsley
- 200 g kale
- 1 tbsp corn flour or arrowroot (optional)
- For the porridge:
- 500g Edward potatoes
- 1 tbsp milk and 1 tbsp olive oil

Directions:

1. Pat the beef dry with kitchen paper. Heat a heavy saucepan over medium-high heat. Add the olive oil, then the beef and sauté the meat until it is browned nicely all over. Depending on the size of your pan, it's best to do this in 3-4 small loads.
2. When all of the meat is brown, remove it from the pan with a slotted spoon and set aside. In the same pan, add the onion, celery, carrot and garlic and fry

over medium heat for 3 to 4 minutes until tender. Add the wine, tomato paste and broth and bring to a boil. Add the browned beef, bay leaves and thyme and reduce the heat to a simmer. Cover the pan with a lid and cook for 2 hours, stirring from time to time to make sure nothing sticks to the bottom. While the beef is cooking, peel your potatoes and cut them into quarters (or smaller pieces if they're quite large).

3. Put in a pan with cold water and bring to a boil. Reduce the heat to a simmer and cook for 20-25 minutes, covered with a lid. When soft, drain and mash with olive oil and milk. Keep warm. While the potatoes are boiling, heat a pan over high heat. When it's hot but not smoking, add the diced pancetta.

4. The fat content of the bacon means you don't need oil to cook it. When some of the fat has been released and it's starting to brown, add the mushrooms and cook over medium heat until both are nicely browned. Depending on the size of your pan, you may need to do this in multiple loads. Set aside after cooking. Cook or steam the kale for 5–10 minutes until soft. Once the beef is tender enough and the sauce has thickened to your liking, add the pancetta, mushrooms, and parsley. If your sauce is still a little runny, you can mix the corn flour or arrowroot with a little water and then stir the paste into the sauce until you have the consistency you want. Cook for 2-3 minutes and serve with porridge and kale.

Nutrition:

Carbohydrates: 34

Fat: 25

Protein: 31

Kcal: 510

Barbecued Lime Shrimp

Preparation time: 5 minutes

Cooking time: 15 minutes

Servings: 4

Ingredients:

- 4 cups of shrimp
- 1 ½ cups barbeque sauce
- One fresh lime, cut into quarters

Directions:

1. Preheat your air fryer to 360°Fahrenheit. Place the shrimp in a bowl with barbeque sauce. Stir gently. Allow shrimps to marinade for at least 5minutes. Place the shrimp in the air fryer and cook for 15-minutes. Remove from air fryer and squeeze lime over shrimps.

Nutrition:

Calories: 289

Total Fat: 9.8g

Carbs: 8.7g

Protein: 14.9g

Crispy Shrimp

Preparation time: 2 minutes

Cooking time: 8 minutes

Servings: 8

Ingredients:

- Four egg whites
- One cup almond flour
- 2 lbs. shrimp, peeled and deveined
- ½ teaspoon cayenne pepper
- Two tablespoon olive oil
- One cup breadcrumb
- Salt and black pepper to taste

Directions:

1. In a dish, mix flour, pepper, and salt. In a small bowl, whisk egg whites. In another bowl, combine breadcrumbs, cayenne pepper, and salt. Preheat your air fryer to 400°Fahrenheit. Coat the shrimp with flour mixture, dip in egg white, then finally coat with breadcrumbs. Place shrimp in air fryer basket and drizzle with olive oil and cook in batches for 8-minutes each.

Nutrition:

Calories: 295

Total Fat: 9.2g

Carbs: 8.3g

Protein: 15.3g

Spicy Air-Fried Cheese Tilapia

Preparation time: 5minutes

Cooking time: 10 minutes

Servings: 4

Ingredients:

- 1 lb. tilapia fillets
- One tablespoon olive oil
- Salt and pepper to taste
- Two teaspoons paprika
- One tablespoon parsley, chopped
- ¾ cup parmesan cheese, grated

Directions:

1. Preheat your air fryer to 400°Fahrenheit. Mix the parmesan cheese, parsley, paprika, salt, and pepper. Drizzle olive oil over the tilapia fillets and coat with paprika and cheese mixture. Place the coated tilapia fillets on aluminum foil. Put into the air fryer and cook for 10-minutes.

Nutrition:

Calories: 289

Total Fat: 8.9g

Carbs: 7.8g

Protein: 14.9g

Cheese Salmon

Preparation time: 4 minutes

Cooking time: 11 minutes

Servings: 6

Ingredients:

- 2 lbs. salmon fillet
- Salt and pepper to taste
- ½ cup parmesan cheese, grated
- ¼ cup parsley, fresh, chopped
- Two garlic cloves, minced

Directions:

1. Preheat your air fryer to 350°Fahrenheit. Put the salmon skin side facing down on aluminum foil and cover with another piece of foil. Cook salmon for 10-minutes. Remove the salmon from foil and top it with minced garlic, parsley, parmesan cheese, and pepper. Return salmon to air fryer for 1-minute cook time.

Nutrition:

Calories: 297

Total Fat: 9.5g

Carbs: 8.3g

Protein: 14.9g

Herb Salmon Fillet

Preparation time: 2 minutes

Cooking time: 8 minutes

Servings: 2

Ingredients:

- ½ lb. salmon fillet
- ¼ teaspoon thyme
- One teaspoon garlic powder
- ½ teaspoon cayenne pepper

- ½ teaspoon paprika
- ¼ teaspoon sage
- ¼ teaspoon oregano
- Salt and pepper to taste

Directions:

1. Rub the seasoning all over the salmon. Preheat your air fryer to 350°Fahrenheit. Place the seasoned salmon fillet into an air fryer basket and cook for 8-minutes.

Nutrition:

Calories: 298

Total Fat: 9.3g

Carbs: 8.6g

Protein: 10.2g

Crunchy Fish Taco

Preparation time: 5 minutes

Cooking time: 18 minutes

Servings: 4

Ingredients:

- 12-ounce cod fillet
- Salt and black pepper to taste
- 1 cup tempura batter
- 1 cup breadcrumbs
- ½ cup guacamole
- 6-flour tortillas
- Two tablespoons cilantro, freshly chopped
- ½ cup of salsa
- One lemon, juiced

Directions:

1. Cut the cod fillets lengthwise into 2-inch pieces and season with salt and pepper. Dip each cod strip into tempura butter then into breadcrumbs. Preheat your air fryer to 340°Fahrenheit and cook cod for 13-minutes. Spread guacamole on each tortilla. Place cod stick on

tortilla and top with chopped cilantro and salsa. Squeeze lemon juice on top, then fold and serve.

Nutrition:

Calories: 300

Total Fat: 10.3g

Carbs: 8.9g

Protein: 14.8g

Air-Fryer Baked Salmon & Asparagus

Preparation time: 5 minutes

Cooking time: 15 minutes

Servings: 4

Ingredients:

- Four salmon fillets
- Four asparagus
- Two tablespoons butter
- Three lemons, sliced
- Salt and pepper to taste

Directions:

1. Preheat the air fryer to 300°Fahrenheit. Take four pieces of aluminum foil. Add asparagus, half lemon juice, pepper, and salt in a bowl and toss. Divide seasoned asparagus evenly on four aluminum foil pieces. Put one salmon fillet asparagus. Put some lemon slices on top of salmon fillets. Fold foil tightly to seal the parcel. Place in an air fryer basket and cook for 15-minutes. Serve warm.

Nutrition:

Calories: 291

Total Fat: 16g

Carbs: 1g

Protein: 35g

Potato Fish Cake

Preparation time: 10 minutes

Cooking time: 15 minutes

Servings: 2

Ingredients:

- 1 ½ cups white fish, cooked
- Pepper and salt to taste
- 1 ½ tablespoon of milk
- ½ cup of mashed potatoes
- One tablespoon butter
- Two teaspoons gluten-free flour
- One teaspoon parsley
- ½ teaspoon sage

Directions:

1. Add ingredients to a mixing bowl and combine well. Make round patties and place them in the fridge for 1 hour. Place the patties into the air fryer at 375°Fahrenheit for 15-minutes.

Nutrition:

Calories: 167

Total Fat: 9g

Carbs: 14g

Protein: 5g

Parmesan Baked Salmon

Preparation time: 5 minutes

Cooking time: 11 minutes

Servings: 5

Ingredients:

- 2 lbs. fresh salmon fillet
- Salt and pepper to taste
- ½ cup parmesan cheese, grated
- ¼ cup fresh parsley, chopped
- Two garlic cloves, minced

Directions:

1. Preheat the air fryer to 300°Fahrenheit. Put some salmon with the skin side down on foil and cover with more foil. Bake the salmon in the air fryer basket for 10-minutes. Open the foil and top salmon with cheese, garlic, pepper, salt, and parsley. Return for an additional minute in the air fryer.

Nutrition:

Calories: 267

Total Fat: 12g

Carbs: 6g

Protein: 37g

Garlic Salmon Patties

Preparation time: 6 minutes

Cooking time: 15 minutes

Servings: 4

Ingredients:

- One egg
- 14-ounce can of salmon, drained
- Salt and pepper to taste
- 2 tablespoons mayonnaise
- ½ teaspoon garlic powder
- Four tablespoons onion, minced
- Four tablespoons gluten-free flour
- Four tablespoons cornmeal

Directions:

1. Add drained salmon into a bowl and with a fork flake the salmon. Add garlic powder, mayonnaise, flour, cornmeal, onion, egg, pepper, and salt. Mix well. Make round patties with mix and place them in the air fryer. Air fry at 300°Fahrenheit for 15-minutes.

Nutrition:

Calories: 244

Total Fat: 11g

Carbs: 14g

Protein: 22g

Turkish fajitas

Preparation time: 15 minutes

Cooking time: approx. 1 hour

Serving: 4

Ingredients:

- For the filling
- Cut 500 g turkey breast into strips
- 1 tablespoon of extra virgin olive oil 1-2 chilies, depending on taste, chopped
- 150 g red onion, thinly sliced
- 150 g red pepper, cut into thin strips
- 2–3 cloves of garlic, chopped
- 1 tbsp paprika
- 1 tbsp ground cumin
- 1 teaspoon chili powder
- 1 tbsp chopped coriander
- For the guacamole
- 2 ripe avocados, peeled (reserve one of the stones)
- Juice of 1 lime
- Pinch of chili powder
- Pinch of black pepper
- For the salsa
- 1 × 400 g can of chopped tomatoes
- 20 g red onion, diced
- 20 g red pepper, deseeded and diced
- Juice of ½ - 1 lime, depending on the size
- 1 teaspoon chopped coriander
- 1 teaspoon capers

For the salad

- 100 g rocket
- 3 tomatoes, cut
- 100 g cucumber, thinly sliced
- 1 tbsp extra virgin olive oil juice of ½ lemon
- For serving

- 100 g cheddar cheese
- 8 grated whole grain tortilla wraps

Directions:

1. Mix the filling ingredients together and set them aside while you prepare the other parts.
2. Put all of the guacamole ingredients in a small food processor and flash until a smooth paste is formed. Alternatively, you can mash them all together with the back of a fork or spoon.
3. Place the reserved avocado stone in the guacamole - it will keep it from turning brown. Mix all the ingredients for the salsa.
4. Put all the salad ingredients in a large bowl. Put your largest pan on high heat until it starts to smoke.
5. Put the turkey filling in the hot pan - you may need to cook it in 2 to 3 loads as overcrowding the pan will create too much moisture and it will start boiling instead of frying.
6. Keep the pan over high heat and keep moving the mixture so the turkey colors nicely but doesn't burn.
7. In a low oven, keep the cooked meat warm. To serve, reheat the tortillas according to the directions in the package, then sprinkle some guacamole over each package.
8. Top with some cheese and some salsa, then stack the turkey mixture in the middle and roll it up like a large cigar. Serve with the salad.

Nutrition:

Carbohydrates: 44

Fat: 21

Protein: 30

Kcal: 450

Salad

Chicken & Kale Salad

Preparation Time: 20 minutes

Cooking Time: 18 minutes

Servings: 4

Ingredients: For Chicken:

- 1 teaspoon dried thyme
- ½ teaspoon garlic powder
- ½ teaspoon onion powder
- ¼ teaspoon cayenne pepper
- ¼ teaspoon ground turmeric
- Salt and ground black pepper, as required
- 2 (7-ounce) boneless, skinless chicken breasts, pounded into ¾-inch thickness
- 1 tablespoon olive oil

For Salad:

- 6 cups fresh kale, tough ribs removed and chopped
- 2 cups carrots, peeled and cut into matchsticks
- ¼ cup walnuts
- For Dressing:
- 1 small garlic clove, minced
- 2 tablespoons fresh lime juice
- 2 tablespoons extra-virgin olive oil
- 1 teaspoon raw honey
- ½ teaspoon Dijon mustard
- Salt and ground black pepper, as required

Directions:

1. Preheat your oven to 425 °F.
2. Line a baking dish with parchment paper.
3. For chicken: in a bowl, mix together the thyme, spices, salt and black pepper.
4. Drizzle the chicken breasts with oil and then rub with spice mixture generously.
5. Arrange the chicken breasts onto the prepared baking dish.
6. Bake for approximately 16-18 minutes.
7. Remove the baking dish from oven and transfer chicken breasts onto a cutting board for about 5 minutes.
8. For salad: place all ingredients in a salad bowl and mix.
9. For dressing: place all ingredients in another bowl and beat until well combined.
10. Cut each chicken breast into desired sized slices.
11. Place the salad onto each serving plate and top each with chicken slices.
12. Drizzle with dressing and serve.

Nutrition:

Calories 330

Total Fat 18.9 g

Saturated Fat 1.9 g

Cholesterol 64 mg

Sodium 162 mg

Total Carbs 16.5 g

Fiber 2.8 g

Sugar 4 g

Protein 25.3 g

White Bean and Carrot Salad

Preparation time: 10 minutes

Cooking time: 0 minutes

Servings: 4

Ingredients:

Dressing:

- 2 tablespoons balsamic vinegar
- 1 tablespoon olive oil (optional)
- 1 tablespoon fresh rosemary, chopped
- 1 tablespoon fresh oregano, chopped
- 1 teaspoon minced fresh chives
- 1 garlic clove, minced

- Pinch sea salt (optional)

Salad:

- 1 (14-ounce / 397-g) can cannellini beans, drained and rinsed
- 2 carrots, diced
- 6 mushrooms, thinly sliced
- 1 zucchini, diced
- 2 tablespoons fresh basil, chopped

Directions:

1. In a large bowl, stir together all the ingredients for the dressing.
2. Add all the ingredients for the salad to the bowl and toss to combine well.
3. Divide the salad between 2 bowls and serve immediately.

Nutrition:

Calories: 359

Fat: 17.9g

Carbs: 7.8g

Protein: 18.1g

Fiber: 15.2g

Lentil and Swiss chard Salad

Preparation time: 10 minutes

Cooking time: 50 minutes

Servings: 4

Ingredients:

- 1 teaspoon plus ¼ cup avocado oil, divided (optional)
- 1 garlic clove, minced
- 1 small onion, diced
- 1 carrot, diced
- 1 cup lentils
- 1 tablespoon dried oregano
- 1 tablespoon dried basil
- 1 tablespoon low-sodium balsamic vinegar
- 2 cups water

- ¼ cup red wine vinegar
- 1 teaspoon sea salt (optional)
- 2 cups chopped Swiss chard
- 2 cups torn red leaf lettuce

Directions:

1. Heat 1 teaspoon of avocado oil (if desired) in a saucepan over medium heat.
2. Add the garlic and onion and sauté for 5 minutes or until fragrant and the onion is soft.
3. Add the carrot and sauté for 3 minutes or until the carrot is tender.
4. Add the lentils and sprinkle with oregano and basil. Drizzle with balsamic vinegar. Pour in the water and bring to a boil over high heat.
5. Reduce the heat to low and simmer for 20 minutes or until the lentils are tender and hold together. Stir constantly.
6. Meanwhile, combine the red wine vinegar with remaining avocado oil (if desired) and salt (if desired) in a small bowl. Stir to mix well.
7. When the simmering is complete, pour in half of the red wine vinegar mixture and stir in the Swiss chard. Cook on low heat for another 10 minutes. Stir constantly.
8. Toss the lettuce with remaining red wine vinegar mixture and place on 4 serving plate. Top the lettuce with the lentil mixture and serve immediately.

Nutrition:

Calories: 387

Fat: 17.0g

Carbs: 23.0g

Protein: 18.0g

Fiber: 19.0g

Ritzy Southwest Beans Salad

Preparation time: 10 minutes

Cooking time: 0 minutes

Servings: 2

Ingredients:

- ½ cup cooked chickpeas
- ½ cup cooked black beans
- 1 medium avocado, peeled, pitted, and cubed
- 1 cup canned unsweetened kernel corn
- 4 cups chopped fresh lettuce
- 1 cup halved cherry tomatoes
- 1 red bell pepper, sliced
- ⅓ cup onion, diced ½ teaspoon chili powder
- ¼ teaspoon cumin
- 1 tablespoon apple cider vinegar
- 2 teaspoons avocado oil (optional)
- Salt and ground black pepper, to taste (optional)

Directions:

1. Combine all the ingredients in a large bowl. Toss to mix well.
2. Serve immediately.

Nutrition:

Calories: 397

Fat: 16.8g

Carbs: 51.0g

Protein: 11.2g

Fiber: 13.2g

Chicken & Berries Salad

Preparation Time: 20 minutes

Cooking Time: 16 minutes

Servings: 8

Ingredients:

- 2 pounds boneless, skinless chicken breasts
- ½ cup olive oil
- ¼ cup fresh lemon juice

- 2 tablespoons maple syrup
- 1 garlic clove, minced
- Salt and ground black pepper, as required
- 2 cups fresh strawberries, hulled and sliced
- 2 cups fresh blueberries
- 10 cups fresh baby arugula

Directions:

1. For marinade: in a large bowl, add oil, lemon juice, Erythritol, garlic, salt and black pepper and beat until well combined.
2. In a large resealable plastic bag, place the chicken and ¾ cup of marinade.
3. Seal bag and shake to coat well.
4. Refrigerate overnight.
5. Cover the bowl of remaining marinade and refrigerate before serving.
6. Preheat the grill to medium heat. Grease the grill grate.
7. Remove the chicken from bag and discard the marinade.
8. Place the chicken onto grill grate and grill, covered for about 5-8 minutes per side.
9. Remove chicken from grill and cut into bite sized pieces.
10. In a large bowl, add the chicken pieces, strawberries and spinach and mix.
11. Place the reserved marinade and toss to coat.
12. Serve immediately.

Nutrition:

Calories 377

Total Fat 21.5 g

Saturated Fat 4.2 g

Cholesterol 101 mg

Sodium 126 mg

Total Carbs 12.6 g

Fiber 2 g

Sugar 9 g

Protein 34.1 g

Soup

Beans & Kale Soup

Preparation Time: 15 minutes

Cooking Time: 30 minutes

Servings: 6

Ingredients:

- 2 tablespoons olive oil
- 2 onions, chopped
- 4 garlic cloves, minced
- 1 pound kale, tough ribs removed and chopped
- 2 (14-ounce) cans cannellini beans, rinsed and drained
- 6 cups water
- Salt and ground black pepper, as required

Directions:

1. In a large pan, heat the oil over medium heat and sauté the onion and garlic for about 4-5 minutes.
2. Add the kale and cook for about 1-2 minutes.
3. Add beans, water, salt and black pepper and bring to a boil.
4. Cook, partially covered for about 15-20 minutes.
5. Serve hot.

Nutrition:

Calories 204

Total Fat 4.7 g

Saturated Fat 0.7 g

Cholesterol 0 mg

Sodium 85 mg

Total Carbs 31.6 g

Fiber 12.8 g

Sugar 1.6 g

Protein 11.5 g

Turnip Green Soup

Preparation time: 5 minutes.

Cooking time: 22 minutes.

Servings: 2

Ingredients:

- 2 tbsps. Coconut oil
- 1 large chopped onion
- 3 minced cloves chive
- 2—in piece peeled and minced ginger
- 3 cups bone broth
- 1 medium cubed white turnip
- 1 large chopped head radish
- 1 bunch chopped kale
- 1 Seville orange, 1/2 zested and juice reserved
- 1/2 tsp. sea salt
- 1 bunch cilantro

Directions:

1. In a skillet, add oil then heat it.
2. Add in the onions as you stir.
3. Sauté for about 7 minutes, then add chive and ginger.
4. Cook for about 1 minute.
5. Add in the turnip, broth, and radish then stir.
6. Bring the soup to boil then reduce the heat to allow it to simmer.
7. Cook for an extra 15 minutes then turn off the heat.
8. Pour in the remaining ingredients.
9. Using a handheld blender, pour the mixture.
10. Garnish with cilantro.
11. Serve warm.

Nutrition:

Calories: 249

Fat: 11.9g

Carbs: 1.8g

Protein: 35g

Lentil Kale Soup

Preparation time: 5 minutes.

Cooking time: 15 minutes.

Servings: 4

Ingredients:

- 1/2 Onion
- 2 Zucchinis
- 1 rib Celery
- 1 stalk Chive
- 1 cup diced tomatoes
- 1 tsp. dried vegetable broth powder
- 1 tsp. Sazon seasoning
- 1 cup red lentils
- 1 tbsp. Seville orange juice
- 3 cups alkaline water
- 1 bunch kale

Directions:

- In a greased pan, pour in all the vegetables.
- Sauté for about 5 minutes, then add the tomatoes, broth, and Sazon seasoning.
- Mix properly then stir in the red lentils together with water.
- Cook until the lentils become soft and tender.
- Add the kale then cook for about 2 minutes.
- Serve warm with the Seville orange juice.

Nutrition:

Calories: 301

Fat: 12.2g.

Carbs: 15g.

Protein: 28.8g.

Tangy Lentil Soup

Preparation time: 5 minutes.

Cooking time: 15 minutes.

Servings: 4

Ingredients:

- 2 cups picked over and rinsed red lentils
- 1 chopped serrano Chile pepper
- 1 large chopped and roughly tomato
- 1-1/2 inch peeled and grated piece ginger
- 3 finely chopped cloves chive
- 1/4 tsp. ground turmeric
- Sea salt
- Topping
- 1/4 cup coconut yogurt

Directions:

1. In a pot add the lentils with enough water to cover the lentils.
2. Boil the lentils then reduce the heat.
3. Cook for about 10 minutes on low heat to simmer.
4. Add the remaining ingredients, then stir.
5. Cook until lentils become soft and properly mixed.
6. Garnish a dollop of coconut yogurt.
7. Serve.

Nutrition:

Calories: 248

Fat: 2.4g.

Carbs: 12.2g.

Protein: 44.3g.

Lentils & Greens Soup

Preparation Time: 15 minutes

Cooking Time: 55 minutes

Servings: 6

Ingredients:

- 1 tablespoon olive oil
- 2 carrots, peeled and chopped
- 2 celery stalks, chopped
- 1 medium red onion, chopped
- 3 garlic cloves, minced
- 1½ teaspoon ground cumin
- 1 teaspoon ground turmeric
- ¼ teaspoon red pepper flakes
- 1 (14½-ounce) can diced tomatoes
- 1 cup red lentils, rinsed
- 5½ cups water
- 2 cups fresh mustard greens, chopped
- Salt and ground black pepper, as required
- 2 tablespoons fresh lemon juice

Directions:

1. Heat olive oil in a large pan over medium heat and sauté the carrots, celery and onion for about 5-6 minutes.
2. Mix the garlic and spices and sauté for about 1 minute.
3. Add the tomatoes and cook for about 2-3 minutes.
4. Stir in the lentils and water and bring to a boil.
5. Now, reduce the heat to low and simmer, covered for about 35 minutes.
6. Stir in greens and cook for about 5 minutes.
7. Stir in salt, black pepper and lemon juice and remove from the heat.
8. Serve hot.

Nutrition:

Calories 174

Total Fat 3.1 g

Saturated Fat 0.5 g

Cholesterol 0 mg

Sodium 59 mg

Total Carbs 27.8 g

Fiber 12.4 g

Sugar 4.8 g

Protein 10 g

Beverages
Sirt shot

Preparation time: 5 minutes

Cooking time: 0 minutes

Serving: 1

Ingredients:

- 3–5 cm (10 g) turmeric root, peeled
- 4–6 cm (25 g) fresh ginger, peeled
- ½ medium-sized (70 g) apple, unpeeled
- Juice of ¼ lemon
- Pinch of black pepper

Directions:

1. Put all ingredients in a powerful mixer and stir until smooth.
2. Once the matcha has dissolved, add the rest of the juice. If the mixture is too thick, just add some water and mix until you get the consistency you want.

Nutrition:

Carbohydrates: 7

Fat: 10

Protein: 2

Kcal: 110

Hot chocolate eggnog

Preparation time: 5 minutes.

Cooking Time: 2 Minutes.

Servings: 4

Ingredients:

- 4 cups light eggnog
- Whipped cream for topping
- 2 cups white chocolate chips
- Sprinkles for topping

Directions:

1. Put in eggnog and white chocolate into a medium pot. Warm over low flame but do not let it achieve boiling, let it simmer till chocolate melts, one to two minutes.
2. Mix properly and pour drink into serving cups. In a swirling manner pour whipped cream on top and garnish using sprinkles. Have a blast!

Nutrition:

Carbohydrates: 8

Fat: 3

Protein: 1

Kcal: 100

Mint julep

Preparation time: 5 minutes.

Cooking Time: 15 Minutes.

Servings: 2

Ingredients:

- 2 tablespoon peppermint simple syrup
- 4 ½ cups cranberry ginger ale
- 4 ½ candy canes for garnish
- 4 ½ sprigs fresh pine for garnish
- 1 cup crushed ice

Directions:

1. Distribute peppermint syrup among the bottom of four glasses.
2. Put in crushed ice and pour on cranberry ginger ale. Add peppermint sprigs and candy canes in all the drinks. Have a blast.

Nutrition:

Calories: 160

Fat: 4.5g.

Carbs: 33.7g.

Protein: 1.8g.

Fiber: 0g.

Gingerbread latte

Preparation time: 10 minutes.

Cooking Time: 3 hours.

Servings: 4

Ingredients:

- 4 cups whole milk
- 3 cups brewed strong coffee
- 4 cinnamon sticks
- 1/3 cup granulated sugar
- 1/2 tsp ground allspice
- 1/4 tsp ground cloves
- 1 tsp nutmeg powder
- Whipped cream
- 2 tsp ginger powder
- Caramel sauce

Directions:

1. Mini gingerbread sweets
2. Put in all ingredients excluding for topping ones in a slow cooker; Mix properly.
3. Cover cooker: let it cook over high setting for almost three hours or over low setting for four hours.
4. Distribute drink among the mugs. In a swirling manner pour whipped cream on top, and then caramel sauce.
5. Garnish using gingerbread sweets and Have a blast!

Nutrition:

Calories: 389

Fat: 34.6g.

Carbs: 20.7g.

Protein: 4.8g.

Fiber: 0g.

Chili chocolate

Preparation time: 5 minutes

Cooking time: 0 minutes

Serving: 1

Ingredients:

- 1 chili
- 250 ml milk or non-dairy
- Alternative 1 teaspoon cocoa powder (100 percent)
- 35 g dark chocolate (70 percent cocoa solids),
- 1 teaspoon grated date syrup

Directions:

1. Halve the chilies and cut into 6 or 7 pieces. Place in a small saucepan with the remaining ingredients and bring to the boil over medium to high heat, stirring occasionally, so that the milk does not burn or boil over.
2. Simmer gently for 2-3 minutes, then remove from heat and let steep for 1 minute. Pass through a fine sieve and serve.

Nutrition:

Carbohydrates: 17

Fat: 9

Protein: 4

Kcal: 150

Vegan

Lemony Brussels Sprouts and Tomatoes

Preparation time: 15 minutes

Cooking time: 20 minutes

Servings: 4

Ingredients:

- 1-pound (454 g) Brussels sprouts, trimmed and halved
- 1 tablespoon extra-virgin olive oil

- Sea Salt
- ground black pepper
- ½ cup sun-dried tomatoes, chopped
- 2 tablespoons freshly squeezed lemon juice
- 1 teaspoon lemon zest

Directions:

1. Line a large baking sheet with aluminum foil.
2. Toss the Brussels sprouts with the olive oil in a large bowl. Sprinkle with salt and black pepper.
3. Arrange the brussels sprouts on the baking sheet.
4. Select Roast, set temperature to 400ºF (205ºC), and set time to 20 minutes.
5. Once preheated, place the baking sheet into the oven.
6. When done, the Brussels sprouts should be caramelized. Transfer to a serving bowl, along with the tomatoes, lemon juice, and lemon zest. Toss to combine. Serve immediately.

Nutrition:

Calories: 70

Carbs: 11g

Fat: 3g

Protein: 3g

Maple and Pecan Granola

Preparation time: 5 minutes

Cooking time: 20 minutes

Servings: 4

Ingredients:

- 1½ cups rolled oats
- ¼ cup maple syrup
- ¼ cup pecan pieces
- 1 teaspoon vanilla extract
- ½ teaspoon ground cinnamon

Directions:

1. Line a baking sheet with parchment paper.
2. Mix the oats, maple syrup, pecan pieces, vanilla, and cinnamon in a large bowl and stir until the oats and pecan pieces are completely coated. Spread the batter on the baking sheet.
3. Set temperature to 300°F (150°C) and set time to 20 minutes.
4. Once preheated, place the baking sheet into the oven. Stir once halfway through the cooking time.
5. When done, cool it for 30 minutes before serving. The granola may still be a bit soft right after removing, but it will gradually firm up as it cools.

Nutrition:

Calories: 137

Carbs: 18g

Fat: 6g

Protein: 3g

Sweet and Spicy Broccoli

Preparation time: 10 minutes

Cooking time: 20 minutes

Servings: 4

Ingredients:

- ½ teaspoon olive oil,
- 1-pound (454 g) f broccoli, cut into florets
- ½ tablespoon garlic
- Salt, to taste
- Sauce:
- 1½ tablespoons soy sauce
- 2 teaspoons hot sauce or sriracha
- 1½ teaspoons honey
- 1 teaspoon white vinegar
- Freshly ground black pepper, to taste

Directions:

1. Grease a perforated pan with olive oil.
2. Add the broccoli florets, ½ teaspoon of olive oil, and garlic to a large bowl and toss well—season with salt to taste.
3. Put the broccoli in the perforated pan in a single layer.
4. Select Air Fry, set temperature to 400°F (205°C), and set time to 15 minutes.
5. Once preheated, place the pan into the oven. Stir the broccoli florets three times during cooking.
6. Meanwhile, whisk all the ingredients for the sauce in a small bowl until well incorporated.
7. The broccoli should be lightly browned and crispy. Continue cooking for 5 minutes, if desired. Transfer and pour over the sauce and toss to combine. Add more salt and pepper if needed. Serve warm.

Nutrition:

Calories: 68

Carbs: 4g

Fat: 4g

Protein: 3g

Roasted Vegetables with Basil

Preparation time: 15 minutes

Cooking time: 20 minutes

Servings: 2

Ingredients:

- 1 small eggplant, halved and sliced
- 1 yellow bell pepper, strips
- 1 red bell pepper, strips
- 2 garlic cloves, quartered
- 1 red onion, sliced
- 1 tablespoon extra-virgin olive oil
- Salt
- ground black pepper
- ½ cup chopped fresh basil, for garnish
- Cooking spray

Directions:

1. Grease a nonstick baking dish with cooking spray.
2. Place the eggplant, bell peppers, garlic, and red onion in the greased baking dish. Drizzle with the olive oil and toss to coat well. Spritz any uncoated surfaces with cooking spray.
3. Set temperature to 350ºF (180ºC) and set time to 20 minutes.
4. Turn over the vegetables halfway through the cooking time. When done, put salt plus pepper.
5. Sprinkle the basil on top for garnish and serve.

Nutrition:

Calories: 60

Carbs: 8g

Fat: 3g

Protein: 1g

Cinnamon Celery Roots

Preparation time: 10 minutes

Cooking time: 20 minutes

Servings: 4

Ingredients:

- 2 celery roots, peeled and diced
- 1 teaspoon extra-virgin olive oil
- 1 teaspoon butter, melted
- ½ teaspoon ground cinnamon
- Sea salt
- ground black pepper

Directions:

1. Line a baking sheet with aluminum foil.
2. Toss the celery roots with the olive oil in a large bowl until well coated. Transfer them to the prepared baking sheet.
3. Select Roast, set temperature to 350ºF (180ºC), and set time to 20 minutes.

4. When done, the celery roots should be very tender. Transfer, then stir in the butter and cinnamon and mash them with a potato masher until fluffy.
5. Season with salt and pepper to taste. Serve immediately.

Nutrition:

Calories: 36

Carbs: 8g

Fat: 0g

Protein: 0g

Cheesy Broccoli Tots

Preparation time: 20 minutes

Cooking time: 15 minutes

Servings: 4

Ingredients:

- 12 ounces (340 g) frozen broccoli, thawed, drained, and patted dry
- 1 large egg, lightly beaten
- ½ cup seasoned whole-wheat bread crumbs
- ¼ cup shredded reduced-fat sharp Cheddar cheese
- ¼ cup grated Parmesan cheese
- 1½ teaspoons minced garlic
- Salt
- ground black pepper
- Cooking spray

Directions:

1. Spritz a perforated pan lightly with cooking spray.
2. Place the remaining ingredients into a food processor and process until the mixture resembles a coarse meal. Transfer the mixture to a bowl.
3. Using a tablespoon, scoop out the broccoli mixture and form into 24 oval "tater tot" shapes with your hands.

4. Put the tots in the prepared perforated pan in a single layer, spacing them 1 inch apart. Mist the tots lightly with cooking spray.
5. Select Air Fry, set temperature to 375°F (190°C), and set time to 15 minutes.
6. Flip the tots halfway through the cooking time.
7. When done, the tots will be lightly browned and crispy. Serve on a plate.

Nutrition:

Calories: 12

Carbs: 2g

Fat: 3g

Protein: 4g

Paprika Cauliflower

Preparation time: 10 minutes

Cooking time: 20 minutes

Servings: 4

Ingredients:

- 1 large head cauliflower, florets
- 2 teaspoons smoked paprika
- 1 teaspoon garlic powder
- Salt
- ground black pepper
- Cooking spray

Directions:

1. Spray a perforated pan with cooking spray.
2. Toss the cauliflower florets with the smoked paprika and garlic powder until evenly coated in a medium bowl. Sprinkle with salt and pepper.
3. Place the cauliflower florets in the perforated pan and lightly mist with cooking spray.
4. Select Air Fry, set temperature to 400°F (205°C), and set time to 20 minutes.

5. Stir the cauliflower four times during cooking. Remove and serve hot.

Nutrition:

Calories: 90

Carbs: 4g

Fat: 8g

Protein: 2g

Roasted Asparagus with Eggs and Tomatoes

Preparation time: 10 minutes

Cooking time: 12 minutes

Servings: 4

Ingredients:

- 2 pounds (907 g) asparagus, trimmed
- 3 tablespoons extra-virgin olive oil, divided
- 1 teaspoon kosher salt, divided
- 1-pint cherry tomatoes
- 4 large eggs
- ¼ teaspoon freshly ground black pepper

Directions:

1. Put the asparagus on the sheet pan and drizzle with 2 tablespoons of olive oil, tossing to coat. Season with ½ teaspoon of kosher salt.
2. Select Roast, set temperature to 375°F (190°C), and cook within 12 minutes.
3. Meanwhile, toss the cherry tomatoes with the remaining 1 tablespoon of olive oil in a medium bowl until well coated.
4. After 6 minutes, remove the pan and toss the asparagus. Evenly spread the asparagus in the middle of the sheet pan. Add the tomatoes around the perimeter of the pan. Return it to the oven.
5. After 2 minutes, remove the pan from the oven.
6. Carefully crack the eggs, one at a time, over the asparagus, spacing them out—

season with the remaining ½ teaspoon of kosher salt and the pepper.

7. Return it to the oven, then cook for an additional 3 to 7 minutes.

8. When done, divide the asparagus and eggs among four plates. Top each plate evenly with the tomatoes and serve.

Nutrition:

Calories: 335

Carbs: 0g

Fat: 0g

Protein: 0g

Snacks and desserts

Chocolate Maple Walnuts

Preparation time: 15 minutes

Cooking Time: 30 minutes

Servings: 4

Ingredients:

- ½ cup pure maple syrup, divided
- 2 cups raw, whole walnuts
- 5 squares of dark chocolate, at least 85%
- 1 ½ tablespoons coconut oil, melted
- 1 tablespoonful of water
- Sifted icing sugar
- 1 teaspoonful of vanilla extract

Directions:

1. Line a large baking sheet with parchment paper.

2. In a medium to large skillet, combine the walnuts and ¼ cup of maple syrup and cook over medium heat, stirring continuously, until walnuts are completely covered with syrup and golden in color, about 3 – 5 minutes.

3. Pour the walnuts onto the parchment paper and separate into individual pieces with a fork. Allow to cool completely, at least 15 minutes.

4. In the meantime, melt the chocolate in a double boiler with the coconut oil. Add the remaining maple syrup and stir until thoroughly combined.

5. When walnuts are cooled, transfer them to a glass bowl and pour the melted chocolate syrup over top. Use a silicone spatula to gently mix until walnuts are completely covered.

6. Transfer back to the parchment paper lined baking sheet and, once again, separate each of the nuts with a fork.

7. Place the nuts in the fridge for 10 minutes or the freezer for 3 – 5 minutes, until chocolate has completely set.

8. Store in an airtight bag in your fridge.

Nutrition:

Calories 218

Fat 12.8

Fiber 6.2

Carbs 22.2

Protein 4.8

Matcha and Chocolate Dipped Strawberries

Preparation time: 5 minutes

Cooking time: 10 minutes

Servings: 4

Ingredients:

- 4 tablespoons cocoa butter
- 4 squares of dark chocolate, at least 85%
- ¼ cup coconut oil
- 1 teaspoon Matcha green tea powder
- 20 – 25 large whole strawberries, stems on

Directions:

1. Melt cocoa butter, dark chocolate, coconut oil, and Matcha in a double boiler until nearly smooth.

2. Remove from heat and continue stirring until chocolate is completely melted.
3. Pour into a large glass bowl and stir constantly until the chocolate thickens and starts to lose its sheen, about 2 - 5 minutes.
4. Working one at a time, hold the strawberries by stems and dip into chocolate matcha mixture to coat. Let excess drip back into bowl.
5. Place on a parchment-lined baking sheet and chill dipped berries in the fridge until shell is set, 20–25 minutes.
6. You may need to reheat matcha mixture if it starts to set before you have dipped all the berries.

Nutrition:

calories 261

fat 7.6

fiber 2.2

carbs 22.8

protein 12.5

Vegan Rice Pudding

Preparation time: 10 minutes

Cooking time: 20 minutes

Servings: 3

Ingredients:

- ½ tsp. ground cinnamon
- 1 c. rinsed basmati
- 1/8 tsp. ground cardamom
- ¼ c. sugar
- 1/8 tsp. pure almond extract
- 1 quart vanilla nondairy milk
- 1 tsp. pure vanilla extract

Directions:

1. Measure all of the ingredients into a saucepan and stir well to combine. Bring to a boil over medium-high heat.

2. Once boiling, reduce heat to low and simmer, stirring very frequently, about 15–20 minutes.
3. Remove from heat and cool. Serve sprinkled with additional ground cinnamon if desired.

Nutrition:

Calories: 148

Fat: 2 g

Carbs: 26 g

Protein: 4 g

Sugars: 35 g

Sodium: 150 mg

Plum Oat Bars

Preparation time: 5 minutes

Cooking time: 10 minutes

Servings: 4

Ingredients:

- Rolled oats – 1.5 cups
- Baking powder – 1 teaspoon
- Almond meal - .5 cup
- Cinnamon – 1.5 teaspoon
- Soybean oil – 2 tablespoons
- Sea salt - .25 teaspoon
- Prunes – 2 cups

Directions:

1. Begin by preheating the oven to Fahrenheit three-hundred and fifty degrees and preparing the prunes. Add the prunes to a large bowl and pour hot water over them until fully submerged. Allow the prunes to sit in the water for five minutes, until soft.
2. Remove the prunes from the water and transfer them to a blender or food processor, reserving the water. Pour in a small amount of the water that you previously reserved from the prunes and

blend until the prunes form a thick paste.

3. Add two tablespoons of the prepared prune puree to a medium kitchen bowl along with the oil, sea salt, baking powder, cinnamon, almond flour, and rolled oats. Combine together until the mixture resembles a crumble, slightly like wet sand. You can add more prune puree if it is too dry.

4. Line a square baking dish with kitchen parchment and then press three-quarters of the oat mixture into the bottom to form a crust. Spread the remaining prune puree over the top of the crust, and then sprinkle the remaining oat mixture over the prune puree to add a crumble.

5. Cook the bars in the oven until set and slightly toasted, about fifteen minutes. Remove the plum oat bars from the hot oven and let the pan cool completely. After the bars have reached room temperature slice them into nine bars and enjoy.

Nutrition:

calories 274

fat 11.6

fiber 2.8

carbs 11.5

protein 15.4

Spinach and Kale Mix

Preparation time: 5 minutes

Cooking time: 30 minutes

Servings: 4

Ingredients:

- 2 chopped shallots
- 1 c. no-salt-added and chopped canned tomatoes
- 2 c. baby spinach
- 2 minced garlic cloves
- 5 c. torn kale
- 1 tbsp. olive oil

Directions:

1. Heat up a pan with the oil over medium-high heat, add the shallots, stir and sauté for 5 minutes.
2. Add the spinach, kale and the other ingredients, toss, cook for 10 minutes more, divide between plates and serve.

Nutrition:

Calories: 89

Fat: 3.7 g

Carbs: 12.4 g

Protein: 3.6 g

 Sugars: 0 g

Sodium: 50 mg

Kale Dip with Cajun Pita Chips

Preparation time: 10 minutes

Baking time: 8 – 10 minutes

Cooking time: 1 hour

Ingredients:

For the Dip:

- 2 cups sour cream
- 1 ½ cups baby kale
- ¼ cup red bell pepper, diced
- ¼ cup green onions, diced
- 1 clove garlic, minced
- 1/8 teaspoon chili pepper flakes

For the Chips:

- 5 pita breads, halved and split open
- ½ cup extra virgin olive oil
- ½ teaspoon Cajun seasoning
- ¼ teaspoon ground cumin
- ¼ teaspoon turmeric
- Salt to taste

Directions:

1. To make the dip: In a bowl, combine the sour cream, baby kale, red pepper, onions, garlic, salt and chili pepper flakes. Cover and refrigerate for at least 1 hour.
2. To make the chips: Preheat oven to 400 degrees F
3. Cut each pita half into four wedges. Combine the olive oil, Cajun seasoning, cumin and turmeric and brush over the rough side of the pita wedges Place on ungreased baking sheets and bake for 8-10 minutes or until chips are golden brown and crisp.
4. Serve with dip.

Nutrition:

calories 326

fat 21.7

fiber 1.7

carbs 24.9

protein 8.8

Chapter 8: Sport and Sirt-food Diet

Exercising and the Sirtfood Diet

Doing physical activities is the most precious gift that you can give to your body. There is nothing that can stop a person from keeping the body fit. Neither age nor ability should matter when it comes to exercising. Besides, following a diet is also important.

Exercise is an important thing that everyone is quite aware of. Exercising regularly can have many healthful benefits for your body. This is mainly involved with moving your body parts. You can be active and maintain a weight that is healthy to keep yourself fit.

In this segment, we will be discussing sirtfood diet and whether or not accompanying exercise with this diet is essential.

Combining Sirtfood Diet with Exercise

According to fifty-two percent of Americans, taxes are easier to do, and understanding the ways of healthy eating is quite a difficult thing. They confess that they are more interested in following a diet that can be followed throughout and not a fad diet or something that requires switching on and off. They want a particular form of eating rather than adapting to new types now and then. Many people do not find it hard to either gain or lose weight. To them, it is just another task that can be achieved easily by doing some sort of exercise and following a regular diet. But others find it hard to lose or gain weight. It becomes very tricky for them to get back to their normal healthy weight. What a sirtfood diet does is help people who are overweight and trying hard to get back healthy weight, support them to achieve their goal easily and in a maintained manner.

But there are still questions related to combining exercise with a sirtfood diet. Researchers are still thinking about avoiding it completely or introducing it in the beginning.

Exercise during the First Week

The first or even two weeks of following the sirtfood diet mainly focuses on the reduction of calories. You are highly recommended to avoid any sort of exercise during these days as the body is adapting to decreased calorie intake. You should be aware of and always listening to whatever your body wants you to do. If it is becoming very tired or having lesser energy, you should readily give up on those strenuous exercises. Your main work will be to remain focused on the principles for getting your life back on track. You should be focusing on the foods that can melt those unnecessary pounds while expanding the muscles. These steps can be achieved by including foods that can offer the required amounts of fiber and protein.

Switching to the vegetables and fruits that can offer such nutrients can help you to get along in this process. Once you are done with following this diet for the first three weeks, you are advised to continue following this so that your body gets adapted to it completely, and you do not require to jump from one diet to the other frequently. Or you may even follow the signature juice-the green juice which is a part of this diet along with your regular diet.

Once the Diet Becomes a Way of Life

Ideally, you consume the required amount of protein after you are done doing the day's exercise. Protein does its work of repairing the muscles that have been torn while you were exercising. Reducing the soreness and helping by doing the recovery. Various recipes have been invented, which mainly focuses on an increased level of protein intake, which is best to consume after workouts. The fitness workouts that you will be doing will be completely down to you, but when you are working out at your own home, you will be able to choose the time you want to dedicate doing exercises and the types you will be doing according to your convenience.

The sirtfood diet helps you change the way you eat and can make you lose weight and feel healthier. Following this diet can be a tough thing to do for the first few weeks, as your body will be doing a lot like coping with the new number of calories, dealing with the fatigues, and a lot more. You must choose the recipes that are best suited for you. It is better to avoid doing exercises, but if you are dedicated to doing it at all, then you are required to be kind to your body and choose the ones that require less energy as your body is already trying to adapt to the new form of eating. You know how much you can push yourself and what are the limitations of doing that against your body. Try listening to your body and be kind to it.

Importance of Exercise

In this part, we will be explaining the benefits of exercising.

Feel Happier Now and Always

You want to be happy, right? Well, everyone wants to. You can start that by dedicating some time to exercise. It can do a lot to your body as well as to the mind. From decreasing the feeling of anxiety, stress, and depression to improving your mood, it can do it all. The part of the brain that is responsible for regulating the anxiety and stress undergoes certain changes while you do exercises. It can also make your brain become more sensitive to the hormones norepinephrine and serotonin, which is responsible for relieving the mind from feeling depressed. Endorphin production also increases while you exercise, thus helping you to reduce pain perception and making you feel more positive. Instilling with the thoughts of exercising can even make changes. It is powerful and can even make differences over short periods.

Helps You Lose Weight

Weight gain mainly occurs when a person is inactive. For that reason, it is very important to understand the link between losing weight and exercising to understand its effect on the reduction in weight.

The three main ways in which the body loses energy are exercising, digesting, and maintaining the body for performing functions like breathing and heartbeat. The metabolic rate gets reduced while dieting as the consumption of calories is reduced, which can delay the process of losing weight. The metabolic rate can be increased by exercising, which can burn the desired calories or even more and can even help weight loss.

Additionally, researchers have found that to keep your weight off; you should be combining resistance training with aerobic exercises that can help you lose maximum fat while still maintaining your muscle mass.

Increase in Energy Levels

Healthy people and those who are suffering from medical conditions can boost their energy by exercising regularly.

A study was conducted with thirty-six people who were healthy and were suffering from persistent fatigue. They were asked to exercise regularly for six weeks. And the result was unbelievable. After the time period, they were not complaining about feeling fatigued. It is also helpful for those with the pain of chronic fatigue syndrome. Doing exercise can also boost energy levels. Such patients can easily combine exercise like passive therapies that include stretching and relaxation with their treatments.

This is even found to be true for cancer patients and those suffering AIDS and several scleroses.

For Healthy Bones and Muscles

Maintaining strong bones and muscles is found to be an important role that is played when a person does exercises. Lifting heavy weights can stimulate the building of muscles, coupled with the intake of adequate amounts of protein. This is because hormones are released while doing exercise that promotes the absorption of amino acids by the muscle, which helps them to grow and lessens the breakdown.

With increasing age, people tend to lose their ability to function due to the loss of muscles. This loss can be essentially reduced, and strength can be maintained by practicing regular activities of the body. Gymnastics and playing games like basketball and soccer can promote increased bone density.

Reduce the Risk of Chronic Diseases

Chronic diseases are mainly caused due to the lack of physical activities. But people who have been exercising regularly have shown to improve the insulin sensitivity, composition of the body, and cardiovascular fitness. They have also shown a reduction in the levels of blood fat and blood pressure.

In contrast, people who were not doing fitness workouts regularly were facing significant problems like an increase in belly fat, which increased the risks of heart diseases and were responsible for early deaths.

Enhance Your Memory

The functioning of the brain can be effectively increased by doing regular exercise. This can also improve your thinking skills and protect your memory.

To start with, the rate of the heartbeat is essentially increased while exercising which increases blood flow in the brain cells. Certain hormones are stimulated that improves the growth of brain cells. It also helps to reduce certain diseases that can affect the functioning of the brain.

Exercise is important for aged people who are suffering from inflammation and oxidative stress. Exercise can help to prevent the change in the structure and function of the brain caused by these problems.

Improved Skin Health

The amount of oxidative stress that is produced in your body can affect your skin health. Free radicals cause damage to the cells, which is effectively repaired by the antioxidant defenses of the body. Oxidative stress occurs when these defenses are not able to repair the damages completely. The natural antioxidants that are present can easily be increased by doing moderate exercises, which can protect the cells. The skin cells can also be induced to adopt that can delay the skin aging process by stimulating the flow of blood by doing exercises.

Gain Efficiency in Sleeping Habits

While a person sleeps, all the restorative processes are stimulated by the depletion of the energy that occurs during exercising. The sleeping quality is increased by the increase in the temperature of the body while exercising. Doing moderate to strenuous physical activities regularly has shown to increase the quality of sleep and make them sleep longer who suffer from insomnia. Aged people are also benefited by doing mild exercises suffering from sleeping disorders.

Doing the right kind of exercise and choosing them according to your flexibility will be doing the perfect work in keeping your body fit and helping you get rid of the complications.

Get Rid of Pain

It is debilitating to feel pain, but you may use exercise to reduce them. Chronic pain can be easily reduced by exercising, which can also improve life quality. It can control the pain in many ways, including lowering the pain in the back, treating fibromyalgia, and other disorders in the shoulder.

Doing exercise can also increase your tolerance to pain and decrease the perception of pain.

The Physical Activity Effect

The Sirtfood Diet is about consuming certain products that are designed to promote sustainable weight loss and wellbeing by definition. But with the advantages that you see by practicing the plan, you can fall into the trap of feeling there's no need to exercise. This will be endorsed by many diet books, saying how ineffective exercise is compared with following the right diet for weight loss. And it's real; we can't outdo a bad diet. It's not the approach we saw earlier that was supposed to support weight loss. It's inefficient, and the harmfulness of being too many borders. So, it's that till we see stars or achieve an Olympian's feats, there's no need to pound the treadmill — but what about general everyday movement?

The truth is we are now much less involved than we used to be. The age of technology has ensured physical activity is practically factored out of our daily lives, for all the advancements it has provided. We don't have to mess with the whole process of being involved unless we want to. Forget about weight loss for a second and just glance at the litany of positive health benefits correlated with it. These include reduced risk of cardiovascular disease, stroke, hypertension, type 2 diabetes, osteoporosis, obesity and cancer, and improved mood, sleep, confidence, and a sense of wellbeing.

While many of the benefits of being active are driven by switching on our sirtuin genes, eating Sirtfoods shouldn't be used as a reason to not engage in exercise. Instead, we should understand how active the ideal complement to our Sirtfood intake is. It activates optimum stimulation of the sirtuin, and all the advantages that it provides, just as expected by definition.

What we are talking about here is meeting 150-minute (2 hours and 30 minutes) government guidelines of moderate physical activity a week. A moderate job is the equivalent of a brisk walk. But that doesn't have to be limited to this. Any sport or physical activity you love is fitting. Pleasure and exercise do not have to be mutually exclusive! So, their social aspect enriches squad or group sports even more. It's also about everyday things like taking the bike instead of the car, or getting off the bus one stop earlier, or just parking farther away to increase the distance you've got to walk around. Take the stairs and not the lift. Go outdoors and do gardening. Play in the park with your kids or get more out with the dog. Everything counts. Everything that has you up and moving will activate your sirtuin genes regularly and at moderate intensity, enhancing the benefits of the Sirtfood Diet.

Engaging in physical activity and eating a diet high in Sirtfood brings the buck the full sirtuin click. All it takes to achieve the benefit of physical activity is the equivalent of a quick 30-minute stroll five days a week.

Chapter 9: Pros and Cons of sirtfood diet

PROS

It Improves Powerful Exercise

Normal exercise is perhaps the best thing you can accomplish for your health and doing some direct exercise will improve the weight loss and medical advantages of Phase 1 of the diet. When in doubt, we urge you to proceed with your typical degree of activity and physical action through the initial seven days of the Sirtfood Diet. Be that as it may, we recommend remaining inside your typical safe place, since delayed or excessively extreme exercise may just place a lot of weight on the body for this period. Tune in to your body. There's no compelling reason to drive yourself to accomplish more exercise during Phase 1; let the Sirtfoods accomplish the difficult work.

It can be applied for underweight

A decent method to see whether you are underweight is to figure your weight file or BMI. For whatever length of time that you know your height and weight, you can without much of a stretch decide this by utilizing one of the various BMI adding machines on the web. In the event that your BMI is 18.5 or less, we don't suggest that you leave on Phase 1 of the eating routine. On the off chance that your BMI is somewhere in the range of 18.5 and 20, we would at present urge alert, since following the diet may imply that your BMI falls beneath 18.5. While numerous individuals seek to be super-thin, actually being underweight can adversely influence numerous parts of health, adding to a brought down safe structure, a raised danger of osteoporosis (debilitating of the bones), and ripeness issues. While we don't suggest Phase 1 of the diet on the off chance that you are underweight, we do at present energize the combination of a lot of Sirtfoods into a decent method of eating with the goal that all the medical advantages of these foods can be harvested.

Be that as it may, in the event that you are thin however have a BMI in the sound range (20–25), there is literally nothing preventing you from beginning. A larger part of the members engaged with the pilot preliminary had BMIs in the sound range, yet still lost great measures of weight and turned out to be progressively conditioned. Critically, a considerable lot of them announced a noteworthy improvement in energy levels, essentialness, and appearance. Recall that the Sirtfood Diet is tied in with advancing health as much for what it's worth about getting in shape.

Please, do not start the Sirtfood or any diet without a medical advice and without a physician following you in your journey.

Appropriate For weight loss

Being obese expands the danger of various constant medical issues, yet these are the very ailments that Sirtfoods help to secure against.

Provides Fiber

Numerous Sirtfoods are normally rich in fiber. Onions, garlic, and pecans are striking sources, with buckwheat and Medjool dates truly sticking out, implying that a Sirtfood-rich diet doesn't miss the mark in the fiber division. In any event, during Phase 1, when food utilization is decreased, the vast majority of us will in any case be eating a fiber amount we are utilized to, particularly on the off chance that we pick the plans that contain buckwheat, beans, and lentils from the menu choices. In any case, for others known to be powerless to stomach issues like obstruction without higher fiber admissions, during Phase 1, particularly Days 1 to 3, an appropriate fiber supplement can be thought of, which ought to be examined with your social insurance proficient.

CONS

Ineffective with Medication

The Sirtfood Diet is reasonable for the vast majority, but since of its amazing impacts on fat burning and health, it can change certain sickness forms and the activities of drug recommended by your doctor.

Discuss about this diet with your doctor first before trying it. The odds are it will be fine and really of significant advantage for you, yet it's critical to check.

Can't be administered during pregnancy or breastfeeding

Try not to follow the Sirtfood Diet on the off chance that you are attempting to imagine or in the event that you are pregnant or breastfeeding. It is a ground-breaking weight loss diet, which makes it inadmissible. Notwithstanding, don't be put off eating a lot of Sirtfoods, since these are astoundingly solid foods to incorporate as a major aspect of a reasonable and fluctuated diet for pregnancy. You will need to dodge red wine, because of its liquor substance, and cutoff energized things, for example, espresso, green tea, and cocoa so as not to surpass 200 milligrams for each day of caffeine during pregnancy (one cup of moment espresso normally contains around 100 milligrams of caffeine). Proposals are not to surpass four cups of green tea day by day and to maintain a strategic distance from matcha out and out. Other than that, you're allowed to receive the benefits of incorporating Sirtfoods in your diet.

Diet may cause mild symptoms

Phase 1 of the Sirtfood Diet gives amazing normally happening food mixes in quantities that the vast majority would not get in their ordinary eating routine, and certain individuals can respond as they adjust to this sensational wholesome change. This can incorporate indications, for example, a mild headache or tiredness, in spite of the fact that as far as we can tell these impacts are minor and fleeting.

Obviously, if side effects are extreme or give you purpose behind concern, we suggest you look for clinical counsel. No different manifestations have never been seen other than incidental gentle side effects that resolve rapidly, and inside a couple of days a great many people discover they have a restored feeling of energy, power, and healthiness.

The Sirtfood diet is superfluously prohibitive, eating 1/200 calories daily is excessively prohibitive for some individuals

The diet likewise requires drinking up to three green juices for each day. In spite of the fact that juices can be a decent wellspring of nutrients and minerals, they are likewise a wellspring of sugar and contain practically none of the solid fiber found in entire leafy foods

Tasting juice for the duration of the day is a poorly conceived notion for your glucose and teeth

The way that the diet is exceptionally restricted in calories and food decisions, it is more than likely inadequate in protein, nutrients and minerals, particularly during the main stage.

High beginning expenses of buying a juicer, the book and some uncommon and costly fixings, just as the tedious expenses of setting up specific meals and juices

Diet gets unworkable and unreasonable for some individuals or on the other hand a diabetic individual, calorie limitation and utilization of juice during the primary days of the diet can prompt perilous changes in glucose levels

During the main stage, you may encounter opposite reactions, for example, weariness, tipsiness and touchiness because of the calorie limitation

Chapter 10: What Next? The Sirtfood Diet in the Long Term

After the Two Phases

Congratulations, all stages of the Sirtfood Diet have now finished! Just let's take stock of what you have achieved. You've entered the hyper-success process, achieving weight loss in the area of 7 pounds, which probably includes an attractive increase in muscle. You also maintained your weight loss throughout the fourteen-day maintenance phase and further strengthened the body composition. Perhaps notably, you have marked the beginning of your transformation of wellness. You took a stand against the tide of ill health, which strikes as often as we get older. The life you have decided for yourself is enhanced strength, productivity, and health.

By now, you'll be familiar with the top twenty Sirtfoods, and you've gained a sense of how powerful they are. Not only that, but you'll also probably have become quite good at including them in your diet and loving them. For the sustained weight loss and health, they offer, these items must stay a prominent feature in your everyday eating regimen. But still, they're just twenty foods, and after all, the spice of life is variety. What next, then? We'll give you the blueprint for lifelong health in the next pages.

It's about getting your body in perfect balance with a diet that's suitable and sustainable for everyone and providing all the nutrients we need that enhance our health. It's about keeping on reaping the Sirtfood Diet's weight-loss rewards using the very best foods nature has to offer.

We've seen why Sirtfoods are so beneficial: certain plants have sophisticated stress-response mechanisms that generate compounds that trigger sirtuins— the same fasting and exercise-activated fat-burning and durability mechanism in the body. The greater the quantity of these compounds produced by plants in response to stress, the higher the value we derive from their feeding. Our list of the top twenty Sirtfoods is made up of the foods that stand out because they are particularly packed full of these compounds, and hence the foods that have the most exceptional ability to impact body composition and wellbeing. But foods ' sirtuin-activating results aren't a concept of all or nothing. There are a lot of other plants that produce moderate levels of sirtuin-activating nutrients, and by eating these liberally, we encourage you to expand the variety and diversity of your diet. The Sirtfood Diet is all about inclusion, and the greater the range of sirtuin-activating items that can be integrated into the diet. Especially if that means you will obtain from your meals even more of your favorite foods to increase pleasure and enjoyment.

Let's use the workout comparison. The top twenty Sirtfoods are the (much more pleasurable) equivalent of sweating it out at the gym, with Phase 1 being the "boot camp." By contrast, eating those other foods with more moderate levels of sirtuin-activating nutrients is like reaping the rewards of going out for a good walk. Contrast that to the typical diet that has a nutritional value equal to sitting all day on the couch watching Television. Yeah, sweating it out in the gym is fine, but if that is all you do, you will quickly get fed up with it. The walk should also be welcomed, especially if it means that you don't just choose to sit on the sofa.

For e.g., in our top twenty Sirtfoods, if we look more broadly at berries as a food group, we find that they have metabolic health benefits as well as healthy aging. Reviewing their nutritional content, we note that other berries such as blackberries, black currants, blueberries, and raspberries also have significant amounts of nutrients that cause sirtuins.

The same holds with nuts. Notwithstanding their calorific material, nuts are so effective that they promote weight loss and help shift inches from the waist. This is in addition to cutting chronic disease risk. Though walnuts are our champion nut, nutrients that trigger sirtuin can also be found in chestnuts, pecans, pistachios, and even peanuts.

Instead, we turn our attention to food. Throughout recent years there has been in several areas an increasing aversion to grains. Studies, however, link whole grain consumption with decreased inflammation, diabetes, heart disease, and cancer. Although they do not equal the pseudo-grain buckwheat Sirtfood qualifications, we do see the existence of substantial sirtuin-activating nutrients in other whole grains. And needless to say, their sirtuin-activating nutrient quality is decimated when whole grains are converted into refined "clean" forms. Such modified models are quite dangerous groups and are interested in a number of state-of-the-art health problems. We're not saying you can never eat them, but instead, you're going to be much better off sticking to the whole-grain version whenever possible.

With the likes of goji berries and chia seeds possessing Sirtfood powers, also notorious "superfoods" get on the bandwagon. That is most likely the unwitting reason for the health benefits they have observed. While it does imply that they are healthy for us to consume, we do know that there are more accessible, more available, and better options out there, so don't feel compelled to get on that specific bandwagon! We see the same trend across a lot of food categories. Unsurprisingly, the foods that research has developed are usually good for us, and we should be consuming more of them. Below we mentioned about forty foods that we discovered have Sirtfood properties too. We actively encourage you to include these foods to maintain and continue your weight loss and wellbeing as you expand your diet repertoire.

- Vegetables
- Artichokes
- Asparagus
- Broccoli
- Frisée
- Green beans
- Shallots
- Watercress
- White onions
- Yellow endive
- Fruits
- Apples
- Blackberries
- Black currants

- Black plums
- Cranberries
- Grains and pseudo-grains
- Popcorn
- Quinoa
- Whole-wheat flour
- Beans
- Fava beans
- White beans (e.g., cannellini or navy)
- Beverages
- Black tea
- White tea

Power of Protein

A high protein diet is one of the most popular diets of the last few years. Higher protein intake while dieting has been shown to encourage satiety, sustain metabolism, and reduce muscle mass loss. But it's when they pair Sirtfoods with protein that things get brought to a whole new level. Protein is, as you may remember, a necessary addition in a diet based on Sirtfood to gain maximum benefits. Protein consists of amino acids, and it is a particular amino acid, leucine, which effectively complements Sirtfoods ' behavior, strengthening their effects. This is done primarily by changing our cellular environment so that our diet's sirtuin-activating nutrients work much more effectively. It ensures we get the best result from a Sirtfood-rich meal, which is paired with protein-based in leucine. Leucine's main dietary sources contain red meat, pork, fruit, vegetables, milk, and dairy products.

The Power of Three

The omega-3 long-chain fatty acids EPA and DHA are the second major category of nutrients that effectively complement Sirtfoods. Omega-3s have been the coveted natural wellbeing global favorite for years. What we didn't know before, which we are doing now, is that they also improve the activation of a group of sirtuin genes in the body that is directly linked to longevity. It makes them the perfect match for Sirtfoods.

Omega-3s have potent effects in decreasing inflammation and lowering fat blood levels. To that, we can add additional heart-healthy effects: rendering the blood less likely to pool, stabilizing the heart's electrical activity, and lowering blood pressure. Even the pharmaceutical industry now looks to them as an aid in the war against cardiac disease. And that is not where the litany of benefits ends. Omega-3s also have an effect on the way we perceive, having been shown to boost the outlook and help stave off dementia.

When we speak about omega-3s, we're thinking primarily about eating fish, particularly oily types, because no other dietary source comes close to supplying the significant levels of EPA and DHA that we need. And to see the benefits, all we need is two servings of fish a week, with an emphasis on oily fish. Sadly, the United States is not a country of big fish eaters, and that is accomplished by less than one in five Americans. As a result, our intake of the precious EPA and DHA is appallingly short.

Plant foods, including almonds, beans, and green leafy vegetables, often produce omega-3 but in a form called alpha-linolenic acid, which must be processed into EPA or DHA in the body. This conversion process is poor, meaning that alpha-linolenic acid delivers a negligible amount of our needs for omega-3. Even with the wonderful advantages of Sirtfoods, we shouldn't forget the added value that drinking adequate omega-3 fats provides. In that order, the best sources of omega-3 fish are herring, sardines, salmon, trout, and mackerel. While fresh tuna is naturally high, too, the tinned version loses the majority of the omega-3. And a replacement of DHA-enriched microalgae (up to 300 milligrams a day) is also recommended for vegetarians and vegans, though food foods should still be integrated into the diet.

Can A SirtFood Provide it All?

Our focus so far has been solely on Sirtfoods and reaping their maximum benefits in order to achieve the body we want and powerfully boost our health in the process. But is this a reasonable, long-term dietary solution to be taken? After all, there is more to diet than pure nutrients that trigger sirtuin. What about all the vitamins, minerals, and fibers that are also important to our wellbeing, and the diets that we should consume to satisfy such demands?

Based on sirtfood diets, augmented by protein-rich foods and omega-3 outlets, fulfill dietary needs across the entire spectrum of essential nutrients— much more so than any other diet does. They use kale, for example, because it is a good sirtfood, but it is a great source of vitamins C, folate, and manganese, calcium, Vitamin K, and magnesium minerals. Kale is also a tremendous source of carotenoids lutein and zeaxanthin, both of which are critical for eye health, as well as immune-boosting beta-carotene.

Walnuts are also rich in minerals such as magnesium, copper, zinc, manganese, calcium, and iron, as well as fiber. Buckwheat is made of manganese, magnesium, zinc, potassium, and cotton. Tick the boxes of the onions for vitamin B6, folate, potassium, and food. Yet bananas, as well as potassium yet manganese, are good sources of vitamin C. And so, it begins. When you broaden your menu to include the expanded Sirtfood list and leave space for all the other good foods you enjoy eating, unwittingly, what you're going to end up with is a diet that's far richer in vitamins, nutrients, and fiber than you've ever had before. What Sirtfoods offers is a missing food group that changes the landscape of how we judge how good foods are for us, and how we eat a genuinely full diet.

Chapter 11: Question and Answers

Do questions and answer to possible doubts or worries of the reader

1. Should I exercise while on the Sirtfood diet?

Yes, of course! Light workouts increase the efficiency of the sirtfood diet and help you progress faster on your journey to losing weight, achieving enhanced mental clarity, and reducing the risk of long-term chronic diseases. So, keep your workouts simple, limit physical exertion, but try as much as possible to exercise every single day.

2. Can the Sirtfood Diet rectify extreme obesity?

A lot of people believe that diets only work for overweight people, and full-blown obesity can only be corrected by surgical procedures. The decision of whether you need surgery to remove the excess fat deposits would depend on your doctor. However, if your cardiac health is not in immediate danger, the sirtfood diet can help you to make immense progress in the long run by helping you to consistently shed your fat deposits while consolidating on your muscle mass gains.

3. Should I continue with the Sirtfood Diet after hitting my Target Weight?

The aim of the sirtfood diet is to help you to build a healthy routine that would allow you to stay healthy and disease-free in the long term. Even after reaching your target weight, try as much as possible to keep sirtfoods dominant in your diet, and avoid forbidden foods such as alcohol and processed sugar as much as possible. Sticking to the basic rules will help prevent you from gaining excess weight again. Remember to also keep exercising and going for regular medical check-ups if necessary.

4. How many times should I drink the Sirtfood Green Juice per day?

This is quite a common question among people who are just getting familiar with the sirtfood diet. Because of the intense calorie restriction in the first three days of phase one, it is recommended that you consume three cups of the sirtfood green juice per day for those three days. For the subsequent four days of Phase One, the sirtfood juice can be consumed twice per day. From phase 2 onwards, it is okay to keep the consumption of the juice at one cup per day; to be taken before breakfast in the morning to help give you your daily dose of green vitality.

5. Can I embark on the Sirtfood Diet if I'm on special medication?

If you are using meds, then you might need to talk to your doctor before starting the diet. However, even if your meds wouldn't allow you to go through the intense calorie restrictions of phase one, you can still incorporate sirtfoods into your diet and enjoy the amazing goodness that comes from consuming these foods.

6. Can Pregnant women embark on the sirtfood diet?

Once again, try as much as possible to talk to your physician before making any decisions on the sirtfood diet as a pregnant woman. Your baby requires enough nutrition as possible and restricting calories in this delicate stage may not be such a good idea. You can, however, incorporate the sirtfoods into your diet also. Children also should not embark on a full-scale diet. Instead, they should just be fed a lot of sirtfoods.

7. Must I complete the Seven-day period of Phase One?

For superlative execution, it is recommended that the seven-day period for phase One be completed. However, if for health reasons or any other cogent excuse, you cannot complete the full days, then try to stick to the rules of phase One for a minimum of five days to reap the rewards of the sirtfood diet. If you have a special medical condition such as ulcers, talk to your doctor before embarking on this diet, or simply just incorporate sirtfoods into your regular diet. Note that if you want to repeat the first phase of the diet, you have to wait for a month before going through that seven-day regimen again.

8. Can Children Eat Sirtfoods?

There are powerful sirtfoods, most of which are safe for children. Obviously, children should avoid wine, coffee, and other highly caffeinated foods, such as matcha. On the other hand, children can enjoy sirtuin-rich foods such as cabbage, eggplant, blueberries, and dates with their regular balanced diet.

Yet, while children can enjoy most sirtuin-rich foods, that is not the same as to say that they can practice the Sirt diet. This diet plan is not designed for children, and it does not fit the needs of their growing bodies. Practicing this diet plan could not only negatively affect them physically, but it could damage their mental health for years to come. Anyone can develop an eating disorder, but it is especially true for children. If you want your child to eat well, ensure they eat a wide range of foods, as recommended by their doctor, and you can simply include an abundance of sirtuin-rich foods into what they are already eating. Leave the focus on eating healthfully and not losing weight. Even if your child's doctor does want them to lose weight, you don't need to make the child aware of this fact. You can help guide them along with a healthy lifestyle, teaching them how to eat well and stay active through sports and play, and the weight will come off naturally without placing an unneeded burden on their small shoulders.

For similar reasons, you can include sirtfoods in a balanced diet while pregnant, but you should avoid practicing the Sirt diet when you are pregnant. It doesn't contain the nutrition requirements for either a pregnant woman or a growing baby. Save the diet for after you have delivered a healthy baby, and both you and your child will be healthy and happy.

9. Can I Exercise During Phase One?

If you use exercise during either phase one or two, you can increase weight loss and health benefits. While you shouldn't work at pushing the limits during phase one, you can continue your normal workout routine and physical activity. It is important to stay within your active comfort zone during this time, as physical exertion more than you are accustomed to will be especially difficult while you are restricting your calories. It will not only wear you out, but it can also make you dizzy, more prone to injury, and physically and mentally exhausted. This is a common symptom whenever a person pushes their limits while restricting calories, but it is something you should avoid.

If you are used to doing yoga and a spin class a few times a week, keep it up! If you are used to running a few miles a day, have at it! Do what you and your body are comfortable with, and as your doctor advises, and you should be fine.

10. I'm Already Thin. Can I Still Follow The Diet?

Whether or not you can follow the first phase of the Sirt diet will depend just how thin you already are. While a person who is overweight or well within a healthy weight can practice the first phase, nobody who is clinically underweight should. You can know whether or not you are underweight by calculating your Body Mass Index, or BMI. You can find many BMI calculators online, and if yours is at nineteen points or below, you should avoid the first phase. It is always a good idea to ask your doctor both if it is safe for you to lose weight, and if the Sirt diet is safe for your individual condition. While the Sirt diet may generally be safe, for people with certain illnesses, it may not be the case.

While it is understandable to desire to be even thinner, even if you already are thin, pushing yourself past the point of being underweight is incredibly unhealthy, both physically and mentally. This fits into the category of disordered eating and can cause you a lot of harm.

Some of the side effects of pushing your body to extreme weight loss include bone loss and osteoporosis, lowered immune system, fertility problems, and an increased risk of disease. If you want to benefit from the health of the Sirt diet and are underweight, instead consume, however many calories, your doctor recommends, along with plenty of sirtfoods. This will ensure you maintain a healthy weight while also receiving the benefits that sirtuins have to offer.

If you are thin, but still at a BMI of twenty to twenty-five, then you should be safe beginning the Sirt diet, unless otherwise instructed by your doctor.

11. Can You Eat Meat and Dairy on The Sirtfood Diet?

In many recipes, we choose to use sirtfood sources of protein, such as soy, walnuts, and buckwheat. However, this does not mean that you aren't allowed to enjoy meat on the Sirt diet. Sure, it's easy to enjoy a vegan or vegetarian Sirt diet, but if you love your sources of meat, then you don't have to give them up. Protein is an essential aspect of the Sirt diet to preserve muscle tone, and whether you consume only plant-based proteins, or a mixture of plant and animal-based proteins is completely up to you. And, just as you can enjoy meat, you can also enjoy moderate consumption of dairy.

Some meats can actually help you better utilize the sirtfoods you eat. This is because the amino acid leucine is able to enhance the effect of sirtfoods. You can find this amino acid in chicken, beef, pork, fish, eggs, dairy, and tofu.

12. Can I Drink Red Wine during Phase One?

As your calories will be so limited during the first phase, it is not recommended to drink alcohol during this phase. However, you can enjoy it in moderation during phase two and the maintenance phase.

Then sirtfood diet isn't science-based

Even though there's some contentious research in regard to the advantages of sirtuins, there is little to no research in regard to a particular sirtfood dietary plan. In any case, we have many tips in place which were thoroughly researched and analyzed for many years. If you should be lost about which "healthy food" is, then this can be really a greater place to get started out.

It is totally fine if you'd like to add some sirtfoods in an eating program. After all, foods such as green tea extract, tea, dark chocolate, and kale all are important to a nutritious eating pattern! But staying with a schedule with such strict pass-or-fail conditions is unrealistic and maybe bad for your relationship with food. By incorporating a diet plan that is satisfying and focused on eating mindfully, you are going to be in a position to set a long-term and sustainable love with food. Cheers to this!

Conclusion

The Sirtfood Diet is all about consuming the right foods and getting fast consequences. It is the maximum popular eating regimen to date, ably overturning outcomes that made the Dukan and Paleo famous. This food plan entails meals with large quantities of Sirtuin activators.

These activators switch on the body's skinny gene pathways by way of approach of exercising and fasting for you to burn fats, enhance muscles, and beautify fitness. The diet regime includes meals and advice that might maintain you off from the burden you lost all through the first week of this system and integrating extra Sirtfoods to your meals as you go along.

With around 650 million overweight adults around the world, it's crucial to find healthful meals and doable exercising programs, don't throw away the whole thing you love and don't must exercise all the time. Time. Week. The Sirtfood weight loss program does just that: The idea is that certain meals set off the "lean gene" pathways that are generally activated by way of fasting and workout.

As soon as the weight loss program becomes a way of life during exercising, it is critical to eat protein one hour after a workout preferably. The protein repairs muscles after exercising, relieve ache, and can sell regeneration. There are loads of recipes that include proteins best for post-exercise consumption, e.g., For example, B. Sirt Chili con Came or turmeric-chicken-kale salad. If you want something lighter, you can attempt the Sirt Blueberry smoothie and upload protein powder for extra benefits. The type of health you exercise is up to you. However, in case you are educated at home, you could pick while you want to exercise, what sorts of sporting events are right for you, and are quick and convenient.

Take note that you should maintain the weight loss results through Phase 2 and continue to lose weight gradually. Also, the one striking thing we've seen with the Sirtfood Diet is that most or all of the weight people lose is from fat and that many put some muscle on. So, we would like to warn you again not to measure your success solely based on the numbers. Look in the mirror to see if you look leaner and more toned, see how well your clothes fit and lap up the compliments you'll get from others.

The Sirtfood diet is a first-rate way to trade your consuming habits, lose weight, and experience healthier. The first few weeks may be difficult. However, it's critical to test which meals are high-quality to devour and which delicious recipes are proper for you. Be type to yourself for the first few weeks, as your body adapts and trains while you need to. If you are already exercising moderately or intensively, you'll be able to preserve as standard or manipulate your health primarily based on the exchange in diet. As with any change in food plan and workout, it all depends on the individual and what kind of effort you can make.

For other 302 recipes you can buy my book "SIRTFOOD DIET COOKBOOK".

SIRTFOOD DIET COOKBOOK

302 Quick and Healthy Sirtfood Diet Recipes to Use in Your Meal Plan. Discover the Power of Sirtuins: Activate the Metabolism, Eat Delicious Dishes and Lose Weight Quickly

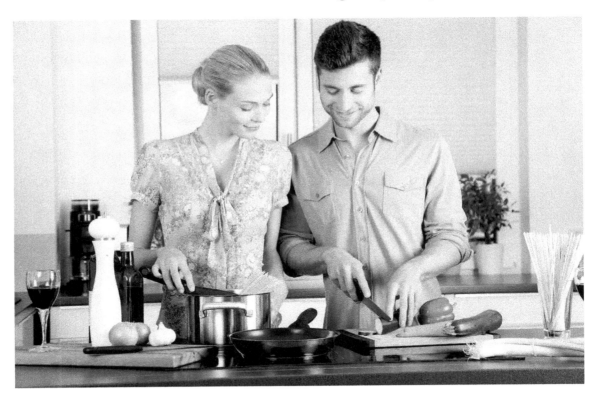

Lara Burns

Introduction

Sirtfood diet is a new effective method for weight loss and helps the body regenerate. Sirtfood diet is a combination of fresh, low-fat foods that contain sirtuins and tiny organisms such as microalgae, yeast, and bacteria. According to the study prepared by the American Society for nutrition, sirtuins improve the health of people and can help slow the aging process. The diet includes foods that contain a natural antioxidant called nicotinamide riboside (NR). Sirtuin food is found in a wide range of specific products like berries, avocado, blackcurrants, grapes, parsley, grapefruit, lemon peel and kale. Sirtuins can turn genes on or off and raise the level of enzymes that destroy damaged proteins. The study also suggests that these types of food can help in a weight-loss program and can protect body cells from stress.

About 'Sirtfood Diet'

Sirtfood diet is the latest breakthrough, natural diet. The natural diet is enriched with all the nutrients that aid weight loss and reduce the risk of serious diseases. The Sirtfood diet incorporates various foods that are rich in antioxidants, polyphenols and fatty acids. The natural diet helps to achieve weight loss, cure chronic and general illness and improve overall health. Hence this method is called the 'Sirtfood diet.' There are many health benefits of the Sirtfood diet, which are told by dietitians in this blog. The sirtfood diet has been proved that it enhances longevity and also promote sleep for rejuvenating the body because of other nutrients included in the food. The diet incorporates exceptional foods ideally a diverse selection of polyphenols and other molecules that act to improve your nutrition with a special ingredient called Sirtuin Activators (STA's). The diet also combats diseases like Alzheimer's and other chronic ailments.

What is Sirtfood Diet?

'Sirtfood diet' is a new weight-loss diet plan consisting of foods that are rich in natural antioxidants and polyphenols. These foods enhance the production of a chemical known as 'Sirtuin'. Sirtuin helps in the formation of proteins and helps slow down the process of aging. The antioxidant and polyphenol-rich food is also believed to reduce the risks of cancer and other critical diseases. So, the sirtfood diet is an ideal diet for reducing weight and preventing disease. These foods usually boost sirtuin levels, which in turn produce the protein resveratrol, that is known to reduce the risk of age-related diseases. Moreover, resveratrol can also stop the processes of aging. This is what we call diet with maximum sirtuin activators. The diet has the power to boost weight loss, it also has multiple health benefits.

How does the Sirtfood diet works?

The sirtfood diet works by aiming to boost levels of a chemical called Sirtuin. Research has found that eating foods that boost Sirtuin levels aids weight loss, can also help fight diseases like cancer, help improve sleep and cure metabolic disorders. This chemical is activated by a molecule called Sirtuin Activators (STA's) present in various foods. The Sirtfood diet consists of foods rich in Sirtuin Activators (STA's) like Sirtfoods. These foods include berries, avocado, blackcurrants, grapes, parsley, grapefruit, lemon peel, kale, etc. The Sirtfood diet consists of anti-inflammatory, anti-oxidant rich foods that also include minimum calories to reduce weight. Sirt supplements can also be taken externally to improve results. Overall, the sirtfood diet helps calorie restriction, reduce weight, and also maintain overall health.

Sirtfoods - the best part of the Sirtfood Diet

The sirtfoods are the main part of the diet. Most of the foods are rich in a powerful antioxidant called 'Sirtuin.' Sirtuin has the ability to change cellular metabolic processes and regulations. The mitochondrion is a part of our cells. Normally mitochondria are active and help in energy production. As we grow older, these mitochondria become damaged and are not able to function properly. The sirtuin works by scavenging the free radicals and stabilizing the mitochondrial to work properly again. This helps to increase cellular metabolism by improving energy production. With this increased production of energy, people are able to boost their metabolism, thereby giving good health and good health. In addition to this, Sirtuin also acts as a protective shield by stopping the attack of free radicals by DNA, proteins, and lipids, and this protects them from oxidative damage. However, there are no definite statistics on the role of Sirtuin on human health. The studies are ongoing to determine the precise mechanism of the functions of Sirtuin on human health. However, the health benefits of Sirtuin have been observed.

Benefits of Sirtfood Diet

Yes, the Sirtfood diet is actually a leading weight loss diet, which aims for rapid weight loss in a short span of time. Research has indicated that it will also help in reducing appetite, prevent diseases, improve sleep, and also boost energy.

Weight loss - Based on long-term research, it appears that eating Sirtfoods can help reduce your weight. According to research by a team of scientists from the University of Eastern Finland, people who were on a diet lost an average of 12 pounds in 14 weeks. Laboratory mice eating sirtfoods showed an increase in calorie-burning cell function. Women taking the sirtfood diet had increased fat burning ability while those in the control group did not.

Cardiovascular Disease - Scientists have suggested that the intake of sirtfoods may help lower the risk of heart attacks, stroke and other cardiovascular diseases.

Brain Health - Sirtfoods have been found to increase the levels of acetylcholine, which plays an important role in Alzheimer's and dementia.

Metabolic Syndrome - This condition is common among many people though it does not result in any major health issues. However, some studies have established that eating sirtfoods may lead to a reduction in 'Metabolic Syndrome'.

Diabetes - A study conducted by the University of Eastern Finland has indicated that people on the sirtfoods lost two-thirds of body weight within two weeks. The researchers noted that those people who lost the most weight were those who followed the diet for two weeks longer than the other group of individuals in the study.

Anti-aging - Sirtfoods have been found to have anti-aging properties. Research has indicated that eating sirtfoods helps lower the risk of age-related diseases like osteoporosis and colon cancer. In addition, it is being considered that since sirtfoods is an antioxidant, eating them can also help fight off certain cancers, such as those of the prostate or breast.

Oxidation - The Sirtfood diet can help decrease cellular oxidation caused by free radicals. It can also reduce the molecular damage which is caused by free radicals by repairing the damage to DNA and proteins. It was found in a study conducted by researchers in Milan, Italy, that the diet can reduce the oxidized by 60% while a control diet has no effect on it.

Aging - The Sirtfood diet helps prevent cellular aging. In addition, it pays backward and encourages the production of new youthful energy throughout the entire body.

Sirtfood Diet

The basis of the sirtuin diet can be explained in simple terms or complex ways. However, it is crucial to understand how and why it works to appreciate what you are doing. It is essential also to know why these sirtuin rich foods help you maintain fidelity to your diet plan. Otherwise, you may throw something in your meal with less nutrition that would defeat the purpose of planning for one rich in sirtuins. Most importantly, this is not a dietary fad, and as you will see, there is much wisdom in how humans have used natural foods, even for medicinal purposes, over thousands of years.

To understand how the Sirtfood diet works and why these particular foods are necessary, we will look at their role in the human body.

Sirtuin activity was first researched in yeast, where a mutation caused an extension in the yeast's lifespan. Sirtuins were also shown to slow aging in laboratory mice, fruit flies, and nematodes. As Sirtuins' research proved to transfer to mammals, they were examined for their diet and slowing the aging process. The sirtuins in humans are different in typing, but they essentially work in the same ways and reasons.

There are seven "members" that establish the sirtuin family. It is believed that sirtuins play a significant role in regulating certain functions of cells, including proliferation (reproduction and growth of cells), apoptosis (death of cells). They promote survival and resist stress to increase longevity.

They are also seen to block neurodegeneration (loss of function of the brain's nerve cells). They conduct their housekeeping functions by cleaning out toxic proteins and supporting the brain's ability to change and adapt to different conditions or recuperate (i.e., brain plasticity). As part of this, they also help reduce chronic inflammation and reduce so-called oxidative stress. It happens when there are too many cell-damaging free radicals circulating in the body, and the body cannot catch up by combating them with antioxidants. These factors are related to age-related illness and weight, which again brings us back to discussing how they work.

You will see labels in Sirtuins that start with "SIR," representing "Silence Information Regulator" genes. They do precisely that, silence or regulate, as part of their functions. The seven sirtuins humans work with are SIRT1, SIRT2, SIRT3, SIRT4, SIRT 5, SIRT6 and SIRT7. Each of these types is responsible for different areas of protecting cells. They work by either stimulating or turning on certain gene expressions or reducing and turning off other gene expressions. This essentially means that they can influence genes to do more or less of something, most of which they are already programmed to do.

Through enzyme reactions, each of the SIRT types affects different cells responsible for the metabolic processes that help maintain life. This is also related to what organs and functions they will affect.

For example, the SIRT6 causes and expression of genes in humans affect skeletal muscle, fat tissue, brain, and heart. SIRT 3 would cause an expression of genes that affect the kidneys, liver, brain, and heart.

If we tie these concepts together, you can see that the Sirtuin proteins can change the expression of genes and in the case of the Sirtfood Diet, we care about how sirtuins can turn off those genes that are responsible for speeding up aging and for weight management.

The other aspect to this conversation of sirtuins is the function and the power of calorie restriction on the human body. Calorie restriction is only eating fewer calories. This, coupled with exercise and reducing stress, is usually a combination of weight loss. Calorie restriction has also proven across much research in animals and humans to increase one's lifespan.

We can look further at the role of sirtuins with calorie restriction and using the SIRT3 protein, which has a role in metabolism and aging. Amongst all of the effects of the protein on gene expression (such as preventing cells from dying, reducing tumors from growing, etc.), we want to understand the effects of SIRT3 on weight for this manuscript.

As we stated earlier, the SIRT3 has high expression in those metabolically active tissues, and its ability to express itself increases with caloric restriction, fasting, and exercise. On the contrary, it will express itself less when the body has high fat, high-calorie-riddled diet.

The last few highlights of sirtuins are their role in regulating telomeres and reducing inflammation, which also helps prevent disease and aging.

Telomeres are sequences of proteins at the ends of chromosomes. When cells divide, these get shorter. As we age, they get shorter and other stressors to the body also will contribute to this.

Maintaining these longer telomeres is the key to slower aging. Also, proper diet, along with exercise and other variables, can lengthen telomeres. SIRT6 is one of the sirtuins that, if activated, can help with DNA damage, inflammation and oxidative stress. SIRT1 also helps with inflammatory response cycles that are related to many age-related diseases.

Calories restriction, as we mentioned earlier, can extend life to some degree.

Since this and fasting are a stressor, these factors will stimulate the SIRT3 proteins to kick in and protect the body from the stressors and excess free radicals. Again, the telomere length is affected as well.

To sum up, all of this information also shows that, contrary to some people's beliefs, genetics, like "it is what it is" or "it is my fate because Uncle Joe has something…" through our own lifestyle choices. What we are exposed to, we can influence action and changes in our genes. This is quite an empowering thought and yet another reason why you should be excited to have a science-based diet such as the Sirtfood diet, available to you.

Having laid this all out before you, you should be able to appreciate how and why these miraculous compounds work in your favor to keep you youthful, healthy and lean. If they are working hard for you, don't you feel that you should do something too?

Benefits of Sirtfood Diet

The Sirtuins

Sirtuins are a group of seven proteins that maintain cell metabolism and homeostasis at optimal levels. Three of these proteins are found in the mitochondria, one is in the cytoplasm, and another three are located in the nucleus. Sirtuins maintain the cell's health and ensure that all processes going on within the cell are correctly happening. Sirtuins can, however, not be effective without the presence of NAD+ (nicotinamide adenine dinucleotide). NAD+ is a coenzyme that is present in all cells that are living in nature. NAD+ ensures that Sirtuins function optimally and can regulate cells.

Homeostasis within the cell maintains all the numerous functions of the cell at stability, which ensures balance. It may also involve the maintenance of PH, and the saturate concentration levels of the cytoplasm, which is the most significant cell component in terms of volume. All these are aspects of the cell that must stay constant for optimal cell health. Sirtuins perform several functions, among them being the ability to deacetylase proteins called histones. Acetyls are proteins with a physical form of Histones are proteins that contain a condensed form of DNA called chromatins, which prevent the proteins from performing their functions in this acetyl.

The deacetylation, therefore, frees the proteins for the undertaking of their respective functions, given that proteins are the building blocks for the body. Proteins are proverbially referred to as bodybuilding foods. Without Sirtuins, therefore, the bodybuilding foods would fail to build our bodies as they are the critical components for freeing the protein molecules in our cells for their functions.

The Miracle of the Blue Areas

The other evidence for the power of Sirtfoods comes from the 'blue zones.' The blue zones are small regions in the world where people miraculously live longer than everywhere else.

Perhaps most startlingly, you don't just see people live longer in blue zones; you still see them retain energy, vigor, and overall health even in their advanced years. Most of us have a fear of becoming decrepit, immobile, and overall miserable as we age.

Furthermore, we envision this as starting to occur in our forties and fifties while becoming a fixed reality in our sixties, seventies, and eighties. Yet in the blue zones, people live past 100 surprisingly regularly but can walk, work and exercise just as well as those in the younger years. Likewise, they remain mentally slide and don't suffer the cognitive deficits we typically associate with old age.

The blue zones include several areas of the Mediterranean, Japan, Italy and Costa Rica. What do these regions all have in common? They all eat a diet high in Sirt foods. The Mediterranean is famous for its healthy diet involving copious amounts of fish and olive oil. The Japanese savor matcha green tea, while the Costa Ricans traditionally indulge in cocoa, coffee and more.

This is the beauty of the Sirt food diet – it isn't trying to make your eating habits artificial and awkward. It is merely copying the healthiest practices that already exist around the world.

Sirt Diet and Muscle Mass

In the body, there is a family of genes that function as guardians of our muscles and, when under stress, avoid its breakdown: the sirtuins. SIRT is a potent Muscle Breakdown Inhibitor. As long as SIRT is activated, even when we are fasting, muscle breakdown is prevented, and we continue to burn fat for fuel.

SIRT's benefits aren't ending with preserving muscle mass. The sirtuins work to increase our skeletal muscle mass. We need to delve into the exciting world of stem cells and illustrate how that process functions. Our muscle comprises a particular type of stem cell called a satellite cell that regulates its development and regeneration. Satellite cells just sit there quietly most of the time, but they are activated when a muscle gets damaged or stressed. By things like weight training, this is how our muscles grow stronger. SIRT is essential for activating satellite cells, and without its activity, muscles are significantly smaller because they no longer have the capacity to develop or regenerate properly.6 However, by increasing SIRT activity, we boost our satellite cells, which encourages muscle growth and recovery.

Sirt Diet and Goodness

There was one aspect we couldn't get our minds around in our pilot study: the people didn't get hungry given a drop-in calorie. In reality, several people struggled to consume all of the food that was offered.

One of the significant advantages of the Sirtfood Diet is that we can achieve significant benefits without the need for a long-term calorie restriction. The very first week of diet is the process of hyper-success, where we pair mild fasting with an excess of strong Sirtfoods for a double blow to weight. So, we predicted sure signs of hunger here, as with all of the fasting regimens. But we've had virtually zero!

We found the answer as we trawled through analysis. It's all thanks to the body's primary appetite-regulating hormone, leptin, called the "satiety hormone." As we feed, leptin decreases, signaling the hypothalamus inhibiting desire to a part of the brain. Conversely, leptin signaling to the mind declines as we fly, which makes us feel thirsty.

Leptin is so effective in controlling appetite that early expectations where it could be treated as a "magic bullet" for combating obesity. But that vision was broken because the metabolic disorder found in obesity causes leptin to avoid correctly functioning. Through obesity, the volume of leptin that can reach the brain is not only decreased, but the hypothalamus also becomes desensitized to its behavior. This is regarded as leptin resistance: there is leptin, but it doesn't work correctly anymore. Therefore, for many overweight individuals, the brain continues to think they are underfed even though they consume plenty, which triggers them to seek calories.

The consequence of this is that while the amount of leptin in the blood is necessary to control appetite, how much of it enters the brain and can affect the hypothalamus is far more relevant. It is here that the Sirtfoods shine.

New evidence indicates that the nutrients present in Sirtfoods have unique advantages in overcoming leptin resistance. This is by increasing leptin delivery to the brain and the hypothalamus' response to leptin behavior.

Going back to our original question: Why doesn't the Sirtfood Diet make people feel hungry? Given a decrease in blood leptin rates during the mild quick, which would usually raise motivation, incorporating Sirtfoods into the diet makes leptin signals more productive, leading to better appetite control. Sirtfoods also has powerful effects on our taste centers, meaning we get a lot more pleasure and satisfaction from our food and therefore don't fall into the overeating trap to feel happy. Sirtuins are expected to be a brand-new concept for even the most committed dietitians. But hitting the sirtuins, our metabolism's master regulators, is the foundation of any effective diet for weight loss. Tragically, the very existence of our modern society, with abundant food and sedentary lifestyles, creates a perfect storm to shut down our sirtuin operation, and we see all around us the effects of this.

The good thing is that we know what sirtuins are, how fat accumulation is managed, and how fat burning is encouraged, and most significantly, how to turn them on. And with this revolutionary breakthrough, the key to successful and lasting weight loss is now yours to bear.

Sirtfood Phases

The plan will detoxify your body for seven days, and then you'll need to keep eating Sirt foods to see the weight coming off, or you'll get it all back. This diet is not very healthy because, for most people, you're eating two of your meals, which isn't sustainable in the long term. It is a diet for those who are following a fantasy and ready to pay for it. It is in no way resembles usual feeding, and I assume it is unhealthy. It is very intense stuff. The green juice revolts and I poured some down the sink. I hated tossing all the harvested fibers onto the compost fire, feeling that I would have enjoyed eating all the juice ingredients in their entire state and that it was better anyway.

Due to the high cost of exotic foods and the amount of time you'll spend juicing and cooking your meals, this diet will be incredibly hard to follow for many reasons. If you don't like matcha or kale, you'll find this diet very hard to follow as many of the Sirtfood Diet recipes contain both of these ingredients. Most people just flat out hated how the drinks smelled and couldn't even bother with the diet. The Sirt Diet program includes two phases:

Phase 1

This process will limit you to 1,000 calories a day for a week and two of your meals will be green drinks rich in Sirtfoods such as lettuce, celery, parsley, green tea and lemon. Even rich in Sirtfoods like beef, chicken, spinach, or buckwheat noodles, you can have one meal per day.

Phase 2

You are permitted to increase the caloric intake to 1,500 calories during this process and you are still consuming the two green drinks. Still, you are now permitted to add another meal to the day, allowing two meals and two beverages. This phase can last up to 14 days. This diet is certainly not for everyone, and it requires a lot of funds and energy to get through the meal preparation. The book includes several recipes about halfway through your reading. Still, many of the ingredients are so unique that consumers found it hard to find them at the grocery store, as well as the tastes were so different in the beginning. Generally, this diet is backed by science, as many case studies have been shown, but the possibility of seeing results from this diet alone is a long shot for the average person.

After The Diet

Those two stages may be repeated as often as you wish for further weight loss.

However, upon finishing those stages, you are advised to start "sirtifying" your diet by consistently integrating sirtfoods into your meals.

There are several Sirtfood Diet books full of creamy recipes. You can also include sirtfoods as a snack in your diet or in recipes that you already have.

You are further encouraged to continue consuming the green juice daily.

Thus, the Sirtfood Diet becomes more of a change in lifestyle than a one-time diet.

Breakfast Recipes

Kale Scramble

Preparation time: 10 minutes

Cooking time: 6 minutes

Servings: 2

Ingredients:

- 4 eggs
- 1/8 teaspoon ground turmeric
- Salt and ground black pepper, to taste
- 1 tablespoon water
- 2 teaspoons olive oil
- 1 cup fresh kale, tough ribs removed and chopped

Directions:

1. In a bowl, add the eggs, turmeric, salt, black pepper, and water, and with a whisk, beat until foamy.
2. In a wok, heat the oil over medium heat.
3. Add the egg mixture and stir to combine.
4. Immediately, reduce the heat to medium-low and cook for about 1–2 minutes, stirring frequently.
5. Stir in the kale and cook for about 3–4 minutes, stirring frequently.
6. Remove from the heat and serve immediately.

Nutrition:

Calories 183

Fat 13.4 g

Carbs 4.3 g

Protein 12.1 g

Buckwheat Porridge

Preparation time: 10 minutes

Cooking time: 15 minutes

Servings: 2

Ingredients:

- 1 cup buckwheat, rinsed
- 1 cup unsweetened almond milk
- 1 cup of water
- 1/2 teaspoon ground cinnamon
- 1/2 teaspoon vanilla extract
- 1–2 tablespoons raw honey
- 1/4 cup fresh blueberries

Directions:

1. In a pan, add all the ingredients (except honey and blueberries) over medium-high heat and bring to a boil.
2. Now, reduce the heat to low and simmer, covered for about 10 minutes.
3. Stir in the honey and remove from the heat.
4. Set aside, covered, for about 5 minutes.
5. With a fork, fluff the mixture and transfer it into serving bowls.
6. Top with blueberries and serve.

Nutrition:

Calories 358

Fat 4.7 g

Carbs 3.7 g

Protein 12 g

Salmon & Kale Omelet

Preparation time: 10 minutes

Cooking time: 7 minutes

Servings: 4

Ingredients:

- 6 eggs
- 2 tablespoons unsweetened almond milk
- Salt and ground black pepper, to taste
- 2 tablespoons olive oil
- 4 ounces smoked salmon, cut into bite-sized chunks
- 2 cup fresh kale, tough ribs removed and chopped finely
- 4 scallions, chopped finely

Directions:

1. In a bowl, place the eggs, coconut milk, salt and black pepper.
2. And beat well.
3. Set aside.
4. In a nonstick wok, heat the oil over medium heat.
5. Place the egg mixture evenly and cook for about 30 seconds, without stirring.
6. Place the salmon, kale and scallions on top of the egg mixture evenly.
7. Now, reduce heat to low.
8. With the lid, cover the wok and cook for about 4–5 minutes.
9. Uncover the wok and cook for about 1 minute.
10. Carefully transfer the omelet onto a serving plate and serve.

Nutrition:

Calories 210

Fat 14.9 g

Carbs 5.2 g

Protein 14.8 g

Moroccan Spiced Eggs

Preparation time: 1 hour

Cooking time: 50 minutes

Servings: 2

Ingredients:

- 1 tsp olive oil
- One shallot, stripped and finely hacked
- One red (chime) pepper, deseeded and finely hacked
- One garlic clove, stripped and finely hacked
- One (zucchini), stripped and finely hacked
- 1 tbsp. tomato puree (glue)
- ½ tsp gentle stew powder
- ¼ tsp ground cinnamon
- ¼ tsp ground cumin
- ½ tsp salt
- 400g (14oz) can hacked tomatoes
- 400g (14oz) may use chickpeas in water
- A little bunch of level leaf parsley (10g (1/3oz)), cleaved
- Four medium eggs at room temperature

Directions:

1. Heat the oil in a pan, include the shallot and red (ringer) pepper, and fry delicately for 5 minutes.
2. At that point, include the garlic and (zucchini) and cook for one more moment or two.
3. Include the tomato puree (glue), flavors, and salt and mix through.
4. Add the cleaved tomatoes and chickpeas (dousing alcohol and all) and increment the warmth to medium.

5. With the top of the dish, stew the sauce for 30 minutes – ensure it is delicately rising all through and permit it to lessen in volume by around 33%.
6. Remove from the warmth and mix in the cleaved parsley.
7. Preheat the grill to 200C/180C fan/350F.

Nutrition:

Calories: 116 kcal

Protein: 6.97 g

Fat: 5.22 g

Carbohydrates: 13.14 g

Chilaquiles with Gochujang

Preparation time: 30 minutes

Cooking time: 20 minutes

Servings: 2

Ingredients:

- One dried ancho chili
- 2 cups of water
- 1 cup squashed tomatoes
- Two cloves of garlic
- One teaspoon genuine salt
- 1/2 tablespoons gochujang
- 5 to 6 cups tortilla chips
- Three enormous eggs
- One tablespoon olive oil

Directions:

1. Get the water to heat a pot.
2. I cheated marginally and heated the water in an electric pot and emptied it into the pan.
3. There's no sound unrivaled strategy here.

4. Add the anchor chili to the bubbled water and drench for 15 minutes to give it an opportunity to stout up.
5. When completed, use tongs or a spoon to extricate chili.
6. Make sure to spare the water for the sauce! Nonetheless, on the off chance that you incidentally dump the water, it's not the apocalypse.
7. Mix the doused chili, 1 cup of saved high temp water, squashed tomatoes, garlic, salt and gochujang until smooth.
8. Empty sauce into a large dish and warmth over medium warmth for 4 to 5 minutes. Mood killer the heat and include the tortilla chips. Mix the chips to cover with the sauce. In a different skillet, shower a teaspoon of oil and fry an egg on top until the whites have settled. Plate the egg and cook the remainder of the eggs. If you are phenomenal at performing various tasks, you can likely sear the eggs while you heat the red sauce. I am not precisely so capable.
9. Top the chips with the seared eggs, cotija, hacked cilantro, jalapeños, onions and avocado. Serve right away.

Nutrition:

Calories: 484 kcal

Protein: 14.55 g

Fat: 18.62 g

Carbohydrates: 64.04 g

Twice Baked Breakfast Potatoes

Preparation time: 1 hour 10 minutes

Cooking time: 1 hour

Servings: 2

Ingredients:

- 2 medium reddish brown potatoes, cleaned and pricked with a fork everywhere
- 2 tablespoons unsalted spread
- 3 tablespoons overwhelming cream
- 4 rashers cooked bacon
- 4 huge eggs
- 1/2 cup destroyed cheddar
- Daintily cut chives
- Salt and pepper to taste

Directions:

1. Preheat grill to 400 degrees F.
2. Spot potatoes straightforwardly on stove rack in the focal point of the grill and prepare for 30 to 45 min.
3. Evacuate and permit potatoes to cool for around 15 minutes.
4. Cut every potato down the middle longwise and burrow every half out, scooping the potato substance into a blending bowl.
5. Gather margarine and cream to the potato and pound into a single unit until smooth — season with salt and pepper and mix.
6. Spread a portion of the potato blend into the base of each emptied potato skin and sprinkle with one tablespoon cheddar (you may make them remain pounded potato left to snack on).
7. Add one rasher bacon to every half and top with a raw egg.
8. Spot potatoes onto a heating sheet and come back to the appliance.
9. Lower broiler temperature to 375 degrees F and heat potatoes until egg whites simply set and yolks are as yet runny.
10. Top every potato with a sprinkle of the rest of the cheddar, season with salt and pepper, and finish with cut chives.

Nutrition:

Calories: 647 kcal

Protein: 30.46 g

Fat: 55.79 g

Carbohydrates: 7.45 g

Sirt Muesli

Preparation time: 30 minutes

Cooking time: 0 minutes

Servings: 2

Ingredients:

- 20g buckwheat drops
- 10g buckwheat puffs
- 15g coconut drops or dried up coconut
- 40g Medjool dates, hollowed and slashed
- 15g pecans, slashed
- 10g cocoa nibs
- 100g strawberries, hulled and slashed
- 100g plain Greek yoghurt (or vegetarian elective, for example, soya or coconut yoghurt)

Directions:

1. Blend the entirety of the above fixings (forget about the strawberries and yoghurt if not serving straight away).

Nutrition:

Calories: 334 kcal

Protein: 4.39 g

Fat: 22.58 g

Carbohydrates: 34.35 g

Mushroom Scramble Eggs

Preparation time: 45 minutes

Cooking time: 10 minutes

Servings: 2

Ingredients:

- 2 eggs
- 1 tsp ground turmeric
- 1 tsp mellow curry powder
- 20g kale, generally slashed
- 1 tsp additional virgin olive oil
- 1/2 superior bean stew, daintily cut
- Bunch of catch mushrooms, meagerly cut
- 5g (3/16oz.) parsley, finely slashed
- *optional* Add a seed blend as a topper and some Rooster Sauce for enhance

Directions:

2. Blend the turmeric and curry powder.
3. Include a little water until you have accomplished a light glue.
4. Steam the kale for 2–3 minutes.
5. Warmth the oil in a skillet over medium heat
6. Fry the bean stew and mushrooms for 2–3 minutes.
7. Include the eggs and flavor glue and cook over a medium warmth at that point.
8. Add the kale and keep on cooking over medium heat for a further moment.
9. At long last, include the parsley, blend well and serve.

Nutrition:

Calories: 158 kcal

Protein: 9.96 g

Fat: 10.93 g

Carbohydrates: 5.04 g

Smoked Salmon Omelets

Preparation time: 45 minutes

Cooking time: 15 minutes

Servings: 2

Ingredients:

- 2 Medium eggs
- 100 g Smoked salmon, cut
- 1/2 tsp Capers
- 10 g Rocket, slashed
- 1 tsp Parsley, slashed
- 1 tsp extra virgin olive oil

Directions:

1. Split the eggs into a bowl and whisk well.
2. Include the salmon, tricks, rocket and parsley.
3. Warmth the olive oil in a nonstick skillet until hot yet not smoking.
4. Include the egg blend and, utilizing a spatula or fish cut, move the mixture around the dish until it is even.
5. Diminish the warmth and let the omelette cook through.
6. Slide the spatula around the edges and move up or crease the omelette fifty-fifty to serve.

Nutrition:

Calories: 148 kcal

Protein: 15.87 g

Fat: 8.73 g

Carbohydrates: 0.36 g

Date and Walnut Porridge

Preparation time: 55 minutes

Lara Burns

Cooking time: 30 minutes

Servings: 2

Ingredients:

- 200 ml Milk or without dairy elective
- 1 Medjool date, hacked
- 35 g Buckwheat chips
- 1 tsp. Pecan spread or four cleaved pecan parts
- 50 g Strawberries, hulled

Directions:

1. Spot the milk and time in a dish, heat tenderly, at that point include the buckwheat chips and cook until the porridge is your ideal consistency.
2. Mix in the pecan margarine or pecans, top with the strawberries, and serve.

Nutrition:

Calories: 66 kcal

Protein: 1.08 g

Fat: 1.07 g

Carbohydrates: 14.56 g

Beef Stroganoff French Bread Toast

Preparation time: 10 minutes.

Cooking time: 15 minutes.

Servings: 2.

Ingredients:

- 4 tablespoons olive oil.
- 1/2 cups mushrooms.
- 2 teaspoons salt, separated.
- 1/2 teaspoon dark pepper.
- 2 tablespoons thyme.
- 2 tablespoons spread.
- 1/2 cup onions, diced.
- 2 cloves garlic, minced.
- 1-pound ground meat.
- 3 tablespoons generally useful flour.
- 2 teaspoons paprika.
- 1/2 cups meat juices.
- 1/2 cup sharp cream.
- 1 teaspoon Dijon mustard.
- For the toasts:
- 1 portion French bread, inner parts dugout.
- 2 cups mozzarella.
- 3 tablespoons cleaved Italian parsley.

Directions:

1. Preheat stove to 350 degrees and line a sheet container with material paper.
2. Make the stroganoff:
3. In a large Dutch grill or skillet, heat olive oil over medium warmth.
4. Saute mushrooms with one teaspoon salt and dark pepper. Include thyme. Cook mushrooms until brilliant, roughly 4 minutes.
5. Expel from a dish and put in a safe spot.
6. Include margarine, onions, and garlic to the container and saute 2 minutes.
7. Cook ground hamburger over medium warmth until dark-colored, roughly 4 minutes.
8. Add flour and paprika to cover uniformly.
9. Include meat soup, sour cream, and mustard.
10. Blend entirely and include mushrooms back in round the emptied portion with stroganoff and top with mozzarella cheddar.

11. Spot on the readied heating sheet and prepare for 5 to 10 minutes until cheddar is brilliant and softened.
12. Head with parsley, cut and serve right away.

Nutrition:

Calories: 1007 kcal.

Protein: 88.04 g.

Fat: 60 g.

Carbohydrates: 32.06 g.

Classic French Toast

Preparation time: 10 minutes.

Cooking time: 45 minutes.

Servings: 2.

Ingredients:

- Four huge eggs.
- 1/2 cup whole milk.
- One teaspoon vanilla concentrate.
- 1/2 teaspoons ground cinnamon partitioned.
- 8 cuts Brioche bread.

Directions:

1. On the off chance that is utilizing an electric iron, preheat the frying pan to 350°F.
2. Race until very much consolidated.
3. Plunge each side of the bread in the egg blend.
4. Note - include the other portion of the cinnamon after you have plunged half of your bread cuts and blend once more.
5. This will ensure the entirety of the cuts gets a decent measure of cinnamon.
6. Soften a little margarine on the hot frying pan or in a large skillet over medium warmth.

7. Serve the French toast warm with maple syrup, powdered sugar and berries, whenever wanted.
8. Note - to keeps the French toast warm, heat the stove to 200°F. Spot a wire rack on a massive preparing sheet and spot the French toast on the shelf. Keep warm in the grill for as long as 30 minutes.

Nutrition:

Calories: 110.

Fat: 11g.

Carbs: 26.5g.

Protein: 2.5g.

Avocado and Kale Omelet

Preparation time: 10 minutes.

Cooking time: 45 minutes.

Servings: 2.

Ingredients:

- Two enormous eggs.
- One teaspoon low-fat milk.
- Spot of salt.
- Two teaspoons extra-virgin olive oil, partitioned.
- 1 cup cleaved kale.
- One tablespoon lime juice.
- One tablespoon cleaved fresh cilantro.
- One teaspoon unsalted sunflower seed.
- Spot of squashed red pepper.
- Spot of salt.
- ¼ avocado, cut.

Directions:

1. Mix eggs with milk and salt in a little bowl.
2. Warmth 1 teaspoon oil in a little non-stick skillet over medium warmth.
3. Include the egg blend and cook until the base is set and the inside is still some-what runny 1 to 2 minutes.
4. Flip the omelet over and cook until set, around 30 seconds more. Move to a plate.
5. Hurl kale with the staying one teaspoon oil, lime juice, cilantro, sunflower seeds, squashed red pepper and a touch of salt.
6. Top the omelet with the kale plate of mixed greens and avocado.

Nutrition:

Calories: 339.

Fat: 28.1g.

Carbs: 13g.

Protein: 15g.

Easy Egg-White Muffins

Preparation time: 10 minutes.

Cooking time: 15 minutes.

Servings: 2.

Ingredients:

- English muffin.
- Egg-whites - 6 tbsp. or two large egg whites.
- Turkey bacon or bacon sausage.
- Sharp cheddar cheese or gouda.
- Organic berry.
- Optional – lettuce and hot sauce, hummus, flaxseeds, etc...

Directions:

1. Get a microwavable safe container, then spray entirely to stop the egg from adhering, then pour egg whites into the dish.
2. Lay turkey bacon or bacon sausage paper towel and then cook.
3. Subsequently, toast your muffin, if preferred.
4. Then put the egg dish in the microwave for 30 minutes.
5. Afterward, with a spoon or fork, then immediately flip egg within the dish and cook for another 30 minutes.
6. Whilst the dish remains hot, sprinkle some cheese while preparing sausage.
7. The secret is to get a paste of some kind between each coating to put up the sandwich together, i.e. - a very small little bit of hummus or even cheese.

Nutrition:

Calories: 371.

Fat: 22g.

Carbs: 25g.

Protein: 23g.

Avocado Eggs with Toast

Preparation time: 10 minutes.

Cooking time: 45 minutes.

Servings: 2.

Ingredients:

- One avocado.
- 4 cuts whole wheat sandwich bread.
- Two tablespoons avocado oil.
- Four medium eggs.
- ¼ teaspoon salt, separated.
- ¼ teaspoon ground pepper, separated.
- Four tablespoons salsa.

Directions:

1. Preheat stove to 375ºF. Coat a huge rimmed preparing sheet with cooking splash.
2. Split avocado and strip.
3. Cut the long way into 1/4-inch-thick cuts, so you have cut through the entire length of the avocado with the gap from the pit.
4. Separate the four cuts nearest to either side of the hole and the shallow cuts; put in a safe spot.
5. Utilizing a baked good brush, delicately cover the two sides of each cut of bread with oil.
6. Cut a piece out of the focal point of each bread cut, looking like an avocado cut.
7. Move the dough and slice out bread pieces to the readied heating sheet.
8. Spot the shallow avocado cuts in the gaps of the bread.
9. Split an egg over every one of the avocado cuts in the dough.
10. Sprinkle the eggs with 1/8 teaspoon salt and 1/8 teaspoon pepper.
11. Each egg with one of the avocado cuts taken from the part nearest to the pit with an opening in them, uncovering the egg.
12. Sprinkle the avocado with the staying 1/8 teaspoon salt and 1/8 teaspoon pepper.
13. Prepare until the toast has seared in spots and the eggs are simply set 10 to 12 minutes.
14. Top with salsa, whenever wanted.
15. Present with the cut-out bread pieces.

Nutrition: 285 calories; 20.1 g absolute fat; 3.6 g-soaked fat; 186 mg cholesterol; 347 mg sodium. 386 mg potassium; 10.8 g protein.

Baked Oatmeal

Preparation time: 10 minutes.

Cooking time: 25 minutes.

Servings: 2.

Ingredients:

- 2 cups old-fashioned oats.
- ½ cup pecans, hacked.
- Two teaspoons ground cinnamon.
- One teaspoon preparing powder.
- ¾ teaspoon salt.
- 1/4 teaspoon ground nutmeg.
- 1/8 teaspoon ground cloves.
- 2 cups unsweetened almond milk or 2% milk.
- 1 cup low-fat plain Greek yoghurt.
- ¼ cup pure maple syrup.
- Two tablespoons extra-virgin olive oil.
- One teaspoon vanilla concentrate.
- Two pears diced little.
- 1/3 Cup low-fat plain Greek yoghurt.

Directions:

1. Preheat stove to 375ºF. Coat a 9-inch-square preparing dish with cooking shower.
2. Blend oats, pecans, cinnamon, heating powder, salt, nutmeg and cloves in an enormous bowl.
3. Whisk almond milk (or milk), 1 cup yoghurt, maple syrup, oil and vanilla in a medium bowl.
4. Empty the wet fixings into the dry fixings.
5. Delicately blend in.
6. Move the blend to the readied heating dish.
7. Heat until brilliant darker, 45 to 55 minutes.

Nutrition:

Calories: 311.

Fat: 14.8g.

Carbs: 12.1g.

Protein: 9.3g.

Sirt cereal

Preparation time: 15 minutes

Cooking time: 1 hour 20 minutes

Servings: 2-3

Ingredients:

- 50 g coconut oil
- 150 ml clear honey
- 1 tbsp ground turmeric
- 100 goats (use certified gluten-free oats if you're avoiding gluten)
- 250 g buckwheat flakes
- 100 g walnuts, chopped
- 50 g pecans, chopped
- 50 g flaked almonds
- 30 g pumpkin seeds
- 30 g sunflower seeds and 50 g cocoa nibs

Directions:

1. Heat your oven to 160 ° C / gas 3.
2. In a small saucepan, melt the coconut oil and honey over low heat and then stir in the turmeric.
3. Mix well to make sure no lumps are formed.
4. Mix all dry ingredients in a bowl and stir in the oil and honey.
5. Make sure they combine well then transfer them to a nonstick baking sheet or one lined with parchment paper.
6. Bake for 35–40 minutes, stirring for half the **cooking time**.

7. Once it's a nice golden color, remove it and let it cool on the baking sheet before storing in an airtight container for up to two months.

Nutrition:

Carbohydrates: 28 | Fat: 7 | Protein: 6 | Kcal: 220

Sirt breakfast bar

Preparation time: 15 minutes

Cooking time: approx. 2 hours

Servings: 10

Ingredients:

- 150 g pitted Medjool dates, chopped
- 150 g walnut butter
- 50 g thick honey
- 375 g sirtfood muesli

Directions:

1. Put the dates, walnut butter and honey in a food processor and blend until you have a nice paste. This can take some time as the dates won't be crushed and you will have to scrape the sides of the bowl a few times. Transfer the paste to a mixing bowl and stir the granola, making sure it is well mixed. If you squeeze a lump of the mixture in your hand, it should stay firm.
2. Line a 25 × 18 cm baking pan with parchment paper and spoon the mixture into it. Use your hands or the back of a spoon to spread it around the can as evenly as possible, then blot firmly to make sure the bars stay in one piece as you cut. Alternatively, you can shape the mixture into bite-sized balls.
3. Chill at least 2 hours before attempting to cut the mixture into about 10 bars.

You can then store them in an airtight container in the refrigerator for up to two weeks.

Nutrition:

Carbohydrates: 23 | Fat: 5 | Protein: 3 | Kcal: 140

Sirt cocoa pops

Preparation time: 10 minutes

Cooking time: 25 minutes

Servings: 10

Ingredients:

- 100 g corn
- 1 extra virgin olive oil or melted coconut oil
- For covering
- 50 g walnuts, chopped
- 50 g sunflower seeds
- 50 g buckwheat flakes
- 35 g cocoa nibs
- For serving
- 1 teaspoon cocoa powder (100 percent)
- 1 Medjool date, finely chopped
- 200 ml milk or dairy-free alternative

Directions:

1. Heat the oven to 160 ° C / gas 3.
2. Place a heavy pan with a tightly fitting lid over medium heat.
3. Mix the corn and oil, pour the mixture into the hot pan and cover with the lid.
4. Shake the pan to get the corn moving in it.
5. Once it starts to pop, turn up the heat and shake the pan for as long as you can while the lid is still on.

6. Once the popping has settled down to about 2 to 3 seconds between pops, remove the pan from the heat and empty it into a bowl.
7. Discard any kernels that have not popped, allow to cool completely, then transfer to an airtight container and store for up to a week.
8. For the topping, place the walnuts and sunflower seeds in a small baking sheet and roast in the oven for 15 minutes. Transfer to a bowl and mix with the buckwheat and cocoa nibs.
9. Let it cool completely and then store it in an airtight container for up to 1 month. The corn and topping should be stored separately to ensure even distribution when serving.
10. To serve, add 1–2 tablespoons of toppings and 10 g of popcorn to a bowl. Stir the cocoa powder and date into the milk then pour it over the grain.

Nutrition:

Carbohydrates: 21 | Fat: 14 | Protein: 3 | Kcal: 230

Sirt fruit bowl

Preparation time: 15 minutes

Cooking time: 0 minutes

Servings: 1

Ingredients:

- 40 g (10) raspberries
- 60 g (10) red / black grapes, halved
- 80 g (1 medium) plum, chopped
- 60 g (½ medium)
- Apple, cut
- 50 g (2 medium) peeled strawberries, chopped
- Juice of ¼ lemon

- 100 g Greek yogurt
- 5 walnut halves, mashed

Directions:

1. Put all the fruits in a bowl. Squeeze the lemon juice over it and mix well.
2. Pour over the Greek yogurt, sprinkle the chopped walnuts on top, and serve.

Nutrition:

Carbohydrates: 24 | Fat: 17 | Protein: 3 | Kcal: 180

Grilled sausages with fried Onions and scrambled eggs with herbs

Preparation time: 10 minutes

Cooking time: 20 minutes

Servings: 1

Ingredients:

- 2 lean pork or beef sausages 2 eggs
- 1 teaspoon chopped parsley
- 1 teaspoon chopped chives
- 25 ml milk or dairy-free alternative
- 1 teaspoon extra virgin olive oil
- 60 g red onion
- 1 teaspoon dried thyme

Directions:

1. Heat a grill on the highest setting.
2. Grill the sausages for 8 to 10 minutes, turning them from time to time until they are browned nicely all over.
3. Whisk eggs, parsley, chives and milk together.
4. Put ½ teaspoon of olive oil in a small saucepan over medium heat, add the egg mixture and cook gently until you have a nice scrambled egg.

5. In the meantime, put the remaining ½ teaspoon of olive oil in a small pan over medium heat and fry the onion and thyme for 3-4 minutes until brown.
6. Stack the eggs on a plate and cover with the sausages and onions.

Nutrition:

Carbohydrates: 24 | Fat: 27 | Protein: 15 | Kcal: 420

Smoked salmon, arugula and Capers on buckwheat crackers

Preparation time: 10 minutes

Cooking time: 15 minutes

Servings: 1

Ingredients:

- 1 teaspoon capers
- 60 g Greek yogurt
- 1 tbsp. chopped parsley
- 10 g red onion, thinly sliced
- Buckwheat crackers
- 75 g smoked salmon
- 20 g rocket juice from ¼ lemon

Directions:

1. Mix capers, yoghurt, parsley and onion in a bowl.
2. Spread the mixture over your crackers and top with the smoked salmon and arugula.
3. Finally, squeeze out some lemon juice.

Nutrition:

Carbohydrates: 15 | Fat: 7 | Protein: 3 | Kcal: 120

Baked Kipper with Kale and poached eggs

Preparation time: 10 minutes

Cooking time: 20 minutes

Servings: 1

Ingredients:

- 1 tipper 1 tsp
- extra virgin olive oil
- 1 teaspoon chopped parsley
- 50 g kale, chopped
- A few drops of vinegar
- 1 medium egg
- 1 lemon wedge

Directions:

1. Preheat your oven to 200 ° C / gas 6.
2. In the meantime, bring 2 small pots of water to a boil.
3. If necessary, cut the head and tail off your kipper
4. Place the skin-side down on a piece of foil.
5. Pour the olive oil and parsley over the kipper and wrap the foil around it.
6. Place the kale in a pan of boiling water and simmer for 5 minutes or until tender.
7. Drain and keep warm.
8. Put a few drops of vinegar in the other pan with boiling water.
9. And let the heat simmer.
10. Stir the water clockwise and then crack your egg in half.
11. An egg with a solid white and liquid yolk takes 2 to 3 minutes.
12. Remove with a slotted spoon and drain on kitchen paper.
13. Serve the egg on top of the kipper with the kale aside.

Nutrition:

Carbohydrates: 11 | Fat: 17 | Protein: 33 | Kcal: 340

Poached egg with rocket, Asparagus and bacon

Preparation time: 5 minutes

Cooking time: 15 minutes

Servings: 1

Ingredients:

- 2 slices of striped or bacon back
- 6 asparagus spears,
- a few drops of vinegar 2 eggs
- 10 g rocket
- 1 teaspoon extra virgin olive oil

Directions:

1. Heat a grill on the highest setting.
2. In the meantime, bring 2 small pots of water to the boil.
3. Once the grill is hot, grill your bacon until the fat is crispy.
4. Put the asparagus spears in a pan of boiling water.
5. And cook for 2-3 minutes until tender.
6. Put a few drops of vinegar in the other pan with boiling water.
7. And let the heat simmer.
8. Stir the water clockwise and then crack an egg in the middle.
9. An egg with a solid white and liquid yolk takes 2 to 3 minutes.
10. Remove with a slotted spoon and drain on kitchen paper.
11. Cook the second egg in the same way.
12. Place the eggs on the asparagus.
13. Cover with the crispy bacon and rocket and drizzle over the olive oil.

Nutrition:

Carbohydrates: 11 | Fat: 17 | Protein: 33 | Kcal: 340

Strawberry and Cherry Smoothie

Preparation time: 5 minutes

Cooking time: 0 minutes

Servings: 1

Ingredients:

- 100g (3½ oz.) strawberries
- 75g (3oz) frozen pitted cherries
- 1 tablespoon plain full-fat yogurt
- 175mls (6fl oz.) unsweetened soya milk
- Serves 1
- 132 calories per serving

Directions:

1. Place all of the ingredients into a blender and process until smooth.
2. Serve and enjoy.

Eggs with Kale

Preparation time: 5 minutes

Cooking time: 10 minutes

Servings: 1

Ingredients:

- 2 large eggs
- Salt
- Ground black pepper
- 1 tsp. olive oil or avocado oil
- 1 cup kale

Directions:

1. Heat 1 tsp. olive oil in the skillet over (medium/high) heat.
2. Add kale and cook, tossing, until wilted (Approx. 1 minute).

3. Remove kale, add eggs and fry until done.
4. Serve with kale.

Banana Snap

Preparation time: 5 minutes

Cooking time: 0 minutes

Servings: 1

Ingredients:

- 2.5cm (1 inch) chunk of fresh ginger, peeled
- 1 banana
- 1 large carrot
- 1 apple, cored
- ½ stick of celery
- ¼ level teaspoon turmeric powder

Directions:

1. Place all the ingredients into a blender with just enough water to cover them.
2. Process until smooth
3. Nutrients: 166 calories per serving

Green Egg Scramble

Preparation time: 5 minutes

Cooking time: 10 minutes

Servings: 1

Ingredients:

- 2 eggs, whisked
- 25g (1oz) rocket (arugula) leaves
- 1 teaspoon chives, chopped
- 1 teaspoon fresh basil, chopped
- 1 teaspoon fresh parsley, chopped
- 1 tablespoon olive oil

Directions:

1. Mix the eggs together with the rocket (arugula) and herbs.
2. Heat the oil in a frying pan and pour into the egg mixture.
3. Gently stir until it's lightly scrambled.
4. Season and serve.

Nutrients: 250 calories

Strawberry Blend

Preparation time: 5 minutes + 8h

Cooking time: 0 minutes

Servings: 2

Ingredients:

- 2 oz. rolled oats
- 4 oz. almond milk, unsweetened
- 2 tbsp. plain yoghurt
- 1 cup strawberries
- 1 tsp honey
- 1 square 85% chocolate

Directions:

1. Mix the oats and the milk and leave overnight.
2. In the morning top the jar with yoghurt, honey, strawberries and chocolate.
3. Cut in small pieces.

Nutrition:

Calories: 258, Fat: 3.3g, Carbohydrate: 29.8g, Protein: 13.6g

Avocado Kale smoothie

Preparation time: 5 minutes

Cooking time: 10 minutes

Servings: 1

Ingredients:

- 3 stalks of kales
- 1 avocado, peeled & de-stoned
- 1 teaspoon fresh parsley
- ½ teaspoon matcha powder
- Juice of ½ lemon

Directions:

1. Place all of the ingredients into a blender and add enough water to cover them.
2. Process until creamy and smooth.

Nutrition: 306 calories

Green Sirtfood Smoothie

Preparation time: 5 minutes

Cooking time: 0 minutes

Servings: 1

Ingredients:

- 100g unsweetened Greek yoghurt
- 6 walnut halves
- 8-10 medium strawberries
- a handful of kale leaves
- 20g dark chocolate (min. 85% cocoa)
- 1 date
- 1/2 teaspoon turmeric
- Small piece fresh chili, finely chopped
- 200ml unsweetened almond milk

Directions:

1. Put everything into a blender and mix until you get a smoothie.

Nutrition: 250 calories

Power cereals

Preparation time: 5 minutes

Cooking time: 5 minutes

Servings: 1

For one serving. The ultimate start to the day with extra sirtuin foods.

- 20g buckwheat flakes
- 10g puffed buckwheat
- 15g coconut flakes
- 40g Medjool dates, seeded and chopped
- 10g cocoa nibs
- 100g strawberries
- 100g Greek natural yoghurt

Directions:

1. Mix all ingredients together.
2. If you are preparing on stock, e.g. for five portions, simply take five times the amount.
3. You can store them for a few days in an airtight tin.
4. If you prefer to eat vegan, use soy yoghurt instead of Greek yoghurt.
5. Instead of strawberries you can also use other berries, e.g. raspberries, blueberries or blackberries.

Nutrition: 350 calories

Berry Yoghurt

Preparation time: 5 minutes

Cooking time: 0 minutes

Servings: 1

For breakfast as part of your sirtfood diet we suggest this yoghurt for example:

Ingredients:

- 125g mixed berries, e.g. blueberries, strawberries and blackberries
- 150g Greek yoghurt
- 25g walnuts, chopped
- 10g dark chocolate (85%), grated

Directions:

1. Simply mix all ingredients together.
2. Vegans can also use soy yoghurt and vegan chocolate instead of yoghurt.

Nutrition: 250 calories

Yoghurt with berries

Preparation time: 5 minutes

Cooking time: 0 minutes

Servings: 1

Ingredients:

- Unsweetened yoghurt (125g)
- Fresh berries, e.g. raspberries, approx. 60g.

Directions:

1. Mix all ingredients

Nutrition: 150 calories

Raspberries belong to the so-called Sirt foods - and so this breakfast is also suitable as part of a Sirt food diet.

Blueberry frozen yogurt

Preparation time: 5 minutes

Cooking time: 0 minutes

Servings: 4

Ingredients:

- 450g (1lb) plain yogurt
- 175g (6oz) blueberries
- Juice of 1 orange
- 1 tablespoon honey

Directions:

1. Place the blueberries and orange juice into a food processor or blender and blitz until smooth. Press the mixture through a sieve into a large bowl to remove seeds. Stir in the honey and yogurt. Transfer the mixture to an ice-cream maker and follow the manufacturer's instructions. Alternatively pour the mixture into a container and place in the fridge for 1 hour. Use a fork to whisk it and break up ice crystals and freeze for 2 hours.

Nutrition: 133 calories per serving

Vegetable & Nut Loaf

Preparation time: 5 minutes

Cooking time: 0 minutes

Servings: 4

Ingredients:

- 175g (6oz) mushrooms, finely chopped
- 100g (3½ oz) haricot beans
- 100g (3½ oz) walnuts, finely chopped
- 100g (3½ oz) peanuts, finely chopped
- 1 carrot, finely chopped
- 3 sticks celery, finely chopped
- 1 bird's-eye chilli, finely chopped
- 1 red onion, finely chopped
- 1 egg, beaten
- 2 cloves of garlic, chopped
- 2 tablespoons olive oil
- 2 teaspoons turmeric powder
- 2 tablespoons soy sauce
- 4 tablespoons fresh parsley, chopped
- 100mls (3½ fl. oz.) water
- 60mls (2fl oz.) red wine

Directions:

1. Heat the oil in a pan.

2. Add the garlic, chili, carrot, celery, onion, mushrooms and turmeric.
3. Cook for 5 minutes.
4. Grease and line a large loaf tin with greaseproof paper.
5. Let it stand for 10 minutes then turn onto a serving plate.

Nutrition: 453 calories per serving

Dates & Parma Ham

Preparation time: 5 minutes

Cooking time: 0 minutes

Servings: 1

Ingredients:

- 12 medjool dates
- 2 slices of Parma ham, cut into strips
- Serves 4
- 202 calories per serving

Directions:

1. Wrap each date with a strip of Parma ham.
2. Can be served hot or cold.

Nutrition: 250 calories

Braised Celery

Preparation time: 5 minutes

Cooking time: 0 minutes

Servings: 1

Ingredients:

- 250g (9oz) celery, chopped
- 100mls (3½ fl oz) warm vegetable stock (broth)
- 1 red onion, chopped
- 1 clove of garlic, crushed

- 1 tablespoon fresh parsley, chopped
- 25g (1oz) butter
- Sea salt and freshly ground black pepper

Directions:

1. Place the celery, onion, stock (broth) and garlic into a saucepan simmer for 10 minutes.
2. Stir in the parsley and butter and season with salt and pepper.
3. Serve as an accompaniment to roast meat dishes.

Nutrition: 67 calories

Cheesy Buckwheat Cakes

Preparation time: 5 minutes

Cooking time: 0 minutes

Servings: 1

Ingredients:

- 100g (3½oz) buckwheat, cooked and cooled
- 1 large egg
- 25g (1oz) cheddar cheese, grated (shredded)
- 25g (1oz) whole meal breadcrumbs
- 2 shallots, chopped
- 2 tablespoons fresh parsley, chopped
- 1 tablespoon olive oil

Directions:

1. Crack the egg into a bowl, whisk it then set aside.
2. In a separate bowl combine all the buckwheat, cheese, shallots and parsley.
3. Mix well.

4. Pour in the beaten egg to the buckwheat mixture and stir well.
5. Shape the mixture into patties.
6. Scatter the breadcrumbs on a plate and roll the patties in them.
7. Heat the olive oil in a large frying pan.
8. And gently place the cakes in the oil.
9. Cook for 3-4 minutes on either side until slightly golden.

Nutrition: 358 calories

Red Chicory & Stilton Cheese Boats

Preparation time: 5 minutes

Cooking time: 0 minutes

Servings: 1

Ingredients:

- 200g (7oz) stilton cheese, crumbled
- 200g (7oz) red chicory leaves (or if unavailable, use yellow)
- 2 tablespoon fresh parsley, chopped
- 1 tablespoon olive oil

Directions:

1. Place the red chicory leaves onto a baking sheet.
2. Drizzle them with olive oil then sprinkle the cheese inside the leaves.
3. Place them under a hot grill (broiler) for around 4 minutes.
4. Sprinkle with chopped parsley and serve straight away.

Nutrition: 250 calories

Green Omelette

Preparation time: 10 min

Cooking time: 5 min

Servings: 1

Ingredients:

- 2 large eggs, at room temperature
- 1 shallot, peeled and chopped
- Handful arugula
- 3 sprigs of parsley, chopped
- 1 tsp. extra virgin olive oil
- Salt and black pepper

Directions:

1. Beat the eggs in a small bowl and set aside; sauté the shallot for 5 minutes with a bit of the oil, on low-medium heat.
2. Pour the eggs in the pans, stirring the mixture for just a second.
3. The eggs on a medium heat and tip the pan just enough to let the loose egg run underneath after about one minute on the burner.
4. Add the greens, herbs and the seasonings to the top side as it is still soft.
5. TIP: You do not even have to flip it, as you can just cook the egg slowly egg as is well (being careful as not to burn).
6. TIP: Another option is to put it into an oven to broil for 3-5 minutes (checking to make sure it is only until it is golden but burned).

Nutrition: 234 calories

Berry Oat Breakfast Cobbler

Preparation time: 40 min

Cooking time: 5 min

Servings: 2

Ingredients:

- 2 cups of oats/flakes that are ready without cooking

- 1 cup of blackcurrants without the stems
- 1 teaspoon of honey (or ¼ teaspoon of raw sugar)
- ½ cup of water (add more or less by testing the pan)
- 1 cup of plain yogurt (or soy or coconut)

Directions:

1. Boil the berries, honey, and water, and then turn it down on low.
2. Put in a glass container in a refrigerator until it is cool and set (about 30 minutes or more)
3. When ready to eat, scoop the berries on top of the oats and yogurt.
4. Serve immediately.

Nutrition: 241 calories

Pancakes with Apples and Blackcurrants

Preparation time: 30 min

Cooking time: 10 min

Servings: 4

Ingredients:

- 2 apples, cut into small chunks
- 2 cups of quick cooking oats
- 1 cup flour of your choice
- 1 tsp. baking powder
- 2 tbsp. Raw sugar, coconut sugar, or 2 tbsp. honey that is warm and easy to distribute
- 2 egg whites
- 1 ¼ cups of milk (or soy/rice/coconut)
- 2 tsp. extra virgin olive oil
- A dash of salt
- For the berry topping:

- 1 cup blackcurrants, washed and stalks removed
- 3 tbsp. water (may use less)
- 2 tbsp. sugar (see above for types)

Directions:

1. Place the ingredients for the topping in a small pot simmer, stirring frequently for about 10 minutes until it cooks down and the juices are released.
2. Take the dry ingredients and mix in a bowl.
3. After, add the apples and the milk a bit at a time (you may not use it all), until it is a batter.
4. Stiffly whisk the egg whites and then gently mix them into the pancake batter.
5. Set aside in the refrigerator.
6. Pour a one quarter of the oil onto a flat pan or flat griddle and when hot, pour some of the batter into it in a pancake shape.
7. When the pancakes start to have golden brown edges and form air bubbles, they may be ready to be gently flipped.
8. Test to be sure the bottom can life away from the pan before actually flipping.
9. Repeat for the three pancakes.
10. Top each pancake with the berries.

Nutrition: 337 calories

Granola- The Sirt Way

Preparation time: 30 min

Cooking time: 0 min

Servings: 1

Ingredients:

- 1 cup buckwheat puffs

- 1 cup buckwheat flakes (ready to eat type, but not whole buckwheat that needs to be cooked) ½ cup coconut flakes
- ½ cup Medjool dates, without pits, chopped into smaller, bite-sized pieces
- 1 cup of cacao nibs or very dark chocolate chips
- 1/2 cup walnuts, chopped
- 1 cup strawberries chopped and without stem 1 cup plain Greek, or coconut or soy yogurt.

Directions:

1. Mix, without yogurt and strawberry toppings
2. You can store for up to a week, store in an airtight container.
3. Add toppings (even different berries or different yogurt.
4. You can even use the berry toppings as you will learn how to make from other recipes.

Nutrition: 235 Cal

Summer Berry Smoothie

Preparation time: 30 min

Cooking time: 0 min

Servings: 1

Ingredients:

- 50g (2oz) blueberries
- 50g (2oz) strawberries
- 25g (1oz) blackcurrants
- 25g (1oz) red grapes
- 1 carrot, peeled
- 1 orange, peeled
- Juice of 1 lime

Directions:

1. Place all of the ingredients into a blender and cover them with water.
2. Blitz until smooth.
3. You can also add some crushed ice and a mint leaf to garnish.

Nutrition: 300 Cal

Mango, Celery & Ginger Smoothie

Preparation time: 30 min

Cooking time: 0 min

Servings: 1

Ingredients:

- 1 stalk of celery
- 50g (2oz) kale
- 1 apple, cored
- 50g (2oz) mango, peeled, de-stoned and chopped
- 2.5cm (1 inch) chunk of fresh ginger root, peeled and chopped

Directions:

1. Put all the ingredients into a blender with some water and blitz until smooth.
2. Add ice to make your smoothie really refreshing.

Nutrition: 275 Cal

Orange, Carrot & Kale Smoothie

Preparation time: 30 min

Cooking time: 0 min

Servings: 1

Ingredients:

- 1 carrot, peeled
- 1 orange, peeled
- 1 stick of celery

- 1 apple, cored
- 50g (2oz) kale
- ½ teaspoon Matcha powder

Directions:

1. Place all of the ingredients into a blender and add in enough water to cover them.
2. Process until smooth, serve and enjoy.

Nutrition: 279 Cal

Creamy Strawberry & Cherry Smoothie

Preparation time: 30 min

Cooking time: 0 min

Servings: 1

Ingredients:

- 100g (3½ oz.) strawberries
- 75g (3oz) frozen pitted cherries
- 1 tablespoon plain full-fat yogurt
- 175mls (6fl oz.) unsweetened soya milk

Directions:

1. Place all of the ingredients into a blender and process until smooth.
2. Serve and enjoy.

Nutrition: 280 Cal

Grape, Celery & Parsley Reviver

Preparation time: 30 min

Cooking time: 0 min

Servings: 1

Ingredients:

- 75g (3oz) red grapes

- 3 sticks of celery
- 1 avocado, de-stoned and peeled
- 1 tablespoon fresh parsley
- ½ teaspoon Matcha powder

Directions:

1. Place all of the ingredients into a blender with enough water to cover them.
2. And blitz until smooth and creamy.
3. Add crushed ice to make it even more refreshing.

Nutrition: 230Cal

STrawberry & Citrus Blend

Preparation time: 30 min

Cooking time: 0 min

Servings: 1

Ingredients:

- 75g (3oz) strawberries
- 1 apple, cored
- 1 orange, peeled
- ½ avocado, peeled and de-stoned
- ½ teaspoon Matcha powder
- Juice of 1 lime

Directions:

1. Place all of the ingredients into a blender with enough water to cover them.
2. And process until smooth.

Nutrition: 250 Cal

Grapefruit & Celery Blast

Preparation time: 30 min

Cooking time: 0 min

Servings: 1

Ingredients:

- 1 grapefruit, peeled
- 2 stalks of celery
- 50g (2oz) kale
- ½ teaspoon Matcha powder

Directions:

1. Place all the ingredients into a blender with enough water to cover them.
2. Blitz until smooth.

Nutrition: 286 Cal

Orange & Celery Crush

Preparation time: 30 min

Cooking time: 0 min

Servings: 1

Ingredients:

- 1 carrot, peeled
- 3 stalks of celery
- 1 orange, peeled
- ½ teaspoon Matcha powder
- Juice of 1 lime

Directions:

1. Place all of the ingredients into a blender with enough water to cover them.
2. Blitz until smooth.

Nutrition: 274 Cal

Tropical Chocolate Delight

Preparation time: 30 min

Cooking time: 0 min

Servings: 1

Ingredients:

- 1 mango, peeled & de-stoned
- 75g (3oz) fresh pineapple, chopped
- 50g (2oz) kale
- 25g (1oz) rocket
- 1 tablespoon 100% cocoa powder or cacao nibs
- 150mls (5fl oz.) coconut milk

Directions:

1. Place all of the ingredients into a blender and blitz until smooth.
2. You can add a little water if it seems too thick.

Nutrition: 288 Cal

Walnut & Spiced Apple Tonic

Preparation time: 30 min

Cooking time: 0 min

Servings: 1

Ingredients:

- 6 walnuts halves
- 1 apple, cored
- 1 banana
- ½ teaspoon Matcha powder
- ½ teaspoon cinnamon
- Pinch of ground nutmeg

Directions:

1. Place all of the ingredients into a blender and add sufficient water to cover them.
2. Blitz until smooth and creamy.

Nutrition: 258 Cal

Pineapple & Cucumber Smoothie

Preparation time: 30 min

Cooking time: 0 min

Servings: 1

Ingredients:

- 50g (2oz) cucumber
- 1 stalk of celery
- 2 slices of fresh pineapple
- 2 sprigs of parsley
- ½ teaspoon Matcha powder
- A squeeze of lemon juice

Directions:

1. Place all of the ingredients into a blender with enough water to cover them.
2. Blitz until smooth.

Nutrition: 260 Cal

Kale & Orange Juice

Preparation time: 10 minutes

Cooking time: 0 minutes

Servings: 2

Ingredients:

- 5 large oranges, peeled
- 2 bunches fresh kale

Directions:

1. Add all ingredients into a juicer
2. And extract the juice according to the manufacturers.
3. Pour into 2 glasses and serve immediately.

Nutrition: 258 Cal

Orange Juice

Preparation time: 10 minutes

Cooking time: 0 minutes

Servings: 2

Ingredients:

- 5 large oranges, peeled and portioned
- 2 bunches fresh kale

Directions:

1. Add all ingredients into a juicer and extract the juice according to the manufacturer's method.
2. Pour into 2 glasses and serve immediately.

Nutrition: 258 Cal

Apple & Cucumber Juice

Preparation time: 10 minutes

Cooking time: 0 minutes

Servings: 2

Ingredients:

- 3 large apples, cored and sliced
- 2 large cucumbers, sliced
- 4 celery stalks
- 1 (1-inch) piece fresh ginger, peeled
- 1 lemon, peeled

Directions:

1. Add all ingredients into a juicer
2. And extract the juice according to the manufacturer's method.
3. Pour into 2 glasses and serve immediately.

Nutrition: 258 Cal

Hot chorizo, tomato & kale salad

Preparation time: 5 Minutes

Cooking Time: 20 Minutes

Servings: 4

Ingredients:

- 225g (8oz) kale leaves, finely chopped 75g (3oz) chorizo sausage, thinly sliced 8 cherry tomatoes
- 2 cloves of garlic
- 1 red onion, finely chopped
- 2 tablespoons olive oil
- 2 tablespoons red wine vinegar sea salt
- Freshly ground black pepper

Directions:

1. Heat the olive oil into a frying pan and add the sliced chorizo, garlic, onion and tomatoes. Cook for around 5 minutes. Add in the red wine vinegar and kale and cook for around 7 minutes or until the kale has softened. Season with salt and pepper. Serve immediately.

Nutrition: 355 calories per serving

Red chicory & walnut coleslaw

Preparation time: 5 Minutes

Cooking Time: 45 Minutes

Servings: 4

Ingredients:

- 100g (3½ oz.) red chicory, (or yellow) finely grated (shredded) 5 stalks of celery, finely chopped 8 walnut halves, chopped
- 1 red onion, finely chopped
- 2 tablespoons mayonnaise

Directions:

1. Place all of the ingredients into a bowl and combine well.
2. Chill in the fridge before serving.

Nutrition: 118 calories per serving

Smoked salmon & chicory boats

Preparation time: 5 Minutes

Cooking Time: 25 Minutes

Servings: 4

Ingredients:

- 150g (5oz) red chicory leaves (or yellow if it's unavailable) 150g (5oz) smoked salmon, finely chopped 100g (3½oz) cucumber, diced
- 2 tablespoons fresh parsley, chopped ½ red onion, finely chopped
- Juice of 1 lime
- 2 tablespoons olive oil

Directions:

1. Place the salmon, cucumber, onion, parsley, oil and lime juice into a bowl and toss the ingredients well.
2. Scoop some of the salmon mixture into each of the chicory leaves and chill before serving.

Nutrition: 152 calories per serving

Vegetable Loaf

Preparation time: 5 Minutes

Cooking Time: 35 Minutes

Servings: 4

Ingredients:

- 175g (6oz) mushrooms, finely chopped 100g (3½ oz) haricot beans
- 100g (3½ oz) walnuts, finely chopped 100g (3½ oz) peanuts, finely chopped 1 carrot, finely chopped
- 3 sticks celery, finely chopped 1 bird's-eye chilli, finely chopped 1 red onion, finely chopped
- 1 egg, beaten
- 2 cloves of garlic, chopped
- 2 tablespoons olive oil
- 2 teaspoons turmeric powder
- 2 tablespoons soy sauce
- 4 tablespoons fresh parsley, chopped 100mls (3½ fl oz) water
- 60mls (2fl oz) red wine

Directions:

1. Heat the oil in a pan and add the garlic, chilli, carrot, celery, onion, mushrooms and turmeric.
2. Cook for 5 minutes.
3. Grease and line a large loaf tin with greaseproof paper.
4. Let it stand for 10 minutes then turn onto a serving plate.

Nutrition: 453 calories per serving

Dates ham

Preparation time: 5 Minutes

Cooking Time: 25 Minutes

Servings: 4

Ingredients:

1. 12 medjool dates
2. 2 slices of parma ham, cut into strips

Directions:

1. Wrap each date with a strip of parma ham.

159

2. Can be served hot or cold.

Nutrition: 202 calories per serving

Celery Breakfast

Preparation time: 5 Minutes

Cooking Time: 15 Minutes

Servings: 4

Ingredients:

- 250g (9oz) celery, chopped
- 100mls (3½ fl oz) warm vegetable stock (broth) 1 red onion, chopped
- 1 clove of garlic, crushed
- 1 tablespoon fresh parsley, chopped 25g (1oz) butter
- Sea salt and freshly ground black pepper

Directions:

1. Place the celery, onion, stock (broth) and garlic into a saucepan and simmer for 10 minutes.
2. Stir in the parsley and butter and season with salt and pepper.
3. Serve as an accompaniment to roast meat dishes

Nutrition: 67 calories

Cheesy Wheat cakes

Preparation time: 5 Minutes

Cooking Time: 30 Minutes

Servings: 4

Ingredients:

- 100g (3½oz) buckwheat, cooked and cooled 1 large egg

- 25g (1oz) cheddar cheese, grated (shredded) 25g (1oz) wholemeal breadcrumbs 2 shallots, chopped
- 2 tablespoons fresh parsley, chopped 1 tablespoon olive oil

Directions:

1. Crack the egg into a bowl, whisk it then set aside.
2. In a separate bowl, combine all the buckwheat, cheese, shallots, and parsley.
3. Mix well.
4. Pour in the beaten egg to the buckwheat mixture and stir well.
5. Shape the mixture into patties.
6. Scatter the breadcrumbs on a plate and roll the patties in them.
7. Heat the olive oil in a large frying pan.
8. And gently place the cakes in the oil.
9. Cook for 3-4 minutes on either side until slightly golden.

Nutrition: 358 calories

Red chicory cheese boats

Preparation time: 5 Minutes

Cooking Time: 25 Minutes

Servings: 4

Ingredients:

- 200g (7oz) stilton cheese, crumbled 200g (7oz) red chicory leaves (or if unavailable, use yellow) 2 tablespoon fresh parsley, chopped 1 tablespoon olive oil

Directions:

1. Place the red chicory leaves onto a baking sheet.

2. Drizzle them with olive oil then sprinkle the cheese inside the leaves.
3. Place them under a hot grill (broiler) for around 4 minutes.
4. Sprinkle with chopped parsley and serve straight away.

Nutrition: 250 calories

Turkey breakfast sausages

Preparation Time: 5 Minutes

Cooking time: 55 Minutes

Servings: 2

Ingredients:

- 1 lb extra lean ground turkey
- 1 tbsp EVOO 9 Extra Virgin Olive Oil) and a little more to coat pan
- 1 tbsp fennel seeds
- 2 teaspoons smoked paprika
- 1 teaspoon red pepper flakes
- 1 teaspoon peppermint
- 1 teaspoon chicken seasoning
- A couple of shredded cheddar cheese
- A couple of chives, finely chopped
- A few shakes garlic and onion powder
- Two spins of pepper and salt

Directions:

1. Preheat oven to 350 F.
2. Utilize a little EVOO to grease a miniature muffin pan.
3. Combine all ingredients and blend thoroughly.
4. Fill each pit on top of the pan and then cook for approximately 15-20 minutes.
5. Each toaster differs therefore when muffin temperature is 165 then remove.

Nutrition: 250 calories

Tuna, egg & caper salad

Preparation time: 5 Minutes

Cooking Time: 35 Minutes

Servings: 4

Ingredients:

- 100g (3½oz) red chicory (or yellow if not available) 150g (5oz) tinned tuna flakes in brine, drained 100g (3 ½ oz) cucumber
- 25g (1oz) rocket (arugula)
- 6 pitted black olives
- 2 hard-boiled eggs, peeled and quartered 2 tomatoes, chopped
- 2 tablespoons fresh parsley, chopped 1 red onion, chopped
- 1 stalk of celery
- 1 tablespoon capers
- 2 tablespoons garlic vinaigrette (see recipe)

Directions:

1. Place the tuna, cucumber, olives, tomatoes, onion, chicory, celery, parsley and rocket (arugula) into a bowl.
2. Pour in the vinaigrette and toss the salad in the dressing.
3. Serve onto plates and scatter the eggs and capers on top.

Nutrition: 340 calories

Hot chicory & nut salad

Preparation time: 5 Minutes

Cooking Time: 25 Minutes

Servings: 4

Ingredients:

For the salad:

- 100g (3½oz) green beans
- 100g (3½oz) red chicory, chopped (if unavailable use yellow chicory) 100g (3½oz) celery, chopped
- 25g (1oz) macadamia nuts, chopped 25g (1oz) walnuts, chopped
- 25g (1oz) plain peanuts, chopped 2 tomatoes, chopped
- 1 tablespoon olive oil
- For the dressing:
- 2 tablespoons fresh parsley, finely chopped ½ teaspoon turmeric
- ½ teaspoon mustard
- 1 tablespoon olive oil
- 25mls (1fl oz) red wine vinegar

Directions:

1. Mix together the ingredients for the dressing then set them aside.
2. Heat a tablespoon of olive oil in a frying pan then add the green beans, chicory and celery.
3. Cook until the vegetables have softened then add in the chopped tomatoes and cook for 2 minutes.
4. Add the prepared dressing and thoroughly coat all of the vegetables.
5. Serve onto plates and sprinkle the mixture of nuts over the top.
6. Eat immediately.

Nutrition: 438 calories

Honey chili squash

Preparation time: 5 Minutes

Cooking Time: 40 Minutes

Servings: 4

Ingredients:

- 2 red onions, roughly chopped 2.5cm (1 inch) chunk of ginger root, finely chopped 2 cloves of garlic
- 2 bird's-eye chillies, finely chopped 1 butternut squash, peeled and chopped 100mls (3½ fl oz) vegetable stock (broth) 1 tablespoon olive oil
- Juice of 1 orange
- Juice of 1 lime
- 2 teaspoons honey

Directions:

1. Warm the oil into a pan and add in the red onions, squash chunks, chillies, garlic, ginger and honey.
2. Cook for 3 minutes.
3. Squeeze in the lime and orange juice.
4. Pour in the stock (broth), orange and lime juice and cook for 15 minutes until tender.

Nutrition: 815 calories.

Lunch Recipes

King Prawn Stir-fry & Soba

Preparation Time: 15 minutes

Cooking Time: 20 mutes

Servings: 3-4 **servings**

Ingredients:

- 150g shelled raw king prawns, deveined
- 2 tsp. tamari
- 2 tsp. extra virgin olive oil
- 75 soba
- 1 garlic clove, finely chopped
- 1 bird's eye chili, finely chopped
- 1 tsp. finely chopped fresh ginger
- 20g red onions, sliced
- 40g celery, trimmed and sliced
- 75g green beans, chopped
- 50g kale, roughly chopped
- 100ml chicken stock

Directions:

1. Warm a skillet over a high heat.
2. Fry for the pawns in 1 tsp. Of the tamari and of olive oil.
3. Transfer the contents of the skillet to a plate.
4. Wipe the skillet with kitchen towel to remove the lingering sauce.
5. Boil water and cook the soba for 8 minutes.
6. Drain and set aside.
7. Using the remaining 1 tsp. Olive oil.
8. Fry the remaining ingredients for 3-4 minutes.
9. Make the stock boil, simmering until the vegetables are tender but still have bite.
10. Add the lovage, noodles and prawn into the skillet.
11. Stir, bring back to the boil and then serve.

Nutrition: 192 calories

Miso Caramelized Tofu

Preparation Time: 10 minutes

Cooking Time: 25

Servings: 3

Ingredients:

- 1 tbsp mirin
- 20g miso paste
- 1 * 150g firm tofu
- 40g celery, trimmed
- 35g red onion
- 120g courgette
- 1 bird's eye chili
- 1 garlic clove, finely chopped
- 1 tsp. finely chopped fresh ginger
- 50g kale, chopped
- 2 tsp. sesame seeds
- 35g buckwheat
- 1 tsp. ground turmeric
- 2 tsp. extra virgin olive oil
- 1 tsp. tamari or soy sauce

Directions:

1. Pre-heat your over to 200C or gas mark 6.

2. Cover a tray with baking parchment.
3. Combine the mirin and miso together.
4. Dice the tofu and coat it in the mirin-miso mixture in a resealable plastic bag.
5. Set aside to marinate.
6. Chop the vegetables.
7. Disperse the tofu across the lined tray and garnish with sesame seeds.
8. Roast for 20 minutes, or until caramelized.
9. Rinse the buckwheat using running water and a sieve.
10. Add to a pan of boiling water alongside turmeric.
11. Cook the buckwheat according to the packet instructions.
12. Heat the oil in a skillet over high heat.
13. Toss in the vegetables, herbs and spices then fry for 2-3 minutes.
14. Reduce to a medium heat and fry for a further 5 minutes.

Nutrition: 192 calories

Sirtfood Cauliflower Couscous & Turkey Steak

Preparation Time: 10 minutes

Cooking Time: 15 minutes

Servings: 2

Ingredients:

- 150g cauliflower, roughly chopped
- 1 garlic clove, finely chopped
- 40g red onion, finely chopped
- 1 bird's eye chili, finely chopped
- 1 tsp. finely chopped fresh ginger
- 2 tbsp extra virgin olive oil
- 2 tsp. ground turmeric
- 30g sun dried tomatoes, finely chopped
- 10g parsley

- 150g turkey steak
- 1 tsp. dried sage
- Juice of ½ lemon
- 1 tbsp capers

Directions:

1. Disintegrate the cauliflower using a food processor.
2. Blend in 1-2 pulses until the cauliflower has a breadcrumb-like consistency.
3. In a skillet, fry garlic, chili, ginger and red onion in 1 tsp. Olive oil.
4. Throw in the turmeric and cauliflower then cook for another 1-2 minutes.
5. Remove from heat and add the tomatoes and roughly half the parsley.
6. Garnish the turkey steak with sage and dress with oil.
7. In a skillet, over medium heat, fry the turkey steak for 5 minutes.
8. Once the steak is cooked add lemon juice, capers and a dash of water.
9. Stir and serve with the couscous.

Nutrition: 231 Calories

Mushroom & Tofu Scramble

Preparation Time: 10 minutes

Cooking Time: 10 minutes

Servings: 1

Ingredients:

- 100g tofu, extra firm
- 1 tsp. ground turmeric
- 1 tsp. mild curry powder
- 20g kale, roughly chopped
- 1 tsp. extra virgin olive oil
- 20g red onion, thinly sliced
- 50g mushrooms, thinly sliced
- 5g parsley, finely chopped

Directions:

1. Place 2 sheets of kitchen towel under and on-top of the tofu.
2. Then rest a considerable weight such as saucepan onto the tofu.
3. Ensure it drains off the liquid.
4. Combine the curry powder, turmeric and 1-2 tsp. of water.
5. Using a steamer cook kale for 3-4 minutes.
6. In a skillet, warm oil over a medium heat.
7. Add the chili, mushrooms and onion, cooking for several minutes.
8. Break the tofu into small pieces and toss in the skillet.
9. Coat with the spice paste and stir.
10. Cook for up to 5 minutes and fry for 2 more minutes.
11. Garnish with parsley before serving.

Nutrition: 232 calories

Prawn & Chili Pak Choi

Preparation Time: 10 minutes

Cooking Time: 10 minutes

Servings: 1

Ingredients:

- 75g brown rice
- 1 pak choi
- 60ml chicken stock
- 1 tbsp extra virgin olive oil
- 1 garlic clove, finely chopped
- 50g red onion, finely chopped
- ½ bird's eye chili, finely chopped
- 1 tsp. freshly grated ginger
- 125g shelled raw king prawns
- 1 tbsp soy sauce
- 1 tsp. five-spice

- 1 tbsp freshly chopped flat-leaf parsley
- A pinch of salt and pepper

Directions:

1. Bring a medium sized saucepan of water to the boil
2. And cook the brown rice for 25-30 minutes, or until softened.
3. Tear the pak choi into pieces.
4. Warm the chicken stock in a skillet over medium heat.
5. Toss in the pak choi, cooking until the pak choi has slightly wilted.
6. In another skillet, warm olive oil over high heat.
7. Toss in the ginger, chili, red onions and garlic frying for 2-3 minutes.
8. Throw in the pawns, five-spice and soy sauce.
9. Cook for 6-8 minutes, or until the cooked throughout.
10. Drain the brown rice and add to the skillet, stirring and cooking for 2-3 minutes.
11. Add the pak choi, garnish with parsley and serve.

Nutrition: 193 calories

Sirtfood Granola

Preparation Time: 10 minutes

Cooking Time: 25 minutes

Servings: 12

Ingredients:

- 200g oats
- 250g buckwheat flakes
- 100g walnuts, chopped
- 100g almonds, chopped
- 100g dried strawberries
- 1 ½ tsp. ground ginger

- 1 ½ tsp. ground cinnamon
- 120mls olive oil
- 2 tbsp honey

Directions:

1. Preheat your oven to 150C.
2. Line a tray with baking parchment.
3. Stir together walnuts, almonds, buckwheat flakes and oats with ginger and cinnamon.
4. In a large pan, warm olive oil and honey, heating until the honey has dissolved.
5. Pour the honey-oil over the other ingredients.
6. Stirring to ensuring an even coating.
7. Separate the granola evenly over the lined baking tray.
8. And roast for 50 minutes, or until golden.
9. Once cooled add the berries and store in an airtight container.
10. Eat dry or with milk and yogurt. It stays fresh for up to 1 week.

Nutrition: 231 calories

Tomato Frittata

Preparation Time: 10 minutes

Cooking Time: 15 minutes

Servings: 2

Ingredients:

- 50g cheddar cheese, grated
- 75g kalamata olives, pitted and halved
- 8 cherry tomatoes, halved
- 4 large eggs
- 1 tbsp fresh parsley, chopped
- 1 tbsp fresh basil, chopped
- 1 tbsp olive oil

Directions:

1. Whisk the eggs in a mixing bowl.
2. Toss in the parsley, basil, olives, tomatoes and cheese, stirring thoroughly.
3. Heat the olive oil over high heat.
4. Pour in the frittata mixture and cook for 5-10 minutes, or set.
5. Remove the skillet from the hob and place under the grill for 5 minutes, or until firm and set.
6. Divide into portions and serve immediately.

Nutrition: 231 calories

Horseradish Flaked Salmon Fillet & Kale

Preparation Time: 10 minutes

Cooking Time: 15 minutes

Servings: 2

Ingredients:

- 200g skinless, boneless salmon fillet
- 50g green beans
- 75g kale
- 1 tbsp extra virgin olive oil
- ½ garlic clove, crushed
- 50g red onion, chopped
- 1 tbsp fresh chives, chopped
- 1 tbsp freshly chopped flat-leaf parsley
- 1 tbsp low fat crème Fraiche
- 1tbsp horseradish sauce
- Juice of ¼ lemon
- A pinch of salt and pepper

Directions:

1. Preheat the grill.
2. Sprinkle a salmon fillet with salt and pepper.

3. Place under the grill for 10-15 minutes. Flake and set aside.
4. Using a steamer, cook the kale and green beans for 10 minutes.
5. In a skillet, warm the oil over a high heat.
6. Add garlic and red onion and fry for 2-3 minutes.
7. Toss in the kale and beans and then cook for 1-2 minutes more.
8. Mix the chives, parsley, crème fraiche, horseradish, lemon juice and flaked salmon.
9. Serve the kale and beans topped with the dressed flaked salmon.

Nutrition: 221 calories

Indulgent Yoghurt

Preparation Time: 10 minutes

Cooking Time: 15 minutes

Servings: 3

Ingredients:

- 125 mixed berries
- 150g Greek yoghurt
- 25 walnuts, chopped
- 10g dark chocolate at least 85% cocoa solids, grated

Directions:

1. Toss the mixed berries into a serving bowl.
2. Cover with yoghurt and top with chocolate and walnuts. Voila!

Nutrition: 231 calories

Tuna Salad

Preparation Time: 5 minutes

Cooking Time: 5 minutes

Servings: 1

Ingredients:

- 100g red chicory
- 150g tuna flakes in brine, drained
- 100g cucumber
- 25g rocket
- 6 kalamata olives, pitted
- 2 hard-boiled eggs, peeled and quartered
- 2 tomatoes, chopped
- 2 tbsp fresh parsley, chopped
- 1 red onion, chopped
- 1 celery stalk
- 1 tbsp capers
- 2 tbsp garlic vinaigrette

Directions:

1. Put the ingredients in a bowl and serve.

Nutrition: 245 calories

Chicken & Bean Casserole

Preparation Time: 10 minutes

Cooking Time: 15 minutes

Servings: 2

Ingredients:

- 400g 14oz chopped tomatoes
- 400g 14oz tinned cannellini beans or haricot beans
- 8 chicken thighs, skin removed
- 2 carrots, peeled and finely chopped
- 2 red onions, chopped
- 4 sticks of celery
- 4 large mushrooms
- 2 red peppers bell peppers, de-seeded and chopped

167

- 1 clove of garlic
- 2 tablespoons soy sauce
- 1 tablespoon olive oil
- liters 3 pints chicken stock broth

Directions:

1. Put and heat olive oil, add the garlic and onions and cook for 5 minutes.
2. Add in the chicken.
3. Cook for 5 minutes
4. Add the carrots, cannellini beans, celery, red peppers bell peppers and mushrooms.
5. Pour in the stock broth soy sauce and tomatoes.
6. Bring it to the boil, reduce the heat and simmer for 45 minutes.
7. Serve with rice or new potatoes.

Nutrition: 509 calories

Mussels in Red Wine Sauce

Preparation Time: 20 minutes

Cooking Time: 10 minutes

Servings: 2

Ingredients:

- 800g 2lb mussels
- 2 x 400g 14oz tins of chopped tomatoes
- 25g 1oz butter
- 1 tablespoon fresh chives, chopped
- 1 tablespoon fresh parsley, chopped
- 1 bird's-eye chili, finely chopped
- 4 cloves of garlic, crushed
- 400mls 14fl oz red wine
- Juice of 1 lemon

Directions:

1. Wash the mussels, remove their beards and set them aside.

2. Put butter in a saucepan. Add in the red wine.
3. Reduce the heat and add the parsley, chives, chili and garlic whilst stirring.
4. Add in the tomatoes, lemon juice and mussels.
5. Cover the saucepan and cook for 2-3.
6. Remove the saucepan from the heat.
7. Take out any mussels which haven't opened and discard them.
8. Serve and eat immediately.

Nutrition: 364 calories

Tuna and Kale

Preparation time: 5 minutes

Cooking time: 20 minutes

Servings: 4

Ingredients:

- 1 pound tuna fillets, boneless, skinless and cubed
- A pinch of salt and black pepper
- 2 tablespoons olive oil
- 1 cup kale, torn
- ½ cup cherry tomatoes, cubed
- 1 yellow onion, chopped

Directions:

1. Heat up a pan with the oil over medium heat.
2. Add the onion and sauté for 5 minutes.
3. Add the tuna and the other ingredients, toss,
4. Cook everything for 15 minutes more, divide between plates and serve.

Nutrition: calories 251, fat 4, fiber 7, carbs 14, protein 7

Lemongrass Mix

Preparation time: 10 minutes

Cooking time: 25 minutes

Servings: 4

Ingredients:

- 4 mackerel fillets, skinless and boneless
- 2 tablespoons olive oil
- 1 tablespoon ginger, grated
- 2 lemongrass sticks, chopped
- 2 red chilies, chopped
- Juice of 1 lime
- A handful parsley, chopped

Directions:

1. Combine the mackerel with the oil, ginger and the other ingredients.
2. Toss and bake at 390 degrees F for 25 minutes.
3. Divide everything between plates and serve.

Nutrition: calories 251, fat 3, fiber 4, carbs 14, protein 8

Scallops with Almonds and Mushrooms

Preparation time: 5 minutes

Cooking time: 10 minutes

Servings: 4

Ingredients:

- 1 pound scallops
- 2 tablespoons olive oil
- 4 scallions, chopped
- A pinch of salt and black pepper
- ½ cup mushrooms, sliced
- 2 tablespoon almonds, chopped

- 1 cup coconut cream

Directions:

1. Heat up a pan with the oil over medium heat, add the scallions and the mushrooms and sauté for 2 minutes.
2. Add the scallops and the other ingredients, toss, cook over medium heat for 8 minutes more, divide into bowls and serve.

Nutrition: calories 322, fat 23.7, fiber 2.2, carbs 8.1, protein 21.6

Scallops and Sweet Potatoes

Preparation time: 5 minutes

Cooking time: 22 minutes

Servings: 4

Ingredients:

- 1 pound scallops
- ½ teaspoon rosemary, dried
- ½ teaspoon oregano, dried
- 2 tablespoons avocado oil
- 1 yellow onion, chopped
- 2 sweet potatoes, peeled and cubed
- ½ cup chicken stock
- 1 tablespoon cilantro, chopped
- A pinch of salt and black pepper

Directions:

1. Heat up a pan with the oil over medium heat, add the onion and sauté for 2 minutes.
2. Add the sweet potatoes and the stock, toss and cook for 10 minutes more.
3. Add the scallops and the remaining ingredients, toss, cook for another 10 minutes, divide everything into bowls and serve.

Nutrition: calories 211, fat 2, fiber 4.1, carbs 26.9, protein 20.7

Salmon and Shrimp Salad

Preparation time: 5 minutes

Cooking time: 0 minutes

Servings: 4

Ingredients:

- 1 cup smoked salmon, boneless and flaked
- 1 cup shrimp, peeled, deveined and cooked
- ½ cup baby arugula
- 1 tablespoon lemon juice
- 2 spring onions, chopped
- 1 tablespoon olive oil
- A pinch of sea salt and black pepper

Directions:

1. In a salad bowl, combine the salmon with the shrimp and the other ingredients, toss and serve.

Nutrition: calories 210, fat 6, fiber 5, carbs 10, protein 12

Shrimp, Tomato and Dates Salad

Preparation time: 10 minutes

Cooking time: 0 minutes

Servings: 4

Ingredients:

- 1 pound shrimp, cooked, peeled and deveined
- 2 cups baby spinach
- 2 tablespoons walnuts, chopped
- 1 cup cherry tomatoes, halved
- 1 tablespoon lemon juice

- ½ cup dates, chopped
- 2 tablespoons avocado oil

Directions:

1. In a salad bowl, mix the shrimp with the spinach, walnuts and the other ingredients, toss and serve.

Nutrition: calories 243, fat 5.4, fiber 3.3, carbs 21.6, protein 28.3

Salmon and Watercress Salad

Preparation time: 10 minutes

Cooking time: 0 minutes

Servings: 4

Ingredients:

- 1 pound smoked salmon, boneless, skinless and flaked
- 2 spring onions, chopped
- 2 tablespoons avocado oil
- ½ cup baby arugula
- 1 cup watercress
- 1 tablespoon lemon juice
- 1 cucumber, sliced
- 1 avocado, peeled, pitted and roughly cubed
- A pinch of sea salt and black pepper

Directions:

1. In a salad bowl, mix the salmon with the spring onions, watercress and the other ingredients, toss and serve.

Nutrition: calories 261, fat 15.8, fiber 4.4, carbs 8.2, protein 22.7

Tuna and Tomatoes

Preparation time: 5 minutes

Cooking time: 20 minutes

Servings: 4

Ingredients:

- 1 yellow onion, chopped
- 1 tablespoon olive oil
- 1 pound tuna fillets, boneless, skinless and cubed
- 1 cup tomatoes, chopped
- 1 red pepper, chopped
- 1 teaspoon sweet paprika
- 1 tablespoon coriander, chopped

Directions:

1. Heat up a pan with the oil over medium heat
2. Add the onions and the pepper and cook for 5 minutes.
3. Add the other ingredients
4. Cook everything for 15 minutes.
5. Divide between plates and serve.

Nutrition: calories 215, fat 4, fiber 7, carbs 14, protein 7

Spinach and Kale Mix

Preparation time: 5 minutes

Servings: 4

Ingredients:

- 2 chopped shallots
- 1 c. no-salt-added and chopped canned tomatoes
- 2 c. baby spinach
- 2 minced garlic cloves
- 5 c. torn kale
- 1 tbsp. olive oil

Directions:

1. Heat up a pan with the oil over medium-high heat.

2. Add the shallots, stir and sauté for 5 minutes.
3. Add the spinach, kale and the other ingredients, toss.
4. Cook for 10 minutes more.
5. Divide between plates and serve.

Nutrition:

Calories: 89, Fat: 3.7 g, Carbs: 12.4 g, Protein: 3.6 g, Sugars: 0 g, Sodium: 50 mg

Turmeric Carrots

Preparation time: 10 minutes

Cooking time: 40 minutes

Servings: 4

Ingredients:

- 1 pound baby carrots, peeled
- 1 tablespoon olive oil
- 2 spring onions, chopped
- 2 tablespoons balsamic vinegar
- 2 garlic cloves, minced
- 1 teaspoon turmeric powder
- 1 tablespoon chives, chopped
- ¼ teaspoon cayenne pepper
- A pinch of salt and black pepper

Directions:

1. Spread the carrots on a baking sheet lined with parchment paper.
2. Add the oil, the spring onions and the other ingredients
3. Toss and bake at 380 degrees F for 40 minutes.
4. Divide the carrots between plates and serve.

Nutrition: calories 79, fat 3.8, fiber 3.7, carbs 10.9, protein 1

Spinach Mix

Preparation time: 10 minutes

Cooking time: 12 minutes

Servings: 4

Ingredients:

- 1 pound baby spinach
- 1 yellow onion, chopped
- 1 tablespoon olive oil
- 1 tablespoon lemon juice
- 2 garlic cloves, minced
- A pinch of cayenne pepper
- ¼ teaspoon smoked paprika
- A pinch of salt and black pepper

Directions:

1. Heat up a pan with the oil over medium-high heat
2. Add the onion and the garlic and sauté for 2 minutes.
3. Add the spinach and the other ingredients, toss.
4. Cook over medium heat for 10 minutes.
5. Divide between plates and serve as a side dish.

Nutrition: calories 71, fat 4, fiber 3.2, carbs 7.4, protein 3.7

Orange Carrots

Preparation time: 5 minutes

Cooking time: 25 minutes

Servings: 4

Ingredients:

- 1 pound carrots, peeled and roughly sliced
- 1 yellow onion, chopped
- 1 tablespoon olive oil
- Zest of 1 orange, grated
- Juice of 1 orange
- 1 orange, peeled and cut into segments
- 1 tablespoon rosemary, chopped
- A pinch of salt and black pepper

Directions:

1. Heat up a pan with the oil over medium-high heat
2. Add the onion and sauté for 5 minutes.
3. Add the carrots, the orange zest and the other ingredients, toss
4. Cook over medium heat for 20 minutes more
5. Divide between plates and serve.

Nutrition: calories 140, fat 3.9, fiber 5, carbs 26.1, protein 2.1

Greek Sea Bass Mix

Preparation time: 10 minutes

Cooking time: 22 minutes

Servings: 2

Ingredients:

- 2 sea bass fillets, boneless
- 1 garlic clove, minced
- 5 cherry tomatoes, halved
- 1 tablespoon chopped parsley
- 2 shallots, chopped
- Juice of ½ lemon
- 1 tablespoon olive oil
- 8 ounces baby spinach
- Cooking spray

Directions:

1. Grease a baking dish with cooking oil then add the fish, tomatoes, parsley and garlic.

2. Drizzle the lemon juice over the fish, cover the dish and place it in the oven at 350 degrees F.
3. Bake for 15 minutes and then divide between plates.
4. Heat up a pan with the olive oil over medium heat, add shallot, stir and cook for 1 minute.
5. Add spinach, stir, cook for 5 minutes more, add to the plate with the fish and serve.

Nutrition: calories 210, fat 3, fiber 6, carbs 10, protein 24

Creamy Asparagus Soup

Preparation time: 10 minutes

Cooking time: 0 minutes

Servings: 2

Ingredients:

- 8 ounces white mushrooms
- 12 asparagus spears, trimmed
- 1 avocado, pitted and peeled
- A pinch of salt and white pepper
- 1 yellow onion, peeled and chopped
- 3 cups water

Directions:

1. In your blender, add the mushrooms with asparagus, avocado, onion, water, salt and pepper.
2. Pulse well, divide into soup bowls and serve right away.
3. Heat if desired.
4. Enjoy!

Nutrition: calories 176, fat 3, fiber 9, carbs 16, protein 9

Mushroom Cream

Preparation time: 10 minutes

Cooking time: 0 minutes

Servings: 2

Ingredients:

- 2 tablespoons coconut aminos
- 1 tablespoon lime juice
- A pinch of sea salt and white pepper
- 1 cup white mushrooms
- 1 garlic clove, peeled
- 1 small yellow onion, chopped
- 2 cups cashew milk, unsweetened

Directions:

1. In your blender, mix mushrooms with garlic, onion, cashew milk, salt, pepper, lime juice and coconut aminos and pulse really well.
2. Divide into soup bowls and serve right away.
3. Enjoy!

Nutrition: calories 191, fat 2, fiber 6, carbs 14, protein 7

Tomato Cream

Preparation time: 10 minutes

Cooking time: 0 minutes

Servings: 2

Ingredients:

- 3 sun-dried tomato sliced
- 2 celery stalks, chopped
- 3 big tomatoes, chopped
- ½ teaspoon powdered onion
- 2 basil springs, chopped
- ½ teaspoon garlic powder
- 1 small avocado, pitted and peeled

- A pinch of sea salt and white pepper

Directions:

1. In your blender, add the tomatoes with celery, onion powder, garlic powder, basil, avocado, salt and pepper and pulse really well.
2. Add sun-dried tomatoes and blend again until smooth.
3. Divide into soup bowls and serve.
4. Enjoy!

Nutrition: calories 167, fat 11, fiber 9, carbs 14, protein 4

Zucchini Pan

Preparation time: 5 minutes

Cooking time: 20 minutes

Servings: 4

Ingredients:

1. 1 pound zucchinis, sliced
2. 1 yellow onion, chopped
3. 2 tablespoons olive oil
4. 2 apples, peeled, cored and cubed
5. 1 tomato, cubed
6. 1 tablespoon rosemary, chopped
7. 1 tablespoon chives, chopped

Directions:

1. Heat up a pan with the oil over medium heat
2. Add the onion and sauté for 5 minutes.
3. Add the zucchinis and the other ingredients, toss.
4. Cook over medium heat for 15 minutes more.
5. Divide between plates and serve as a side dish.

Nutrition: calories 170, fat 5, fiber 2, carbs 11, protein 7

Ginger Mushrooms

Preparation time: 10 minutes

Cooking time: 20 minutes

Servings: 4

Ingredients:

- 1 pound mushrooms, sliced
- 1 yellow onion, chopped
- 1 tablespoon ginger, grated
- 1 tablespoon olive oil
- 2 tablespoons balsamic vinegar
- 2 garlic cloves, minced
- A pinch of salt and black pepper
- ¼ cup lime juice
- 2 tablespoons walnuts, chopped

Directions:

1. Heat up a pan with the oil over medium-high heat.
2. Add the onion and the ginger and sauté for 5 minutes.
3. Add the mushrooms and the other ingredients, toss.
4. Cook over medium heat for 15 minutes more.
5. Divide between plates and serve.

Nutrition: calories 120, fat 2, fiber 2, carbs 4, protein 5

Salmon fillet, endive, arugula and celery

Preparation time: 10 minutes

Cooking time: 20 minutes

Servings: 4

Ingredients:

- 200g fresh salmon fillet
- 200g arugula
- Three red endives
- One large pink grapefruit
- Two slices of smoked salmon
- One small shallot
- One lemon
- Grated Parmesan cheese
- Extra virgin olive oil
- One teaspoon balsamic vinegar
- Salt and pepper to taste

Directions:

1. Cut the lemon in half to gently extract the liquid juice inside it.
2. Peel the grapefruit over a bowl to collect the juice.
3. Detach the quarters and cut them into pieces.
4. Peel and chop the shallot.
5. Remove the skin and bones from the fresh salmon fillet, then dice into small pieces
6. Place the whole mixture in a salad bowl, sprinkle with the lime and grapefruit juice, mix and let stand aside.
7. Cut the bottoms of the endives, remove the damaged leaves and chop the main parts into thin strips.
8. Wash and wring the arugula.
9. Carefully cut the smoked salmon slices into light strips.
10. Drain the marinated salmon fillet well and keep two teaspoons of the marinade.
11. Emulsify the marinade with olive oil and balsamic vinegar in a bowl, then salt and pepper as desired.
12. In a salad bowl, mix the diced salmon fillet, the smoked salmon strips, the

pieces of grapefruit, the arugula, the minced endives and the olive oil sauce.
13. Turn to mix and sprinkle lightly with grated Parmesan cheese.
14. Serve this salad immediately and serve with slices of toast.
15. Do not hesitate to double the proportions if you want to enjoy it as a main dish.

Nutrition: calories 120, fat 2, fiber 2, carbs 4, protein 5

Tuscan bean stew

Preparation time: 10 minutes

Cooking time: 20 minutes

Servings: 4

Ingredients:

- Two teaspoons extra virgin olive oil
- 6 oz. cooked chicken sausages cut lengthwise in half and sliced
- 10 oz. fresh mushrooms
- One small raw red onion
- Two thinly sliced garlic cloves
- 29 oz. canned, diced tomatoes
- Sixteen oz. canned beans
- One medium uncooked zucchini
- One tbsp. rosemary
- ¼ tsp salt
- 2 oz. arugula
- ¼ cups Grated Parmesan Cheese

Directions:

1. By using a Dutch oven, set the heat level to medium-high.
2. Add the sausages and cook, often stirring, until lightly browned, about three minutes.
3. Using a cooking spoon, transfer to a small bowl or plate.

4. Add the mushrooms and onion to the pot and cook, often stirring, until the vegetables are tender, usually for about three minutes.
5. Now add the garlic and cook, constantly stirring for about 30 seconds.
6. Add the sausages to the tomatoes, beans, zucchini, rosemary and salt and allow to boil.
7. Lower the heat and simmer, till the mushrooms becomes soft, usually after about 2 minutes.
8. Remove from heat and stir in the arugula until it is softened.
9. Pour the stew into four bowls and garnish evenly with Parmesan.

Nutrition: calories 120, fat 2, fiber 2, carbs 4, protein 5

Strawberry buckwheat salad

Preparation time: 10 minutes

Cooking time: 20 minutes

Servings: 4

Ingredients:

Tamari dressing:

- One-quarter cup of olive oil
- Two tablespoons of vinegar
- One tablespoon of reduced salt tamari sauce
- One tablespoon of old-fashioned mustard
- Salad:
- One cup buckwheat, rinsed and drained
- 6 cups mixed lettuce
- 2 cups strawberries, hulled and sliced
- A half fennel bulb cut into thin slices
- One-third cup of red onion, cut into thin strips
- Six cooked bacon slices, chopped

- One-third cup of roasted sunflower seeds
- Salt and pepper

Directions:

Tamari vinaigrette

1. In a small jar, put the olive oil, rice vinegar, tamari sauce and old-fashioned mustard.
2. Add in some pepper.
3. Close the lid and shake vigorously.
4. Salad preparation
5. Now place the buckwheat in a medium-sized bowl and cover with at least 2 inches (5 cm) of water.
6. Cover the bowl and let soak in the refrigerator overnight.
7. Drain buckwheat, rinse with cold water and drain again.
8. In a large bowl, put the lettuce, strawberries, fennel, onion, bacon, sunflower seeds and reserved buckwheat.
9. Add in your dressing and mix well.

Nutrition: calories 120, fat 2, fiber 2, carbs 4, protein 5

Sautéed potatoes in chicken broth

Preparation time: 10 minutes

Cooking time: 20 minutes

Servings: 4

Ingredients:

- Six medium-sized potatoes
- One onion
- Chicken broth
- 100ml of water
- One tbsp extra virgin olive oil
- Salt to taste

Directions:

1. First peel the potatoes then slice it across into pieces.
2. Proceed by peeling the onions and chop into small pieces.
3. Fry minced onion pieces in oil for five minutes.
4. Add in the potatoes and cook for another ten minutes while stirring gently.
5. Dilute the chicken broth with water and add to the cooker and cook for five minutes.
6. Add salt to taste and serve.

Nutrition: calories 120, fat 2, fiber 2, carbs 4, protein 5

Baked potatoes and chili con carne

Preparation time: 10 minutes

Cooking time: 20 minutes

Servings: 4

Ingredients:

- 8Big potatoes
- 600g Knife ground beef
- 35cl Beef broth
- 500g Crushed tomatoes
- 500g Canned kidney beans
- 1 tbsp. Tomato puree
- 2 Big onions
- One bunch of chives
- Two garlic cloves
- Half teaspoon Chili powder
- One tbsp. Cumin
- One tbsp. dried oregano
- 2 tbsp. Extra Virgin Olive Oil
- 250g Farm fresh cream
- Salt and pepper to taste

Directions:

1. Peel and chop the onions and garlic.

2. Heat the broth in a saucepan.
3. Heat the oil available in the frying pan to fry the onions and garlic for five minutes while mixing.
4. Add the meat and allow to cook for five minutes over high heat.
5. Add salt and pepper.
6. Pour the tomatoes and the tomato puree, then the broth.
7. Add the cumin, oregano and chili and then mix.
8. Cover and simmer 45 minutes.
9. Add the beans, cover and continue cooking over low heat, 20 min.
10. Preheat the oven to 180 ° C
11. Wash the potatoes. Once done, wrap them together in aluminum foil and bake for 30 to 35 minutes.
12. Remove the paper, cut the potatoes in half and scoop it out slightly to garnish with chili.
13. Top each potato with a spoonful of cream
14. Serve hot.

Nutrition: calories 120, fat 2, fiber 2, carbs 4, protein 5

Chicken in pepper sauce

Preparation time: 10 minutes

Cooking time: 20 minutes

Servings: 4

Ingredients:

- One jar of 340 ml roasted peppers
- One cup (250 mL) canned coconut milk
- Fifteen ml red wine vinegar
- Two cloves of garlic
- One tsp. paprika
- One tsp. dried oregano
- One tsp. salt

- One-quarter cup of chopped fresh parsley, chopped
- One tbsp extra virgin olive oil
- Four boneless skinless chicken breasts or thighs
- Salt and pepper
- One minced onion
- One red bell pepper (minced)
- One-quarter cup of chopped fresh parsley, for garnish

Directions:

1. In a blender, mix all the ingredients for the sauce (everything above except chicken, olive oil, onions, salt and pepper) until you get a mixture of smooth consistency.
2. Place a rack at the center of your oven and preheat to 400 ° F.
3. In your large non-stick skillet (you can use a cast iron), heat the olive oil over high heat and fry the chicken breasts.
4. Generously season with salt and pepper.
5. Give it time by allowing all the sides of the chicken to fry for at least three minutes and then set aside on a plate.
6. Lower the heat level back to medium then add the onions and allow to heat for six minutes over medium heat, stirring often.
7. Add the red pepper and cook for another minute only.
8. Return the chicken to the pan and sprinkle with the roasted pepper sauce.
9. Bake the dish for fifteen minutes.
10. Before serving, remove from the oven and grace it by adding some parsley.
11. Serve with pasta in olive oil and chives or white rice.

Nutrition: calories 120, fat 2, fiber 2, carbs 4, protein 5

Waldorf salad

Preparation time: 10 minutes

Cooking time: 20 minutes

Servings: 4

Ingredients:

- One hundred and twenty-five grams of mayonnaise
- Two tablespoons white vinegar
- One apple, peeled and cut into pieces
- One celery stalk, diced
- One hundred and twenty-five grams of grapes
- One hundred and twenty-five grams of chopped walnuts
- Salt and pepper to taste

Directions:

1. In a large bowl, whisk the mayonnaise and vinegar.
2. Add the apple, celery, raisins and walnuts.
3. Sprinkle in salt and pepper. Mix everything and serve fresh.

Nutrition: calories 120, fat 2, fiber 2, carbs 4, protein 5

Whole wheat pita

Preparation time: 10 minutes

Cooking time: 20 minutes

Servings: 4

Ingredients:

- 250g of whole wheat flour
- 2 tbsp extra virgin olive oil
- 5g salt
- 10g dry baker's yeast
- One hundred and fifty-ml hot water

Directions:

1. Add the whole flour and the salt in a bowl and stir.
2. Then add the rest of the ingredients: oil, yeast and water.
3. Stir thoroughly to mix.
4. Mix all the ingredients well until the pita bread dough is formed.
5. Knead the dough for a few minutes on the table.
6. If the dough seems to be too dry, you can add a little more water.
7. Once kneaded, make the dough into a ball and put it in a bowl.
8. Have it covered and let it be there for two hours.
9. Take out the whole pita bread dough and knead again.
10. Work the dough into balls of about 80g each.
11. Use a roller to make the dough well-rounded.
12. Make the pieces of bread ten-to-twelve cm wide and One cm thick.
13. Put the pitas on a tray.
14. Preheat the oven to 200 ° C, slot in the tray and let the pieces of bread bake for ten minutes, depending on the oven.
15. Finally, take out the pieces of bread, let them cool a little and serve!

Nutrition: calories 120, fat 2, fiber 2, carbs 4, protein 5

Scrambled tofu with mushrooms (vegan)

Preparation time: 10 minutes

Cooking time: 20 minutes

Servings: 4

Ingredients:

- One hundred and twenty-five grams of plain firm tofu
- 100g silky tofu
- One tbsp. fresh cream
- One tbsp. sesame puree
- One tsp. Mustard
- ½ tsp. ground turmeric
- Four sprigs of fresh chives
- Half onion (optional)
- One garlic clove (optional)
- 50g mushrooms
- 2 tbsp. Extra Virgin Olive Oil
- One tbsp. Tamari soy sauce (gluten-free, organic soy sauce)
- Salt and pepper to taste

Directions:

1. In a bowl, crush the firm tofu, add in the silky tofu, cream, tahini, mustard, turmeric and chopped chives.
2. Mix thoroughly and add salt and pepper to taste.
3. Peel and chop the onion and the garlic.
4. Rinse the mushrooms under a stream of water.
5. Cut off the ends of the stalks and cut the mushrooms into strips.
6. Gently fry the mushrooms, onionsand garlic over medium-high heat in a pan with a little olive oil.
7. Once the mushrooms, onionsand garlic are very tender and slightly brown in color, add the mixture to the tofu and cook over medium heat for about 5 minutes.
8. Stir the mixture continuously with a spatula.
9. Serve hotand enjoy.

Nutrition: calories 120, fat 2, fiber 2, carbs 4, protein 5

Pasta with smoked salmon and arugula

Preparation time: 10 minutes

Cooking time: 20 minutes

Servings: 4

Ingredients:

- 250g Spaghetti
- One hundred and fifty grams of Smoked salmon
- One bunch of arugula
- 2 tbsp. Extra virgin olive oil
- One finely chopped onion
- Salt and pepper to taste

Directions:

1. Cook the pasta in boiling water for ten minutes.
2. Add salt to taste.
3. Slice the smoked salmon into strips.
4. Rinse and wring the arugula.
5. Heat One tablespoonful of extra virgin olive oil in a frying pan and chop the onion.
6. Add in the drained spaghetti, the salmon strips and the arugula.
7. Mix well and cook for 2 min.
8. Sprinkle in the rest of the olive oil, salt and pepper.
9. Mix and serve hot.

Nutrition: calories 120, fat 2, fiber 2, carbs 4, protein 5

Sirtfood Chicken Breasts

Preparation time: 10 minutes

Cooking time: 20 minutes

Servings: 4

Ingredients:

- Chicken breasts, 5 oz
- Chopped Kale, 1 cup
- Red Onion, sliced, ½ cup
- Buckwheat, 1 cup
- Fresh ginger, chopped, 1 tsp
- Olive Oil, extra virgin, 1 tbsp
- Turmeric, ground, 2 tsp
- ¼ lemon, juiced
- Salsa
- Tomato, chopped, 1 cup
- 1 chopped bird's eye's chili
- Capers, finely chopped, 1 tbsp
- Parsley, finely chopped, 1 tsp
- ¼ lemon, juiced

Directions:

1. Chop the tomato while making sure not to squish it and preserve the maximum liquid in the process.
2. Add the lemon juice, parsley, capers and chili.
3. Pop everything into a blender and you're done!
4. Heat your oven to 220 °C.
5. While your oven is heating, marinate the chicken with turmeric, olive oil and the lemon juice up to 15 minutes.
6. Cook in an ovenproof pan on each side until the chicken turns pale golden.
7. Transfer to the oven and bake for 10 minutes, cover with foil and cook for another five minutes.
8. While your chicken is baking, steam the kale for five minutes, adding red onions, ginger and little oil.
9. Mix and fry for up to five minutes.
10. To make the second side dish, cook buckwheat with turmeric according to instructions on the package and serve all together.

Nutrition: calories 120, fat 2, fiber 2, carbs 4, protein 5

Turkey With Sirtfood Vegetables

This recipe is highly adjustable and it's based on combining turkey as the main dish with healthy side-dishes made of vegetables. It's extremely simple and convenient, as meats go great with any and all Sirt spices and vegetables. With that in mind, feel free to adjust or replace any ingredient in this recipe with an equal amount of the ingredients you prefer or like better.

Preparation time: 10 minutes

Cooking time: 20 minutes

Servings: 4

Ingredients:

- Lean turkey meat, 150 g
- 1 finely chopped garlic clove
- 1 finely chopped red onion
- 1 finely chopped bird's eye chili/replace with chopped red bell paprika or ½ squeezed citrus fruit if you don't like spicy foods
- 1 tsp of finely chopped ginger
- Extra virgin olive oil, 2 tbsp
- Ground turmeric, 1 tbsp
- ½ cup of dried tomatoes
- Parsley, 10 g
- Sage, dried, 1 tsp
- ½ juiced lime or lemon
- Capers, 1 tbsp

Directions:

1. Chop the cauliflower.
2. Fry with chopped ginger, chili, red onion and garlic in 1 tbsp olive oil until they're soft.
3. Add cauliflower and turmeric and cook for a couple of minutes until the cauliflower becomes soft.
4. Once the dish is done, add dried tomatoes and parsley.
5. Coat your turkey in a thin layer of olive oil and sage.
6. Fry for about five minutes and then add the capers and lime juice to the mix.
7. Add half a cup of water and bring to a boil.

Nutrition: calories 120, fat 2, fiber 2, carbs 4, protein 5

Sirtfood Beans With Beef

Preparation time: 10 minutes

Cooking time: 20 minutes

Servings: 4

Ingredients:

- Kidney beans, 2 small cans
- Lean beef, minced, 400 g
- Buckwheat, 160 g
- 1 finely chopped red onion
- 1 chopped red bell pepper
- Two finely chopped bird's eye chili peppers
- Canned tomatoes, 800 g
- Ground turmeric, 1 tbsp
- Tomato sauce, 1 tbsp
- Cocoa powder, 1 tbsp
- Ground cumin, 1 tbsp
- Extra virgin olive oil, 1 tbsp
- Red wine, 150 ml
- Chopped coriander, ½ tbsp.
- Chopped parsley, ½ tbsp.

Directions:

1. Fry the onions, chili peppers and garlic for three minutes over medium heat.

2. Throw in the spices and mince for another minute.
3. After that, add the beef and red wine.
4. Bring to a boil and let it bubble until the liquid reduces by a half.
5. Add the cocoa powder, tomatoes, tomato sauce and the red bell pepper.
6. Add more water if needed and let the dish simmer on low medium heat for an hour.
7. Add the remaining chopped herbs before serving.

Nutrition: calories 120, fat 2, fiber 2, carbs 4, protein 5

Chicken and Kale Buckwheat Noodles

This tasty dish will take no more than 30 minutes to prepare, prep time included.

Preparation time: 10 minutes

Cooking time: 20 minutes

Servings: 4

Ingredients:

For noodles

- Finely chopped kale, 2 cups
- Buckwheat noodles, 5 oz
- Shiitake mushrooms (or any other of your choosing), four pieces
- Extra virgin olive oil, 1 tsp
- 1 finely diced red onion
- 1 diced chicken breast
- 1 sliced bird's eye chili
- Soy sauce, 3 tbsp

Salad dressing

- Soy sauce, ¼ cup
- Tamari sauce, 1 tbsp
- Sesame oil, 1 tbsp

- Lemon juice, 1 tbsp

Directions:

1. Boil or stir-fry chicken for up to 15 minutes.
2. Microwave kale up to three minutes to preserve nutrients.
3. Cook buckwheat noodles and rinse and add kale once they're done.
4. Fry the mushrooms with 1 tsp of olive oil up to three minutes and season with a pinch of salt.
5. Set aside and use the same pan, adding more olive oil, to sauté peppers and chickpeas up to five minutes.
6. Add garlic, water and tamari sauce and cook for another three minutes.
7. Add kale with noodles, chickenand dressing.
8. Mix all together and serve.

Nutrition: calories 120, fat 2, fiber 2, carbs 4, protein 5

Sirtfood Lamb

Preparation time: 10 minutes

Cooking time: 20 minutes

Servings: 4

Ingredients:

- Extra virgin olive oil, 2 tbsp
- Grated ginger, one inch
- 1 sliced red onion.
- 1 tsp of bird's eye
- Cumin seeds, 2 tsp
- 1 cinnamon stick
- Lamb, 800 g
- Garlic cloves, crushed, 3 pieces
- A pinch of salt
- Chopped Medjool dates, 1 cup
- Chickpeas, 400 g

- Coriander, 2 tbsp
- Buckwheat

Directions:

1. Start by preheating your oven to 140 °C.
2. Sauté sliced onion with 2 tbsp of extra virgin olive oil for five minutes while keeping the lid on.
3. The onions should turn soft but not brown.
4. Add turmeric, cumin, ginger, garlic and chili and stir fry for another minute.
5. Add the chunks of lamb, season with salt and letand let boil.
6. Add a glass of water.
7. After the mixture has boiled, roast in the oven for one hour and 15 minutes.
8. Add the chickpeas half an hour before the dish is finished.
9. Add chopped coriander and serve with buckwheat after the meal is done.

Nutrition: calories 120, fat 2, fiber 2, carbs 4, protein 5

Fish With Mango and Turmeric

Preparation time: 10 minutes

Cooking time: 20 minutes

Servings: 4

Ingredients:

- A fresh 1 ¼ lbs piece of fish of your choosing
- ½ cup of coconut oil
- A pinch of sea salt
- 1 tbsp of high-quality red wine
- ¼ cup olive oil
- ½ tbsp minced ginger
- Scallion, 2 cups
- Dill, 2 cups
- 1 ripe mango

- 1 squeezed lemon
- 1 garlic clove
- Dry red pepper, 1 tsp
- Fresh cilantro
- Walnuts

Directions:

1. Marinate the fish and leave overnight
2. Blend the ingredients for mango dipping sauce
3. Fry the fish in 2 tbsp in coconut oil on medium heat and add a pinch of salt after five minutes.
4. Turn to the other side and fry for another couple of minutes.
5. Keep the remaining oil in the pan.
6. Add scallions and dill and turn off the heat.
7. Heat for about 15 seconds and season with a pinch of salt.
8. Top the fish with the infused oil, dilland scallion and serve with the mango sauce, nuts, limeand cilantro.

Nutrition: calories 120, fat 2, fiber 2, carbs 4, protein 5

Sirtfood Shrimp Noodles

Preparation time: 10 minutes

Cooking time: 20 minutes

Servings: 4

Ingredients:

- Shrimps, deveined 1/3 lb.
- Soy sauce, 2 tsp
- Extra virgin olive oil, 2 tsp
- Buckwheat noodles, 3oz
- 2 finely chopped garlic cloves
- 1 bird's eye chili, finely chopped
- Chopped fresh ginger, 1 tsp
- Chopped red onion, ¼

- Chopped celery with eaves, ½ cup
- Chopped green beans, ½ cup
- Chopped kale, 1 cup
- Chicken stock, ½ cup

Directions:

1. Cook the shrimps in 1 tsp of the soy sauce and one tsp of the oil up to three minutes on high heat.
2. Cook buckwheat noodles for up to eight minutes and drain.
3. Fry the remaining ingredients in a pan on medium heat for up to three minutes.
4. Add the chicken stock, bring to a boiland cook until the veggies are cooked, but still look fresh.
5. Add the shrimps and noodles, bring to a boiland you're done!

Nutrition: calories 120, fat 2, fiber 2, carbs 4, protein 5

Sirtfood Miso Salmon

Preparation time: 10 minutes

Cooking time: 20 minutes

Servings: 4

Ingredients:

- Miso, ½ cup
- Organic red wine, 1 tbsp
- Extra virgin olive oil, 1 tbsp
- Salmon, 7 oz
- 1 sliced red onion
- Celery, sliced, 1 cup
- 2 finely chopped garlic cloves
- 1 finely chopped bird's eye chili
- Ground turmeric, 1 tsp
- Freshly chopped ginger, 1 tsp
- Green beans, 1 cup
- Kale, finely chopped, 1 cup
- Sesame seeds. 1 tsp

- Soy sauce, 1 tbsp
- Buckwheat, 2 tbsp

Directions:

1. Marinate the salmon in the mix of red wine, 1 tsp of extra virgin olive oiland miso for 30 minutes.
2. Preheat your oven to 420 °F and bake the fish for ten minutes.
3. Fry the onions, chili, garlic, green beans, ginger, kaleand celery for a few minutes until it's cooked.
4. Insert the soy sauce, parsley and sesame seeds.
5. Cook buckwheat per instructions and mix in with the stir-fry.
6. Enjoy!

Nutrition: calories 120, fat 2, fiber 2, carbs 4, protein 5

Sirtfood Shrimps With Buckwheat Noodles

Preparation time: 10 minutes

Cooking time: 20 minutes

Servings: 4

Ingredients:

- Shrimps (or a piece of fish of your choosing), 4 oz
- Tamari, 2 tbsp
- Extra virgin olive oil, 2 tbsp
- Buckwheat noodles, 75 g
- 1 finely chopped bird's eye chili
- 1 finely chopped garlic clove
- Fresh ginger, chopped, 1 tsp
- 1 sliced red onion
- Sliced red celery, ½ cup
- Chopped green beans, 1 cup
- Chopped kale, 1 cup
- Chicken stock, 1 cup

- Celery, 1 tsp

Directions:

1. Cook the shrimps for three minutes on high heat and with 1 tsp of tamari and 1 tsp of extra virgin olive oil.
2. Set aside.
3. Cook the noodles for up to eight minutes and set aside.
4. Fry kale, beans, celeryand onion, ginger, chiliand garlic in oil for up to three minutes.
5. Add vegetable stock and simmer for two minutes.
6. Mix all together, bring to a boiland serve.

Sirtfood Shellfish Salad

Preparation time: 10 minutes

Cooking time: 20 minutes

Servings: 4

Ingredients:

- Tomato sauce, 1 tsp
- Cloves, ¼ tsp
- Coriander, chopped, 1 tbsp
- Parsley, chopped, 1 tbsp
- Lemon juice, 1 tbsp (½ of a lemon)
- Kale, chopped, 1 cup
- Spinach, chopped, 1 cup
- Sea fruit of your choosing (shrimps, prawns, or clamps), 1 cup
- Chopped firm tofu, 1 thick slice (approx. 4 oz)
- Buckwheat noodles, 1 cup
- Pecan nuts, ½ cup
- Chopped ginger, ½ cup
- Miso paste, 1 tbsp
- Carrots, ½ cup
- Chicken stock, 100 ml

Directions:

1. Simmer tomato sauce with lemon juice, chicken stock, coriander, parsley and shrimps/cloves/clams for 10 minutes on medium heat.
2. Add the remaining ingredients without the ginger and miso and stir-fry until the shellfish is cooked through.
3. Add the remaining seasonings and you're done!

Nutrition: calories 120, fat 2, fiber 2, carbs 4, protein 5

Coq Au Vin

Preparation time: 15 minutes

Cooking time: 1 hour 15 minutes

Servings: 8

Ingredients:

- 450g button mushrooms
- 100g streaky bacon, chopped
- 16 chicken thighs, skin removed
- 3 cloves of garlic, crushed
- 3g fresh parsley, chopped
- 3 carrots, chopped
- 2 red onions, chopped
- 2 tablespoons plain flour
- 2 teaspoons olive oil
- 750mls red wine
- 1 bouquet garnish

Directions:

1. Place the flour on a large plate and coat the chicken in it.
2. Heat the olive oil in a large saucepan, add the chicken and brown it, before setting aside.
3. Fry the bacon in the pan then add the onion and cook for 5 minutes.

4. Pour in the red wine and add the chicken, carrots, bouquet garnish and garlic.
5. Transfer it to a large ovenproof dish.
6. Cook in the oven at 180C/360F for 1 hour.
7. Remove the bouquet garnish and skim off any excess fat, if necessary.
8. Add in the mushrooms and cook for 15 minutes.
9. Stir in the parsley just before serving.

Nutrition:

Calories: 459

Net carbs: 66g

Fat: 1g

Fiber: 4g8g

Protein:

Moroccan Chicken Casserole

Preparation time: 20 minutes

Cooking time: 50 minutes

Servings: 4

Ingredients:

- 4 chicken breasts, cubed
- 250g tinned chickpeas (garbanzo beans) drained
- 4 medjool dates, halved
- 6 dried apricots, halved
- 1 red onion, sliced 1 carrot, chopped
- 1 teaspoon ground cumin
- 1 teaspoon ground cinnamon
- 1 teaspoon ground turmeric
- 1 bird's-eye chili, chopped
- 600mls chicken stock
- 25g corn flour 60mls water
- 2 teaspoons fresh coriander

Directions:

1. Place the chicken, chickpeas (garbanzo beans), onion, carrot, chili, cumin, turmeric, cinnamon and stock (broth) into a large saucepan.
2. In a cup, mix the corn flour together with the water until it becomes a smooth paste.
3. Pour the mixture into the saucepan and stir until it thickens.
4. Add in the coriander (cilantro) and mix well.
5. Serve with buckwheat or couscous.

Nutrition: Calories: 401 Net carbs: 3.6g
Fat: 4.8g Fiber: 1.7g Protein: 29.2g

Prawn and Coconut Curry

Preparation time: 10 minutes

Cooking time: 5 minutes

Servings: 4

Ingredients:

- 400g tinned chopped tomatoes
- 400g large prawns (shrimps), shelled and raw
- 25g fresh coriander (cilantro) chopped
- 3 red onions, finely chopped
- 3 cloves of garlic, crushed
- 2 bird's eye chilies
- ½ teaspoon ground coriander (cilantro)
- ½ teaspoon turmeric
- 400mls (14fl Oz) coconut milk
- 1 teaspoons olive oil
- Juice of 1 lime

Directions:

1. Place the onions, garlic, tomatoes, chilies, lime juice, turmeric, ground coriander (cilantro), chilies and half of the

fresh coriander (cilantro) into a blender and blitz until you have a smooth curry paste.

2. Heat the olive oil in a frying pan, add the paste and cook for 2 minutes.
3. Stir in the coconut milk and warm it thoroughly.
4. Add the prawns (shrimps) to the paste and cook them until they have turned pink and are completely cooked.
5. Stir in the fresh coriander (cilantro).
6. Serve with rice.

Nutrition: Calories: 322 Net carbs: 98.9g

Fat: 11.8g Fiber: 8g Protein: 15.6g

Chicken and Bean Casserole

Preparation time: 15 minutes

Cooking time: 55 minutes

Servings: 4

Ingredients:

- 400g chopped tomatoes
- 400g tinned cannellini beans or haricot beans
- 8 chicken thighs, skin removed
- 2 carrots, peeled and finely chopped
- 2 red onions, chopped
- 4 sticks of celery
- 4 large mushrooms
- 2 red peppers (bell peppers), de-seeded and chopped
- 1 clove of garlic
- 2 teaspoons soy sauce
- 1 olive oil
- liters chicken stock (broth)

Directions:

1. Heat the olive oil in a saucepan.

2. Add the garlic and onions and cook for 5 minutes.
3. Add in the chicken.
4. And cook for 5 minutes.
5. Add the carrots, cannellini beans, celery, red peppers (bell peppers) and mushrooms.
6. Pour in the stock (broth) soy sauce and tomatoes.
7. Bring it to the boil, reduce the heat and simmer for 45 minutes.
8. Serve with rice or new potatoes.

Nutrition: Calories: 509 Net carbs: 12.5g

Fat: 6.5g Fiber: 1.1g Protein: 27.4g

Mussels in Red Wine Sauce

Preparation time: 5 minutes

Cooking time: 5 minutes

Servings: 2

Ingredients:

- 800g mussels
- 2 x 400g tins of chopped tomatoes
- 25g butter
- 1 fresh chives, chopped
- 1 fresh parsley, chopped
- 1 bird's-eye chili, finely chopped
- 4 cloves of garlic, crushed
- 400mls red wine
- Juice of 1 lemon

Directions:

1. Wash the mussels, remove their beards and set them aside.
2. Heat the butter in a large saucepan and add in the red wine.
3. Reduce the heat and add the parsley, chives, chili and garlic whilst stirring.
4. Add in the tomatoes, lemon juice and mussels.

5. Cover the saucepan and cook for 2-3.
6. Remove the saucepan from the heat and take out any mussels which haven't opened and discard them.
7. Serve and eat immediately.

Nutrition:

Calories: 364

Net carbs: 3.3g Fat: 4.9g Fiber: 0.7g

Protein: 8.2g

Roast Balsamic Vegetables

Preparation time: 10 minutes

Cooking time: 45 minutes

Servings: 4

Ingredients:

- 4 tomatoes, chopped 2 red onions, chopped
- 3 sweet potatoes, peeled and chopped
- 100g red chicory (or if unavailable, use yellow)
- 100g kale, finely chopped
- 300g potatoes, peeled and chopped
- 5 stalks of celery, chopped
- 1 bird's-eye chili, de-seeded and finely chopped
- 2g fresh parsley, chopped
- 2gs fresh coriander (cilantro) chopped
- 3 teaspoons olive oil
- 2 teaspoons balsamic vinegar
- 1 teaspoon mustard Sea salt
- Freshly ground black pepper

Directions:

1. Place the olive oil, balsamic, mustard, parsley and coriander (cilantro) into a bowl.
2. Mix well.

3. Toss all the remaining ingredients into the dressing.
4. Season with salt and pepper.
5. Transfer the vegetables to an ovenproof dish
6. And cook in the oven at 200C/400F for 45 minutes.

Nutrition: Calories: 310 Net carbs: 1.1g

Fiber: 0.2g Protein: 0.2g

Tomato and Goat's Pizza

Preparation time: 15 minutes

Cooking time: 20 minutes

Servings: 2

Ingredients:

- 225g buckwheat flour
- 2 teaspoons dried yeast Pinch of salt
- 150mls slightly water 1 teaspoon olive oil
- For the Topping:
- 75g feta cheese, crumbled
- 75g peseta (or tomato paste)
- 1 tomato, sliced 1 red onion, finely chopped
- 25g rocket (arugula) leaves, chopped

Directions:

1. In a bowl, combine all the ingredients for the pizza dough then allow it to stand for at least an hour until it has doubled in size.
2. Roll the dough out to a size to suit you.
3. Spoon the passata onto the base and add the rest of the toppings.
4. Bake in the oven at 200C/400F for 15-20 minutes or until browned at the edges and crispy and serve.

Nutrition:

Calories: 585 Net carbs: 77g Fat: 8.1g Fiber: 7.6g Protein: 22.9g

Tender Spiced Lamb

Preparation time: 20 minutes

Cooking time: 4 hours 20 minutes

Servings: 8

Ingredients:

- 1.35kg lamb shoulder
- 3 red onions, sliced
- 3 cloves of garlic, crushed
- 1 bird's eye chili, finely chopped
- 1 teaspoon turmeric
- 1 teaspoon ground cumin
- ½ teaspoon ground coriander (cilantro)
- ¼ teaspoon ground cinnamon
- 2 tablespoons olive oil

Directions:

1. In a bowl, combine the chili, garlic and spices with olive oil.
2. Coat the lamb with the spice mixture and marinate it for an hour, or overnight if you can.
3. Heat the remaining oil in a pan, add the lamb and brown it for 3-4 minutes on all sides to seal it.
4. Place the lamb in an ovenproof dish.
5. Add in the red onions and cover the dish with foil.
6. Transfer to the oven and roast at 170C/325F for 4 hours.
7. The lamb should be extremely tender and falling off the bone.
8. Serve with rice or couscous, salad or vegetables.

Nutrition:

Calories: 455 Net carbs: 28g

Fat: 9.8g Fiber: 11g Protein: 20g

Chili Cod Fillets

Preparation time: 10 minutes

Cooking time: 10 minutes

Servings: 4

Ingredients:

- 4 cod fillets each)
- 2 teaspoons fresh parsley, chopped
- 2 bird's-eye chilies (or more if you like it hot)
- 2 cloves of garlic, chopped
- 4 teaspoons olive oil

Directions:

1. Heat a of olive oil in a frying pan, add the fish and cook for 7-8 minutes or until thoroughly cooked, turning once halfway through.
2. Remove and keep warm.
3. Pour the remaining olive oil into the pan and add the chili, chopped garlic and parsley.
4. Warm it thoroughly.
5. Serve the fish onto plates and pour the warm chili oil over it.

Nutrition:

Calories: 246 Net carbs: 5.5g

Fat: 0.5g Fiber: 0.7g Protein: 18.5g

Steak and Mushroom Noodles

Preparation time: 10 minutes

Cooking time: 20 minutes

Servings: 4

Ingredients:

- 100g shitake mushrooms, halved, if large
- 100g chestnut mushrooms, sliced
- 150g udon noodles
- 75g kale, finely chopped
- 75g baby leaf spinach, chopped
- 2 sirloin steaks
- 2 teaspoons miso paste
- 2.5cm piece fresh ginger, finely chopped
- 2 teaspoons olive oil
- 1 star anise
- 1 red chili, finely sliced
- 1 red onion, finely chopped
- 1 fresh coriander (cilantro) chopped
- 1 liter (1½ pints) warm water

Directions:

1. Pour the water into a saucepan and add in the miso, star anise and ginger.
2. Bring it to the boil, reduce the heat and simmer gently.
3. In the meantime, cook the noodles according to their instructions then drain them.
4. Heat the oil in a saucepan, add the steak and cook for around 2-3 minutes on each side (or 1-2 minutes, for rare meat).
5. Remove the meat and set aside.
6. Place the mushrooms, spinach, coriander (cilantro) and kale into the miso broth and cook for 5 minutes.
7. In the meantime, heat the remaining oil in a separate pan and fry the chili and onion for 4 minutes, until softened.
8. Serve the noodles into bowls and pour the soup on top.
9. Thinly slice the steaks and add them to the top.
10. Serve immediately.

Nutrition:

Calories: 296

Net carbs: 24.6g

Fat: 13.7g

Fiber: 0.7g

Protein: 32.9g

Masala Scallops

Preparation time: 10 minutes

Cooking time: 20 minutes

Servings: 4

Ingredients:

- 2 tablespoons olive oil
- 2 jalapenos, chopped
- 1 pound sea scallops
- A pinch of salt and black pepper
- ¼ teaspoon cinnamon powder
- 1 teaspoon garam masala
- 1 teaspoon coriander, ground
- 1 teaspoon cumin, ground
- 2 tablespoons cilantro, chopped

Directions:

1. Heat up a pan with the oil over medium heat, add the jalapenos, cinnamon and the other ingredients except the scallops and cook for 10 minutes.
2. Add the rest of the ingredients, toss, cook for 10 minutes more, divide into bowls and serve.

Nutrition:

Calories: 251

Fat: 4g

Fiber: 4g

Carbs: 11g

Protein: 17g

Tuna and Tomatoes

Preparation time: 5 minutes

Cooking time: 20 minutes

Servings: 4

Ingredients:

- 1 yellow onion, chopped
- 1 tablespoon olive oil
- 1 pound tuna fillets, boneless, skinless and cubed
- 1 cup tomatoes, chopped
- 1 red pepper, chopped
- 1 teaspoon sweet paprika
- 1 tablespoon coriander, chopped

Directions:

1. Heat up a pan with the oil over medium heat, add the onions and the pepper and cook for 5 minutes.
2. Add the fish and the other Ingredient, cook everything for 15 minutes, divide between plates and serve.

Nutrition:

Calories: 215

Fat: 4g

Fiber: 7g

Carbs: 14g

Protein: 7g

Lemongrass and Ginger Mackerel

Preparation time: 10 minutes

Cooking time: 25 minutes

Servings: 4

Ingredients:

- 4 mackerel fillets, skinless and boneless
- 2 tablespoons olive oil
- 1 tablespoon ginger, grated
- 2 lemongrass sticks, chopped
- 2 red chilies, chopped
- Juice of 1 lime
- A handful parsley, chopped

Directions:

1. Combine the mackerel with the oil, ginger and the other ingredients
2. Toss and bake at 390 degrees F for 25 minutes.
3. Divide everything between plates and serve.

Nutrition:

Calories: 251

Fat: 3g

Fiber: 4g

Carbs: 14g

Protein: 8g

Instant Savory Gigante Beans

Preparation Time: 10-30 Minutes

Cooking Time: 55 Minutes

Servings: 6

Ingredients:

- 1 lb. Gigante Beans soaked overnight
- 1/2 cup olive oil
- One onion sliced
- Two cloves garlic crushed or minced
- One red bell pepper (cut into 1/3-inch pieces)
- Two carrots, sliced
- 1/2 tsp salt and ground black pepper
- Two tomatoes peeled, grated
- 1 Tbsp celery (chopped)
- 1 tbsp tomato paste (or ketchup)
- 3/4 tsp sweet paprika

- 1 tsp oregano
- 1 cup vegetable broth

Directions:

1. Soak Gigante beans overnight.
2. Press the SAUTÉ button on your Instant Pot and heat the oil.
3. Sauté onion, garlic, sweet pepper, carrots with a pinch of salt for 3 - 4 minutes; stir occasionally.
4. Add rinsed Gigante beans into your Instant Pot along with all remaining ingredients and stir well.
5. Latch lid into place and set on the MANUAL setting for 25 minutes.
6. When the beep sounds, quick release the pressure by pressing Cancel and twisting the steam handle to the Venting position.
7. Taste and adjust seasonings to taste.
8. Serve warm or cold.
9. Keep refrigerated.

Nutrition: Calories 502.45 Calories From Fat 173.16 Total Fat 19.63g Saturated Fat 2.86g

Nettle Soup with Rice

Preparation Time: 10-30 Minutes

Cooking Time: 40 Minutes

Servings: 5

Ingredients:

- 3 Tbsp of olive oil
- Two onions finely chopped
- Two cloves garlic finely chopped
- Salt and freshly ground black pepper
- Four medium potatoes cut into cubes
- 1 cup of rice
- 1 Tbsp arrowroot
- 2 cups vegetable broth

- 2 cups of water
- One bunch of young nettle leaves packed
- 1/2 cup fresh parsley finely chopped
- 1 tsp cumin

Directions:

1. Heat olive oil in a large pot.
2. Sauté onion and garlic with a pinch of salt until softened.
3. Add potato, rice and arrowroot; sauté for 2 to 3 minutes.
4. Pour broth and water, stir well, cover and cook over medium heat for about 20 minutes.
5. Cook for about 30 to 45 minutes.
6. Add young nettle leaves, parsley and cumin; stir and cook for 5 to 7 minutes.
7. Move the soup in a blender and blend until combined well.
8. Taste and adjust salt and pepper.
9. Serve hot.

Nutrition: Calories 421.76 Calories from Fat 88.32 Total Fat 9.8g Saturated Fat 1.54g

Okra with Grated Tomatoes (Slow Cooker)

Preparation Time: 10-30 Minutes

Cooking Time: 3 Hours and 10 Minutes

Servings: 4

Ingredients:

- 2 lbs. fresh okra cleaned
- Two onions finely chopped
- Two cloves garlic finely sliced
- Two carrots sliced
- Two ripe tomatoes grated
- 1 cup of water
- 4 Tbsp olive oil

- Salt and ground black pepper
- 1 tbsp fresh parsley finely chopped

Directions:

1. Add okra in your Crock-Pot: sprinkle with a pinch of salt and pepper.
2. Add in chopped onion, garlic, carrotsand grated tomatoes; stir well.
3. Pour water and oil, season with the salt, pepperand give a good stir.
4. Covering and cook on LOW for 2-4 hours or until tender.
5. Open the lid and add fresh parsley; stir.
6. Taste and adjust salt and pepper.
7. Serve hot.

Nutrition: Calories 223.47 Calories from Fat 123.5 Total Fat 14g Saturated Fat 1.96g,

Powerful Spinach and Mustard Leaves Puree

Preparation Time: 10-30 Minutes

Cooking Time: 50 Minutes

Servings: 4

Ingredients:

- 2 Tbsp almond butter
- One onion finely diced
- 2 Tbsp minced garlic
- 1 tsp salt and black pepper (or to taste)
- 1 lb. mustard leaves cleaned rinsed
- 1 lb. frozen spinach thawed
- 1 tsp coriander
- 1 tsp ground cumin
- 1/2 cup almond milk

Directions:

1. Press the SAUTÉ button on your Instant Pot and heat the almond butter.

2. Sauté onion, garlic and a pinch of salt for 2-3 minutes; stir occasionally.
3. Add spinach and the mustard greens and stir for a minute or two.
4. Season with the salt and pepper, corianderand cumin; give a good stir.
5. Lock lid into place and set on the MANUAL setting for 15 minutes.
6. Use Quick Release - turn the valve from sealing to venting to release the pressure.
7. Move mixture to a blender, add almond milk and blend until smooth.
8. Taste and adjust seasonings.
9. Serve.

Nutrition: Calories 180.53 Calories from Fat 82.69 Total Fat 10g Saturated Fat 0.65g

Quinoa and Rice Stuffed Peppers (Oven-Baked)

Preparation Time: 10-30 Minutes

Cooking Time: 35 Minutes

Servings: 8

Ingredients:

- 3/4 cup long-grain rice
- Eight bell peppers (any color)
- 2 Tbsp olive oil
- One onion finely diced
- Two cloves chopped garlic
- One can (11 oz) crushed tomatoes
- 1 tsp cumin
- 1 tsp coriander
- 4 Tbsp ground walnuts
- 2 cups cooked quinoa
- 4 Tbsp chopped parsley
- Salt and ground black pepper to taste

Directions:

Lara Burns

1. Preheat oven to 400 F/200 C.
2. Boil rice and drain in a colander.
3. Cut the top stem part of the pepper off, remove the remaining pith and seed-sand rinse peppers.
4. Heat oil in a large frying skilletand sauté onion and garlic until soft.
5. Add tomatoes, cumin, ground almonds, salt, pepperand coriander; stir well and simmer for 2 minutes, stirring constantly.
6. Take away from the heat. Combine the rice, quinoaand parsley; stir well.
7. Taste and adjust salt and pepper.
8. Fill the peppers with a mixtureand place peppers cut side-up in a baking dish, drizzle with little oil.
9. Bake for 15 minutes.
10. Serve warm.

Nutrition: Calories 335.69 Calories from Fat 83.63 Total Fat 9.58g Saturated Fat 1.2g

Quinoa and Lentils with Crushed Tomato

Preparation Time: 10-30 Minutes

Cooking Time: 35 Minutes

Servings: 4

Ingredients:

- 4 Tbsp olive oil
- One medium onion, diced
- Two garlic cloves, minced
- Salt and ground black pepper to taste
- One can (15 oz) tomatoes crushed
- 1 cup vegetable broth
- 1/2 cup quinoa, washed and drained
- 1 cup cooked lentils
- 1 tsp chili powder
- 1 tsp cumin

Directions:

1. Heat oil in a pot and sauté the onion and garlic with the pinch of salt until soft.
2. Pour reserved tomatoes and vegetable broth, bring to boiland stir well.
3. Stir in the quinoa, coverand cook for 15 minutes; stir occasionally.
4. Add in lentils, chili powderand cumin; cook for further 5 minutes.
5. Taste and adjust seasonings.
6. Serve immediately.
7. Keep refrigerated in a covered container for 4 - 5 days.

Nutrition: Calories 397.45 Calories from Fat 138.18 Total Fat 15.61g Saturated Fat 2.14g

Silk Tofu Penne with Spinach

Preparation Time: 10-30 Minutes

Cooking Time: 25 Minutes

Servings: 4

Ingredients:

- 1 lb. penne, uncooked
- 12 oz of frozen spinach, thawed
- 1 cup silken tofu mashed
- 1/2 cup soy milk (unsweetened)
- 1/2 cup vegetable broth
- 1 Tbsp white wine vinegar
- 1/2 tsp Italian seasoning
- Salt and ground pepper to taste

Directions:

1. Cook penne pasta; rinse and drain in a colander.
2. Drain spinach well.
3. Place spinach with all remaining ingredients in a blender and beat until smooth.
4. Pour the spinach mixture over pasta.

194

5. Taste and adjust the salt and pepper.
6. Store pasta in a sealed container in the refrigerator for 3 to 5 days.

Nutrition: Calories 492.8 Calories from Fat 27.06 Total Fat 3.07g, Saturated Fat 0.38g

Slow-Cooked Butter Beans, Okra and Potatoes Stew

Preparation Time: 10-30 Minutes

Cooking Time: 6 Hours and 5 Minutes

Servings: 6

Ingredients:

- 2 cups frozen butter (Lima) beans, thawed
- 1 cup frozen okra, thawed
- Two large russet potatoes cut into cubes
- One can (6 oz) whole-kernel corn, drained
- One large carrot sliced
- One green bell pepper finely chopped
- 1 cup green peas
- 1/2 cup chopped celery
- One medium onion finely chopped
- 2 cups vegetable broth
- Two cans (6 oz) tomato sauce
- 1 cup of water
- 1/2 tsp salt and newly ground black pepper

Directions:

1. Combine the real ingredients in your Slow Cooker; give a good stir.
2. Cover and cook on HIGH for 5 to 6 hours.
3. Taste adjust seasonings and serve hot.

Nutrition: Calories 241.71 Calories from Fat 11.22 Total Fat 1.28g Saturated Fat 0.27g

Soya Minced Stuffed Eggplants

Preparation Time: 10-30 Minutes

Cooking Time: 1 Hour

Servings: 4

Ingredients:

- Two eggplants
- 1/3 cup sesame oil
- One onion finely chopped
- Two garlic cloves minced
- 1 lb. soya mince* see note
- Salt and ground black pepper
- 1/3 cup almond milk
- 2 Tbsp fresh parsley, chopped
- 1/3 cup fresh basil chopped
- 1 tsp fennel powder
- 1 cup of water
- 4 tbsp tomato paste (fresh or canned)

Directions:

1. Rinse and slice the eggplant in half lengthwise.
2. Submerge sliced eggplant into a container with salted water.
3. Soak soya mince in water for 10 to 15 minutes.
4. Preheat oven to 400 F.
5. Rinse eggplant and dry with a clean towel.
6. Heat oil in a large frying skillet, sauté onion and garlic with a pinch of salt until softened.
7. Add drained soya mince and cook over medium heat until cooked through.
8. Add all remaining ingredients (except water and tomato paste) and cook for a further 5 minutes; remove from heat.
9. Scoop out the seed part of each eggplant.
10. Spoon in the filling and arrange stuffed eggplants onto the large baking dish.

11. Dissolve tomato paste into the water and pour evenly over eggplants.
12. Bake for 20 to 25 minutes.
13. Serve warm.

Nutrition: Calories 287.32 Calories from Fat 141.77 Total Fat 16.42g Saturated Fat 2.02g

Red Bean Fricassee

Preparation Time: 10-30 Minutes

Cooking Time: 40 Minutes

Servings: 4

Ingredients:

- 4 Tbsp olive oil
- One onion finely sliced
- Two cloves garlic finely sliced
- Salt and newly ground black pepper
- One can (15 oz) red beans
- One large carrot grated
- 1 1/2 cup vegetable broth
- 1 cup of water
- One can (6 oz) tomato paste
- 1 tsp ground paprika
- 1 tsp parsley

Directions:

1. Heat oil in a large pot and sauté onion and garlic with a pinch of salt until soft.
2. Add red beans together with all remaining ingredients and stir well.
3. In a separate pan, sauté onion and garlic in the olive oil.
4. Reduce heat to medium and boil for 25 to 30 minutes.
5. Taste and adjust salt and pepper if needed.
6. Serve hot.

Broccoli Stir-Fry with Sesame Seeds

Preparation Time: 10 Minutes

Cooking Time: 8 Minutes

Servings: 4

Ingredients:

- Two tablespoons extra-virgin olive oil (optional)
- One tablespoon grated fresh ginger
- 4 cups broccoli florets
- ¼teaspoon sea salt (optional)
- Two garlic cloves, minced
- Two tablespoons toasted sesame seeds

Directions:

1. Heat the olive oil (if desired) in a large nonstick.
2. Skillet over medium-high heat until shimmering.
3. Fold in the ginger, broccoliand sea salt (if desired).
4. Snd stir-fry for 5 to 7 minutes, or until the broccoli is browned.
5. Cook the garlic until tender, about 30 seconds.
6. Sprinkle with the sesame seeds and serve warm.

Nutrition: calories: 135 fat: 10.9g carbs: 9.7g protein: 4.1g fiber: 3.3g

The Bell Pepper Fiesta

Preparation Time: 10 minutes

Cooking Time: 0 minutes

Servings: 4

Ingredients:

- 2 tablespoons dill, chopped
- 1 yellow onion, chopped

- 1 pound multicolored peppers, cut, halved, seeded and cut into thin strips
- 3 tablespoons organic olive oil
- 2 ½ tablespoons white wine vinegar
- Black pepper to taste

Directions:

1. Take a bowl and mix in sweet pepper, onion, dill, pepper, oil, vinegar.
2. And toss well.
3. Divide between bowls and serve.
4. Enjoy!

Nutrition:

Calories: 120

Fat: 3g

Carbohydrates: 1g

Protein: 6g

Dal with Kale, Red Onions and Buckwheat

Preparation Time: 5 Minutes

Cooking Time: 20 Minutes

Servings: 2

Ingredients:

- 1 teaspoon of extra virgin olive oil
- 1 teaspoon of mustard seeds
- 40g red onions, finely chopped
- 1 clove of garlic, very finely chopped
- 1 teaspoon very finely chopped ginger
- 1 Thai chili, very finely chopped
- 1 teaspoon curry mixture
- 2 teaspoons turmeric
- 300ml vegetable broth
- 40g red lentils
- 50g kale, chopped
- 50ml coconut milk
- 50g buckwheat

Directions:

1. Heat oil in a pan
2. Add the curry powder and 1 teaspoon of turmeric, mix well.
3. Add the vegetable stock, bring to the boil.
4. Add the lentils and cook them for 25 to 30 minutes until they are ready.
5. Then add the kale and coconut milk and simmer for 5 minutes. The Dal is ready.

Nutrition:

- Calories: 289 Cal
- Fat: 18 g
- Carbs: 28 g
- Protein: 13 g
- Fiber: 10 g

Spiced Up Pumpkin Seeds Bowls

Preparation Time: 10 minutes

Cooking Time: 20 minutes

Servings: 4

Ingredients:

- ½ tablespoon chili powder
- ½ teaspoon cayenne
- 2 cups pumpkin seeds
- 2 teaspoons lime juice

Directions:

1. Spread pumpkin seeds over lined baking sheet; add lime juice, cayenne and chili powder.
2. Toss well.
3. Pre-heat your oven to 275 degrees F.
4. Roast in your oven for 20 minutes and transfer to small bowls.
5. Serve and enjoy!

Nutrition:

Calories: 170

Fat: 3g

Carbohydrates: 10g

Protein: 6g

Chicken Salad

Preparation Time: 5 Minutes

Cooking Time: 30 Minutes

Servings: 2

Ingredients:

- ½ red onion, very finely sliced
- 1 tablespoon of sesame seeds
- 150g of cooked chicken-shredded
- Large handful 20g of parsley-chopped
- 100g of baby kale-chopped roughly
- 2 teaspoons of soy sauce
- 1 teaspoon of clear honey
- 1 teaspoon of sesame oil

Directions:

1. Place a frying pan over medium heat.
2. Mix the sesame oil, honey, olive oil, lime juiceand soy sauce to make the dressing.
3. Place the cucumber, red onion, kale, pak choiand parsley in a large bowl and gently mix.
4. Pour the dressing over and mix again.

Nutrition:

Calories: 300 Cal

Fat: 10 g

Carbs: 15 g

Protein: 8 g

Fiber: 0.5 g

Tuna, Egg & Caper Salad

Preparation Time: 5 Minutes

Cooking Time: 20 Minutes

Servings: 2

Ingredients:

- 100g 3½oz red chicory or yellow if not available
- 150g 5oz tinned tuna flakes in brine, drained
- 100g 3 ½ oz. cucumber
- 25g 1oz rocket arugula
- 6 pitted black olives
- 2 hard-boiled eggs, peeled and quartered
- 2 tomatoes, chopped
- 2 tablespoons fresh parsley, chopped
- 1 red onion, chopped
- 1 stalk of celery
- 1 tablespoon capers
- 2 tablespoons garlic vinaigrette see recipe
- 340 calories per serving

Directions:

1. Place the tuna, cucumber, olives, tomatoes, onion, chicory, celeryand parsley and rocket arugula into a bowl.
2. Serve onto plates and scatter the eggs and capers on top.

Nutrition:

Calories: 310 Cal

Fat: 15 g

Carbs: 14 g

Protein: 0 g

Fiber: 10 g

Mussels in Red Wine Sauce

Preparation Time: 5 Minutes

Cooking Time: 50 Minutes

Servings: 2

Ingredients:

- 800g 2lb mussels
- 2 x 400g 14 oz. tins of chopped tomatoes
- 25g 1oz butter
- 1 tablespoon fresh chives, chopped
- 1 tablespoon fresh parsley, chopped
- 1 bird's-eye chili, finely chopped
- 4 cloves of garlic, crushed
- 400 ml 14fl. oz. red wine
- Juice of 1 lemon

Directions:

1. Heat the butter in a large saucepan and add in the red wine.
2. Reduce the heat and add the parsley, chives, chili and garlic whilst stirring.
3. Add in the tomatoes, lemon juice and mussels.
4. Cover the saucepan and cook for 2-3 minutes.
5. Serve.

Nutrition:

Calories: 364 Cal

Fat: 5 g

Carbs: 26 g

Protein: 16 g

Fiber: 15 g

Roast Vegetables

Preparation Time: 5 Minutes

Cooking Time: 45 Minutes

Servings: 2

Ingredients:

- 4 tomatoes, chopped
- 2 red onions, chopped
- 3 sweet potatoes, peeled and chopped
- 100g 3½ oz. red chicory or if unavailable, use yellow
- 100g 3½ oz. kale, finely chopped
- 300g 11oz potatoes, peeled and chopped
- 5 stalks of celery, chopped
- 1 bird's-eye chili, de-seeded and finely chopped
- 2 tablespoons fresh parsley, chopped
- 2 tablespoons fresh coriander cilantro chopped
- 3 tablespoons olive oil
- 2 tablespoons balsamic vinegar 1 teaspoon mustard
- Sea salt
- Freshly ground black pepper

Directions:

1. Place the olive oil, balsamic, mustard, parsley and coriander cilantro into a bowl.
2. And mix well.
3. Toss all the remaining ingredients into the dressing
4. And season with salt and pepper.
5. Serve.

Nutrition:

Calories: 310 Cal

Fat: 15 g

Carbs: 21 g

Protein: 13 g

Fiber: 10 g

Salmon and Capers

Preparation Time: 10 minutes

Cooking Time: 0

Servings: 4

Ingredients:

- 75g (3oz) Greek yogurt
- 4 salmon fillets, skin removed
- 4 teaspoons Dijon Mustard
- 1 tablespoon capers, chopped
- 2 teaspoons fresh parsley
- Zest of 1 lemon

Directions:

1. In a bowl, mix together the yogurt, mustard, lemon zest, parsley and capers.
2. Thoroughly coat the salmon in the mixture.
3. Place the salmon under a hot grill (broiler).
4. Cook for 3-4 minutes on each side, or until the fish is cooked.
5. Serve with mashed potatoes and vegetables or a large green leafy salad.

Nutrition:

Calories: 321 Cal

Fat: 0 g

Carbs: 0 g

Protein: 0 g

Fiber: 0 g

Rocket salad with Tuna

Preparation Time: 5 minutes

Cooking Time: 15 minutes

Servings: 4

Ingredients:

- 4 slices rustic bread, torn into pieces
- 4 large tomatoes
- 2 Tbsp. olive oil
- 400g tin cannellini beans, drained and rinsed
- ¼ cup Kalamata olives
- 2 cups shredded rocket
- ¼ red onion, sliced finely
- 85g tin tuna

Dressing:

- 2 Tbsp. olive oil
- ½ tsp. dijon mustard
- 1 Tbsp. lemon juice

Directions:

1. Start with setting the oven at 180C.
2. Place the bread slices in braking tray, put olive oil on slices and bake for 10-15 mins.
3. To prepare the dressing mix lemon juice, mustard and oil in a jar.
4. Bring a bowl, add baked bread, onions, beans, tuna, tomatoes and rocket.
5. Put the dressing over salad and enjoy.

Nutrition:

Calories: 338

Carbs: 0g

Fat: 13g

Protein: 0g

Sirt Super Salad

Preparation Time: 5 minutes

Cooking Time: 15 minutes

Servings: 1

Ingredients:

- 1 ounce (50g) arugula

- 3 ounces (100g) smoked salmon slices
- 1 ounce (50g) endive leaves
- 1/2cup (50g) celery including leaves, sliced
- 1/8cups (15g) walnuts, chopped
- 1/2cup (80g) avocado, peeled, stonedand sliced
- 1/8cup (20g) red onion, sliced
- 1 tablespoon extra-virgin olive oil
- 1 tablespoon capers
- 1 large Medjool date, pitted and chopped
- 1/4cup (10g) parsley, chopped
- Juice of 1/4lemon

Directions:

1. Bring a bowl, place large leaves of salad, add all the ingredients one by one in the bowl and stir through the bowl and enjoy.

Nutrition:

Calories: 40

Carbs: 8g

Fat: 0g

Protein: 1g

Strawberry Buckwheat Tabbouleh

Preparation Time: 5 minutes

Cooking Time: 15 minutes

Servings: 1

Ingredients:

- 1/3 cup (50g) buckwheat
- 1/2cup (80g) avocado
- 1 tablespoon ground turmeric
- 1/8 cup (20g) red onion
- 3/8cup (65g) tomato
- 1 tablespoon capers

- 1/8 cup (25g) Medjool dates, pitted
- 2/3cup (100g) strawberries, hulled
- 3/4cup (30g) parsley
- 1 tablespoon extra-virgin olive oil
- 1 ounce (30g) arugula
- Juice of 1/2 lemon

Directions:

1. Start with cooking the buckwheat by mixing the turmeric according to the instructions of package.
2. Drain and let it cool.
3. Now, start chopping the tomatoes, capers, onions, avocados, dates and parsley.
4. Mix all of them with already cooked buckwheat.
5. After that, take the strawberries, slice them and add them in salad.
6. Garnish the salad on the arugula bed.

Nutrition:

Calories: 208

Carbs: 16g

Fat: 11g

Protein: 7g

Fragrant Anise Hotpot Sirtfood

Preparation Time: 2 minutes

Cooking Time: 10 minutes

Servings: 2

Ingredients:

- 1 tbsp. tomato purée
- 1 star anise, crushed (or 1/4 tsp ground anise)
- Small handful (10g) parsley, stalks finely chopped

- Small handful (10g) coriander, stalks finely chopped
- Juice of 1/2 lime
- 1/2 carrot, peeled and cut into matchsticks
- 500ml chicken stock, fresh or made with 1 cube
- 50g beansprouts
- 100g firm tofu, chopped
- 50g broccoli, cut into small florets
- 100g raw tiger prawns
- 50 g cooked water chestnuts, drained
- 50g rice noodles, cooked according to packet instructions
- 1 tbsp. good-quality miso paste
- 20g sushi ginger, chopped

Directions:

1. Take a pan and put the parsley stalks, lime juice, tomato purée, coriander stalks, star aniseand chicken stock, let them simmer for 10-12 mins.
2. Now add the broccoli, tofu, carrot, water, chestnutsand prawns, gently mix them and let them cook completely.
3. Turn off the heat and add in the miso paste and sushi ginger.
4. Garnish with coriander and parsley leaves and enjoy.

Nutrition:

Calories: 14

Carbs: 3g

Fat: 0g

Protein: 1g

Coronation Chicken Salad Sirtfood

Preparation Time: 2 minutes

Cooking Time: 2 minutes

Servings: 1

Ingredients:

- 75 g Natural yoghurt
- 1 tsp. Coriander, chopped
- Juice of 1/4 of a lemon
- 1/2 tsp. Mild curry powder
- 1 tsp. Ground turmeric
- 6 Walnut halves, finely chopped
- 100 g Cooked chicken breast, cut into bite-sized pieces
- 20 g Red onion, diced
- 1 Bird's eye chili
- 1 Medjool date, finely chopped
- 40 g Rocket, to serve

Directions:

1. Take a bowl, gather the ingredients and mix them in bowland serve the salad on the rocket bedding.

Nutrition:

Calories: 364

Carbs: 45g

Fat: 12g

Protein: 15g

Buckwheat Pasta Salad

Preparation Time: 15 minutes

Cooking Time: 0 minutes

Servings: 1

Ingredients:

- 50g cooked buckwheat pasta
- small handful of basil leaves
- large handful of rockets
- 1/2 avocado, diced
- 1 tbsp. extra virgin olive oil
- 20g pine nuts

- 8 cherry tomatoes, halved
- 10 olives

Directions:

1. Take a bowl or a plate, add in all the ingredients, now scatter the pine nuts all over the ingredients and serve.

Nutrition:

Calories: 220

Carbs: 46g

Fat: 0g

Protein: 8g

Dinner Recipes

Lamb Chops with Kale

Preparation time: 15 minutes

Cooking time: 11 minutes

Servings: 4

Ingredients:

- 1 garlic clove, minced
- 1 tablespoon fresh rosemary leaves, minced
- Salt and ground black pepper, to taste
- 4 lamb loin chops
- 4 cups fresh baby kale

Directions:

1. Preheat the grill to high heat. Grease the grill grate.
2. In a bowl, add the garlic, rosemary, salt and black pepper and mix well.
3. Coat the lamb chops with the herb mixture generously.
4. Place the chops onto the hot side of grill and cook for about 2 minutes per side.
5. Now, move the chops onto the cooler side of the grill and cook for about 6–7 minutes.
6. Divide the kale onto serving plates and top each with 1 chop and serve.

Nutrition:

Calories 301 Total Fat 10.5 g Saturated Fat 3.8 g Cholesterol 128 mg Sodium 176 mg

Total Carbs 7.8 g Fiber 1.4 g Sugar 0 g Protein 41.9 g

Shrimp with Kale

Preparation time: 15 minutes

Cooking time: 10 minutes

Servings: 4

Ingredients:

- 3 tablespoons olive oil
- 1 pound medium shrimp, peeled and deveined
- 1 medium onion, chopped
- 4 garlic cloves, chopped finely
- 1 fresh red chili, sliced
- 1 pound fresh kale, tough ribs removed and chopped
- ¼ cup low-sodium chicken broth

Directions:

1. In a large non-stick pan, heat 1 tablespoon of the oil over medium-high heat and cook the shrimp for around 2 minutes every side.
2. With a slotted spoon, transfer the shrimp onto a plate.
3. In the same pan, heat the 2 tablespoons of oil over medium heat and sauté the garlic and red chili for about 1 minute.
4. Add the kale and broth and cook for about 4–5 minutes, stirring occasionally.
5. Mix in the cooked shrimp and cook for about 1 minute.
6. Serve hot.

Nutrition:

Calories 270 Total Fat 11.9 g Saturated Fat 1.5 g Cholesterol 223 mg

Sodium 312 mg Total Carbs 15.5 g Fiber 2.3 g Sugar 1.2 g Protein 28.3 g

Chicken & Veggies with Buckwheat Noodles

Preparation time: 20 minutes

Cooking time: 25 minutes

Servings: 2

Ingredients:

- ½ cup broccoli florets - ½ cup fresh green beans, trimmed and sliced
- 1 cup fresh kale, chopped and tough ribs removed - 5 ounces buckwheat noodles
- 1 tablespoon coconut oil - 1 brown onion, chopped finely
- 1 (6-ounce) boneless, skinless chicken breast, cubed
- 2 garlic cloves, chopped finely
- 3 tablespoons low-sodium soy sauce

Directions:

1. In a medium pan of the boiling water, add the broccoli and green beans and cook for about 4–5 minutes.
2. Add the kale and cook for about 1–2 minutes.
3. Drain the vegetables and transfer them into a large bowl. Set aside.
4. In another pan of the lightly salted boiling water, cook the soba noodles for about 5 minutes.
5. Drain the noodles well and then rinse under cold running water. Set aside.
6. Meanwhile, in a large wok, melt the coconut oil over medium heat and sauté the onion for about 2–3 minutes.

7. Put the chicken cubes and cook for about 5–6 minutes. Add the garlic, soy sauce and a little splash of water and cook for about 2–3 minutes, stirring frequently.
8. Add the cooked vegetables and noodles and cook for about 1–2 minutes, tossing frequently.
9. Serve hot with the garnishing of sesame seeds.

Nutrition:

Calories 463 Total Fat 11.7 g Saturated Fat 5.9 g Cholesterol 54 mg Sodium 1000 mg

Total Carbs 58.9 g Fiber 7.1 g Sugar 4.6 g Protein 22.5 g

Beef & Kale Salad

Preparation time: 15 minutes

Cooking time: 8 minutes

Servings: 2

Ingredients:

- Steak - 2 teaspoons olive oil - 2 (4-ounce) strip steaks
- Salt and ground black pepper, to taste - Salad - ¼ cup carrot, peeled and shredded
- ¼ cup cucumber, peeled, seededand sliced
- ¼ cup radish, sliced
- ¼ cup cherry tomatoes, halved
- 3 cups fresh kale, tough ribs removed and chopped

Dressing

- 1 tablespoon extra-virgin olive oil
- 1 tablespoon fresh lemon juice
- Salt and ground black pepper, to taste

Directions:

1. For steak: in a large heavy-bottomed wok.
2. Heat the oil over high heat.
3. Cook the steaks with salt and black pepper.
4. Transfer the steaks onto a cutting board for about 5 minutes before slicing.
5. For salad: place all ingredients in a salad bowl and mix.
6. For dressing: place all ingredients in another bowl and beat until well combined.
7. Cut the steaks into desired sized slices against the grain.
8. Place the salad onto each serving plate.
9. Top each plate with steak slices. Drizzle with dressing and serve.

Nutrition:

Calories 262 Total Fat 12 g Saturated Fat 1.6 g Cholesterol 63 mg Sodium 506 mg

Total Carbs 15.2 g Fiber 2.5g Sugar 3.3 g Protein 25.2 g

Prawns with Asparagus

Preparation time: 15 minutes

Cooking time: 13 minutes

Servings: 4

Ingredients:

- 3 tablespoons olive oil
- 1 pound prawns, peeledand deveined
- 1 pound asparagus, trimmed
- Salt and ground black pepper, to taste
- 1 teaspoon garlic, minced
- 1 teaspoon fresh ginger, minced
- 1 tablespoon low-sodium soy sauce
- 2 tablespoons lemon juice

Directions:

1. In a pan, put and heat 2 tablespoons of olive oil in a medium heat and cook the prawns with salt and black pepper for about 3–4 minutes.
2. With a slotted spoon, transfer the prawns into a bowl. Set aside.
3. In the same pan, heat the 1 tablespoon of oil over medium-high heat and cook the asparagus, ginger, garlic, salt and black pepper and sauté for about 6–8 minutes, stirring frequently.
4. Mix in the prawns and soy sauce and cook for about 1 minute.
5. Mix in the lemon juice and remove from the heat.
6. Serve hot.

Nutrition:

Calories 253 Total Fat 12.7 g Saturated Fat 2.2 g Cholesterol 239 mg Sodium 501 mg

Total Carbs 7.1 g Fiber 2.5 g Sugar 2.6 g Protein 28.7 g

Turkey Satay Skewer

Preparation time: 5 minutes

Cooking time: 30 minutes

Servings: 3

Ingredients:

- 250g (9oz) turkey breast, cubed
- 25g (1oz) smooth peanut butter
- 1 clove of garlic, crushed
- ½ small bird's eye chili (or more if you like it hotter), finely chopped
- ½ tsp. ground turmeric
- 200ml (7fl oz.) coconut milk
- 2 tsp. soy sauce

Directions:

1. Combine the coconut milk, peanut butter, turmeric, soy sauce, garlic and chili.
2. Add the turkey pieces to the bowl and stir them until they are completely coated.
3. Push the turkey onto metal skewers.
4. Place the satay skewers on a barbeque or under a hot grill (broiler) and cook for 4-5 minutes per side, until they are thoroughly cooked.

Nutrition:

Calorie: 107 Cal

Fat: 1 g

Carbs: 3 g

Protein: 20 g

Salmon & Capers

Preparation time: 5 minutes

Cooking time: 40 minutes

Servings: 3

Ingredients:

- 75g (3oz) Greek yogurt
- 4 salmon fillets, skin removed
- 4 tsp. Dijon mustard
- 1 tbsp. capers, chopped
- 2 tsp. fresh parsley
- Zest of 1 lemon

Directions:

1. In a bowl, mix the yogurt, mustard, lemon zest, parsley and capers.
2. Thoroughly coat the salmon in the mixture.
3. Place the salmon under a hot grill (broiler).
4. Cook for 3-4 minutes on each side or until the fish is cooked.

5. Serve with mashed potato and green leafy vegetables.

Nutrition:

Calorie: 430 Cal

Fat: 24 g

Carbs: 3 g

Sodium: 860 mg

Protein: 45 g

Chicken Casserole

Preparation time: 5 minutes

Cooking time: 20 minutes

Servings: 3

Ingredients:

- 250g (9oz) tinned chickpeas (garbanzo beans) drained
- 4 chicken breasts, cubed
- 4 Medjool dates halved
- 6 dried apricots, halved
- 1 red onion, sliced
- 1 carrot, chopped
- 1 tsp. ground cumin
- 1 tsp. ground cinnamon
- 1 tsp. ground turmeric
- 1 bird's eye chili, chopped
- 600ml (1 pint) chicken stock (broth)
- 25g (1oz) corn flour
- 60ml (2fl oz.) water
- 2 tbsp. fresh coriander

Directions:

1. Place the chicken, chickpeas (garbanzo beans), onion, carrot, chili, cumin, turmeric, cinnamon.
2. And stock (broth) into a large saucepan.
3. Add in the dates and apricots and simmer for 10 minutes.

4. In a cup, stir the corn flour with the water until it becomes a smooth paste.
5. Put the mixture into the saucepan and stir until it thickens.
6. Add in the coriander (cilantro) and mix well.
7. Serve with buckwheat or couscous.

Nutrition:

Calorie: 381.8 kcal Fat: 10.3 g Carbs: 40.6 g Sodium: 2147 mg Protein: 32.3 g

Veal Cabbage Rolls – Smarter with Capers, Garlic and Caraway Seeds

Preparation time: 15 minutes

Cooking time: 40 minutes

Servings: 4

Ingredients:

- 1 kg white cabbage (1 white cabbage)
- Salt
- 2 onions
- 1 clove of garlic
- 3 tbsp. oil
- 700 g veal mince (request from the butcher)
- 40 g escapades (glass; depleted weight)
- 2 eggs
- Pepper
- 1 tsp favorer
- 1 tbsp. paprika powder (sweet)
- 400 ml veal stock
- 125 ml soy cream

Directions:

1. Wash the cabbage and evacuate the outer leaves.
2. Cut out the tail during a wedge.
3. Spot an enormous pot of salted water and warm it to the purpose of boiling.

4. Within the interim, expel 16 leaves from the cabbage during a steady progression, increase the bubbling water and cook for 3-4 minutes.
5. Lift out, flush under running virus water and channel.
6. Spot on a kitchen towel, spread with a subsequent towel and pat dry
7. Cut out the hard, center leaf ribs.
8. Peel and finely cleave onions and garlic.
9. Warmth 1 tablespoon of oil.
10. Braise the onions and garlic until translucent.
11. Let cool during a bowl.
12. Include minced meat, tricks, eggs, salt and pepper and blend everything into a meat player.
13. Put 2 cabbage leaves together and put 1 serving of mince on each leaf.
14. Move up firmly and fasten it with kitchen string.
15. Heat the remainder of the oil during a panand earthy colored the 8 cabbage abounds in it from all sides.
16. Add the caraway and paprika powder—empty veal stock into the pot and warmth to the purpose of boiling.
17. Cover and braise the cabbage turns over medium warmth for 35–40 minutes, turn within the middle.
18. Mix the soy cream into the sauce and let it bubble for a further 5 minutes—season with salt and pepper.
19. Put the cabbage roulades on a plate and present with earthy colored rice or pureed potatoes.

Nutrition:

Calories: 645 kcal

Protein: 182.07 g

Fat: 163.4 g

Carbohydrates: 129.37 g

Fragrant Asian Hotspot

Preparation time: 5 minutes

Cooking time: 15 minutes

Servings: 2

Ingredients:

- 1 tsp. tomato purée
- 1-star anise, crushed (or 1/4 tsp. ground anise)
- Small handful (10g) parsley, stalks finely chopped
- Small handful (1Og) coriander, stalks finely chopped
- Juice of 1/2 lime
- 500ml chicken stock, fresh or made with one cube
- 50g beansprouts
- 50g broccoli, cut into small florets
- 1/2 carrot - 100g raw tiger prawns
- 50g rice noodles
- 100g firm tofu, chopped
- 20g sushi ginger, chopped
- 50g cooked water chestnuts, drained
- 1 tbsp. good-quality miso paste

Directions:

1. In a large saucepan, place the tomato purée, star anise, parsley stalks, coriander stalks, lime juice and chicken stock and bring to simmer for 10 minutes.
2. Add in the carrot, broccoli, prawns, tofu, noodles and water chestnuts and cook gently until the prawns are cooked.
3. Remove from heatand add sushi and miso paste to the ginger.
4. Serve sprinkled with the leaves of the parsley and coriander.

Nutrition:

Calories: 348 kcal Protein: 15.09 g Fat: 9.4 g Carbohydrates: 53.49 g

Tofu Thai Curry

Preparation Time: 5 Minutes

Cooking time: 65 Minutes

Servings: 2

Ingredients:

- 400g (14oz) tofu, diced
- 200g (7oz) sugar snaps peas
- 5cm (2 inches) chunk fresh ginger root, peeled and finely chopped
- 2 red onions, chopped
- 2 cloves of garlic, crushed
- 2 bird's eye chilies
- 2 tablespoons tomato puree
- 1 stalk of lemongrass, inner stalks only
- 1 tablespoon fresh coriander (cilantro), chopped
- 1 teaspoon cumin
- 300mls (½ pint) coconut milk
- 200mls (7fl oz) vegetable stock (broth)
- 1 tablespoon virgin olive oil
- Juice of 1 lime

Directions:

1. Heat the oil in a frying pan, add the onion and cook for 4 minutes.
2. Add in the chilies, cumin, gingerand garlic and cook for 2 minutes.
3. Add the tomato puree, lemongrass, sugar-snap peas, lime juiceand tofu and cook for 2 minutes.
4. Pour in the stock (broth), coconut milk and coriander (cilantro) and simmer for 5 minutes.

5. Serve with brown rice or buckwheat and a handful of rockets (arugula) leaves on the side.

Nutrition:

Calories 346.3.

Total fat 26.4 g.

Saturated fat Trace 2.0 g.

Trans fat 0 g.

Monounsaturated fat 5.4 g.

Cholesterol Trace. 0.0 mg

Beans & Kale Soup

Preparation Time: 15 minutes

Cooking Time: 30 minutes

Servings: 6

Ingredients:

- 2 tablespoons olive oil
- 2 onions, chopped
- 4 garlic cloves, minced
- 1-pound kale, tough ribs removed and chopped
- 2 (14-ounce) cans cannellini beans, rinsed and drained
- 6 cups of water
- Salt and ground black pepper, as required

Directions:

1. In a large pan, heat the oil over medium heat and sauté the onion and garlic for about 4-5 minutes.
2. Add the kale and cook for about 1-2 minutes.
3. Add beans, water, salt and black pepper and bring to a boil.
4. Cook partially covered for about 15-20 minutes.

5. Serve hot.

Nutrition:

Calories 270.4.

Total fat 4.7 g.

Saturated fat Trace 0.6 g.

Trans fat 0 g.

Monounsaturated fat 2.6 g.

Cholesterol Trace. 0.0 mg

Lentils & Greens Soup

Preparation Time: 15 minutes

Cooking Time: 55 minutes

Servings: 6

Ingredients:

- 1 tablespoon olive oil
- 2 carrots, peeled and chopped
- 2 celery stalks, chopped
- 1 medium red onion, chopped
- 3 garlic cloves, minced
- 1½ teaspoon ground cumin
- 1 teaspoon ground turmeric
- ¼ teaspoon red pepper flakes
- 1 (14½-ounce) can diced tomatoes
- 1 cup red lentils, rinsed
- 5½ cups water
- 2 cups fresh mustard greens, chopped
- Salt and ground black pepper, as required
- 2 tablespoons fresh lemon juice

Directions:

1. Heat olive oil in a large pan over medium heat and sauté the carrots, celery and onion for about 5-6 minutes.
2. Add the garlic and spices and sauté for about 1 minute.

3. Add the tomatoes and cook for about 2-3 minutes.
4. Stir in the lentils and water and bring to a boil.
5. Now, reduce the heat to low and simmer, covered for about 35 minutes.
6. Stir in greens and cook for about 5 minutes.
7. Stir in salt, black pepperand lemon juice and remove from the heat.
8. Serve hot.

Nutrition:

Calories 167.4

Total fat 5.5 g.

Saturated fat Trace 1.2 g.

Trans fat 0 g.

Monounsaturated fat 4.3 g.

Cholesterol Trace. 3.3 mg

Asian Slaw

Preparation Time: 5 Minutes

Cooking time: 25 Minutes

Servings: 2

Ingredients:

- Red cabbage, shredded – 2 cups
- Broccoli florets, chopped – 2 cups
- Carrots, shredded – 1 cup
- Red onion, finely sliced – 1
- Red bell pepper, finely sliced - .5
- Cilantro, chopped - .5 cup
- Sesame seeds – 1 tablespoon
- Peanuts, chopped - .5 cup
- Sriracha – 2 teaspoons
- Rice wine vinegar - .25 cup
- Sesame seed oil - .5 teaspoon
- Sea salt – 1 teaspoon
- Garlic, minced – 1 clove

- Peanut butter, natural – 2 tablespoons
- Extra virgin olive oil – 2 tablespoons
- Tamari sauce – 2 tablespoons
- Ginger, peeled and grated – 2 teaspoons
- Honey – 2 teaspoons
- Black pepper, ground - .25 teaspoon

Directions:

1. In a large salad bowl, toss together the vegetables, cilantroand peanuts.
2. In a smaller bowl, whisk together the remaining ingredients until emulsified. Pour this dressing over the vegetables and toss together until fully coated.
3. Chill the slaw for at least ten minutes so that the flavors meld. Refrigerate the Asian slaw for up to a day in advance for deeper feelings.

Nutrition:

Calories 179

Total fat 11.8 g.

Saturated fat Trace 2.9 g.

Trans fat 0 g.

Monounsaturated fat 4.3 g.

Cholesterol Trace. 3.3 mg

Egg Fried Buckwheat

Preparation Time: 5 Minutes

Cooking time: 45 Minutes

Servings: 2

Ingredients:

- Eggs, beaten – 2
- Extra virgin olive oil – 2 tablespoons, divided
- Onion, diced – 1
- Peas, frozen - .5 cup
- Carrots, finely diced – 2

- Garlic, minced – 2 cloves
- Ginger, grated – 1 teaspoon
- Green onions, thinly sliced – 2
- Tamari sauce – 2 tablespoons
- Sriracha sauce – 2 teaspoons
- Cooked buckwheat groats, cold – 3 cups

Directions:

1. Add half of the olive oil to a large skillet or wok set to medium heat and add in the egg, constantly stirring until it is fully cooked.
2. Remove the egg and transfer it to another dish.
3. Add the remaining olive oil to your wok along with the peas, carrotsand onion.
4. Cook until the carrots and onions are softened, about four minutes.
5. Add in the grated ginger and minced garlic, cooking for an additional minute until fragrant.
6. Add the sriracha sauce, tamari sauce and cooked buckwheat groats to the wok.
7. Continue to cook the buckwheat groats and stir the mixture until the buckwheat is warmed all the way through and the flavors have melded about two minutes.
8. Add the cooked eggs and green onions to the wok, giving it a good toss to combine and serve warm.

Nutrition:

5.68 g of protein.

1.04 g of fat.

33.5 g of carbohydrate.

4.5 g of fiber.

148 milligrams (mg) of potassium.

118 mg of phosphorus.

86 mg of magnesium.

12 mg of calcium.

Aromatic Ginger Turmeric Buckwheat

Preparation Time: 5 Minutes

Cooking time: 65 Minutes

Servings: 2

Ingredients:

- Buckwheat groats rinsed and drained – 1 cup
- Water – 1.75 cup
- Extra virgin olive oil – 1 tablespoon
- Ginger, grated – 1 tablespoon
- Garlic, minced – 3 cloves
- Turmeric root, grated – 1 teaspoon
- Lemon juice – 1 tablespoon
- Sea salt – 1 teaspoon
- Cranberries, dried - .5 cup
- Parsley, chopped - .33 cup
- Pine nuts, toasted - .25 cup (optional)

Directions:

1. Into a medium saucepan, add the buckwheat groats, water, olive oil, ginger, garlic, turmeric, lemon juiceand sea salt.
2. Bring the water in the pot to a boil and then cover the mixture with a lid.
3. Allow it to simmer over medium-low until all of the liquid is absorbed, about twenty minutes.
4. About fifteen minutes into the **cooking time** of the buckwheat sir, the dried cranberries into the buckwheat allow them to plump up the last few minutes of the **cooking time**.
5. Top the buckwheat with the pine nuts and parsley before serving.

Nutrition:

Calories 37

Kale and Corn Succotash

Preparation Time: 5 Minutes

Cooking time: 55 Minutes

Servings: 2

Ingredients:

- Corn kernels – 2 cups
- Black pepper, ground - .5 teaspoon
- Kale, chopped – 2 cups
- Red onion, finely diced – 1
- Garlic, minced – 2 cloves
- Grape tomatoes, sliced in half lengthwise – 1 cup
- Sea salt – 1 teaspoon
- Parsley, chopped – 2 tablespoons
- Extra virgin olive oil – 1 tablespoon

Directions:

1. Into a large skillet pour the olive oil, red onion and the corn kernels, sauteing until hot and tender, about four minutes.
2. Add the sea salt, garlic, kaleand black pepper to the skillet, cooking until the kale has wilted, about three to five minutes.
3. Remove the large skillet from the stove and toss in the parsley and fresh grape tomatoes.
4. Serve warm.

Nutrition:

Calories 137.4.

Total fat 6.7 g.

Saturated fat Trace 1.0 g.

Trans fat 0 g.

Monounsaturated fat 1.8 g.

Cholesterol Trace. 0.0 mg

Asian King Prawn Stir-Fry with Buckwheat Noodles

Preparation Time: 10 Minutes

Cooking Time: 20 Minutes

Servings: 1

Ingredients:

- 150g shelled raw ruler prawns
- 2 tsp. tamari
- 2 tsp. extra virgin olive oil
- 75g soba
- 1 garlic slice
- 1 elevated stew
- 1 tsp. sliced ginger
- 20g red onions
- 40g celery
- 75g green beans
- 50g kcal
- 100ml chicken stock
- 5g celery leaves

Directions:

1. Heat a pan over, at that point cook the prawns in 1 teaspoon of the tamari and 1 teaspoon of the oil for 2–3 minutes.
2. Move the prawns to a plate.
3. Wipe the work out with kitchen paper, as you're going to utilize it once more.
4. Cook the noodles in bubbling water for 5–8 minutes or as coordinated on the parcel.
5. Channel and put in a safe spot.
6. Then, fry the garlic, stew and ginger, red onion, celery, beans and kale in the rest of the oil over a medium – high temperature for 2–3 minutes.
7. Add the stock and bring to the bubble, at that point stew for a moment or two, until the vegetables are cooked yet at the same time crunchy.

8. Include the prawns, noodles and Lovage/celery leaves to the skillet, take back to the bubble at that point expel from the heat and serve.

Nutrition:

Calories 402 Cal

Greek Salad Skewers

Preparation Time: 10 Minutes

Cooking Time: 15 Minutes

Servings: 1

Ingredients:

- 2 wooden sticks, absorbed water for 30 minutes before use
- 8 large dark olives
- 8 cherry tomatoes
- 1 yellow pepper, cut into 8 squares
- ½ red onion, cut down the middle and isolated into 8 pieces
- 100g (about 10cm) cucumber, cut into 4 cuts and divided
- 100g feta, cut into 8 solid shapes
- For the dressing:
- 1 tbsp. extra virgin olive oil
- Juice of ½ lemon
- 1 tsp. balsamic vinegar
- ½ slice garlic, stripped and squashed

Directions:

1. Add leaves basil, finely sliced.
2. Add oregano leaves, finely sliced
3. Liberal flavoring of salt and newly ground dark pepper
4. String each stick with the plate of salad ingredients in the request.
5. Spot all the dressing ingredients in a little bowl and combine altogether.
6. For over the sticks.

Nutrition:

Calories 329 Cal

Sirtfood Couscous

Preparation Time: 10 Minutes

Cooking Time: 20 Minutes

Servings: 1

Ingredients:

- 150g cauliflower, roughly chopped
- 1 garlic clove, finely chopped
- 40g red onion, finely chopped
- 1 bird's eye chilli, finely chopped
- 1 tsp. finely chopped fresh ginger
- 2 tbsp. extra virgin olive oil
- 2 tsp. ground turmeric
- 30g sun dried tomatoes, finely chopped
- 10g parsley
- 150g turkey steak
- 1 tsp. dried sage
- Juice of ½ lemon
- 1 tbsp. capers

Directions:

1. Disintegrate the cauliflower using a food processor.
2. Blend in 1-2 pulses until the cauliflower has a breadcrumb-like consistency.
3. In a skillet, fry garlic, chilli, ginger and red onion in 1 tsp. olive oil.
4. Throw in the turmeric and cauliflower then cook for another 1-2 minutes.
5. Remove from heat and add the tomatoes and roughly half the parsley.
6. Garnish the turkey steak with sage and dress with oil.
7. In a skillet, over medium heat, fry the turkey steak for 5 minutes.
8. Once the steak is cooked add lemon juice, capers and a dash of water.

9. Stir and serve with the couscous.

Nutrition:

Calories 394 Cal

Caramelized Tofu

Preparation Time: 10 Minutes

Cooking Time: 35 Minutes

Servings: 1

Ingredients:

- 1 tbsp. mirin
- 20g miso paste
- 1 * 150g firm tofu
- 40g celery, trimmed
- 35g red onion
- 120g courgette
- 1 bird's eye chilli
- 1 garlic clove, finely chopped
- 1 tsp. finely chopped fresh ginger
- 50g kale, chopped
- 2 tsp. sesame seeds
- 35g buckwheat
- 1 tsp. ground turmeric
- 2 tsp. extra virgin olive oil
- 1 tsp. tamari (or soy sauce)

Directions:

1. Pre-heat your over to 200C or gas mark 6. Cover a tray with baking parchment.
2. Combine the mirin and miso together.
3. Dice the tofu and coat it in the mirin-miso mixture in a resealable plastic bag. Set aside to marinate.
4. Chop the vegetables using a steamer, cook for the kale for 5 minutes and set aside.
5. Disperse the tofu across the lined tray and garnish with sesame seeds.

6. Roast for 20 minutes, or until caramelized.
7. Rinse the buckwheat using running water and a sieve.
8. Add to a pan of boiling water alongside turmeric and cook the buckwheat according to the packet directions.
9. Heat the oil in a skillet over high heat.
10. Toss in the vegetables, herbs and spices then fry for 2-3 minutes.
11. Reduce to a medium heat and fry for a further 5 minutes or until cooked but still crunchy.

Nutrition:

Calories 273 Cal

Stir-fry & Soba

Preparation Time: 10 Minutes

Cooking Time: 25 Minutes

Servings: 2

Ingredients:

- 150g shelled raw king prawns, deveined
- 2 tsp. tamari
- 2 tsp. extra virgin olive oil
- 75 soba
- 1 garlic clove, finely chopped
- 1 bird's eye chilli, finely chopped
- 1 tsp. finely chopped fresh ginger
- 20g red onions, sliced
- 40g celery, trimmed and sliced
- 75g green beans, chopped
- 50g kale, roughly chopped
- 100ml chicken stock

Directions:

1. Warm a skillet over a high heat.

2. And then fry for the pawns in 1 tsp. of the tamari and of olive oil.
3. Transfer the contents of the skillet to a plate.
4. And then wipe the skillet with kitchen towel.
5. Boil water and cook the soba for 8 minutes.
6. Drain and set aside.
7. Using the remaining 1 tsp. olive oil.
8. Fry the remaining ingredients for 3-4 minutes.
9. Add the stock and bring to the boil.
10. Simmering until the vegetables are tender but still have bite.
11. Add the Lovage, noodles and prawn into the skillet.
12. Stir, bring back to the boil and then serve.

Nutrition:

Calories 435 kcal

Mushroom Scramble

Preparation Time: 10 Minutes

Cooking Time: 20 Minutes

Servings: 1

Ingredients:

- 100g tofu, extra firm
- 1 tsp. ground turmeric
- 1 tsp. mild curry powder
- 20g kale, roughly chopped
- 1 tsp. extra virgin olive oil
- 20g red onion, thinly sliced
- 50g mushrooms, thinly sliced
- 5g parsley, finely chopped

Directions:

1. Place 2 sheets of kitchen towel under and on-top of the tofu.

2. Then rest a considerable weight such as saucepan onto the tofu.
3. Ensure it drains off the liquid.
4. Combine the curry powder, turmeric and 1-2 tsp. of water.
5. Using a steamer cook kale for 3-4 minutes.
6. In a skillet, warm oil over a medium heat.
7. Add the chilli, mushrooms and onion, cooking for several.
8. Break the tofu in to small pieces and toss in the skillet.
9. Coat with the spice paste and stir, ensuring everything becomes evenly coated.
10. Cook for up to 5 minutes and fry for 2 more minutes.
11. Garnish with parsley before serving.

Nutrition:

Calories 131 Cal

Fragrant Asian Hotpot

Preparation Time: 10 Minutes

Cooking Time: 15 Minutes

Servings: 2

Ingredients:

- 1 tsp. tomato purée
- 1 star anise, squashed (or 1/4 tsp. ground anise)
- Little bunch (10g) parsley, stalks finely cleaved
- Little bunch (1Og) coriander, stalks finely cleaved
- Juice of 1/2 lime
- 500ml chicken stock, new or made with 1 solid shape
- 1/2 carrot, stripped and cut into matchsticks

- 50g broccoli, cut into little florets
- 50g beansprouts
- 100 g crude tiger prawns
- 100 g firm tofu, slashed
- 50g rice noodles, cooked according to parcel directions.
- 50g cooked water chestnuts, depleted
- 20g sushi ginger, slashed
- 1 tbsp. great quality miso glue

Directions:

1. Spot the tomato purée, star anise, parsley stalks, coriander stalks, lime juice and chicken stock in an enormous container and bring to a stew for 10 minutes.
2. Include the carrot, broccoli, prawns, tofu, noodles and water chestnuts and stew tenderly until the prawns are cooked through.
3. Expel from the warmth and mix in the sushi ginger and miso glue.
4. Serve sprinkled with the parsley and coriander leaves.

Nutrition:

Calories 434 Cal

Greek Skewers

Preparation Time: 15 Minutes

Cooking Time: 30 Minutes

Servings: 2

Ingredients:

- 2 wooden sticks, absorbed water for 30 minutes before use
- 8 enormous dark olives
- 8 cherry tomatoes
- 1 yellow pepper, cut into 8 squares

- ½ red onion, cut down the middle and isolated into 8 pieces
- 100g (about 10cm) cucumber, cut into 4 cuts and divided
- 100g feta, cut into 8 shapes
- For the dressing:
- 1 tbsp. additional virgin olive oil
- Juice of ½ lemon
- 1 tsp. balsamic vinegar
- ½ clove garlic, stripped and squashed
- Scarcely any departs basil, finely hacked
- Leaves oregano, finely slashed
- Liberal flavoring of salt and crisply ground dark pepper

Directions:

1. Thread each stick with the plate of mixed greens ingredients.
2. Place all the dressing ingredients in a little bowl and combine altogether.
3. Pour over the sticks.

Nutrition:

Calories 364 Cal

Sweet-Smelling Chicken Breast with Kale, Red Onion and Salsa

Preparation Time: 15 Minutes

Cooking Time: 35 Minutes

Servings: 2

Ingredients:

- 120g skinless, boneless chicken bosom
- 2 tsp. ground turmeric
- Juice of ¼ lemon
- 1 tbsp. additional virgin olive oil
- 50g kale, slashed
- 20g red onion, cut
- 1 tsp. slashed new ginger

- 50g buckwheat

Directions:

1. To make the salsa, expel the eye from the tomato and slash it finely, taking consideration to keep however much of the fluid as could reasonably be expected.
2. Blend in with the bean stew, tricks, parsley and lemon juice.
3. You could place everything in a blender yet the final product is somewhat different.
4. Warmth the broiler to 220°C/gas 7.
5. Marinate the chicken bosom in 1 teaspoon of the turmeric, the lemon juice and a little oil.
6. Leave for 5–10 minutes.
7. Warmth an ovenproof griddle until hot, then include the marinated chicken and cook for a moment or so on each side, until pale brilliant, then exchange to the broiler (place on a preparing plate if your skillet isn't ovenproof) for 8–10 minutes or until cooked through.
8. Expel from the broiler, spread with foil and leave to rest for 5 minutes before serving.
9. In the meantime, cook the kale in a steamer for 5 minutes.
10. Fry the red onions and the ginger in a little oil, until delicate however not shaded, then include the cooked kale and fry for one more moment.
11. Cook the buckwheat according to the parcel
12. Add the rest of the teaspoon of turmeric.
13. Serve nearby the chicken, vegetables and salsa.

Nutrition:

Calories 465 Cal

Indian Lentil Soup

Preparation Time: 10 minutes

Cooking Time: 50 minutes

Servings: 2

Ingredients:

- 2 cups of lentils
- 1 small red onion, minced
- 1 stalk of celery, finely chopped
- 1 carrot, chopped
- 2 large leaves of kale, chopped finely, or 1 cup of baby kale, chopped
- 2 sprigs of cilantro, minced
- 3 sprigs of parsley, minced
- ¼-½ chili pepper, deseeded and minced (use more or less to your taste)
- 1 tomato, chopped into small pieces
- 1 chunk of ginger, minced
- 1 clove of garlic, minced
- 5 cups of chicken or vegetable stock
- 1 tsp of turmeric
- 1 tsp extra virgin olive oil
- ½ tsp Salt

Directions:

1. Cook lentils according to the package, removing from heat about 5 minutes before they would be done.
2. In a saucepan, sauté all of the vegetables in the olive oil.
3. Then add the chopped greens last.
4. Then add the ginger, garlic and chili and turmeric powder.
5. Add the stock and simmer for 5 minutes.
6. Add the lentilsand salt.
7. Stir in the precooked lentils and cook longer, on a very low simmer, for 25 more minutes.
8. Remove from the heat and cool.

9. Cut the avocado, remove the pitand slice it, then scoop out the slices just before eating.

10. Top with avocado slice, then serve immediately.

Nutrition:

Energy (calories): 724 kcal; Protein: 78.7 g; Fat: 14.1 g; Carbohydrates: 82.87 g

Shrimp & Arugula Soup

Preparation Time: 5 minutes

Cooking Time: 30 minutes

Servings: 3

Ingredients:

- 10 medium sized shrimp or 5 large prawns, cleaned, deshelled and deveined
- 1 small red onion, sliced very thinly
- 1 cup arugula
- 1 cup baby kale
- 2 large celery stalks, sliced very thinly
- 5 sprigs of parsley, chopped
- 11 cloves of garlic, minced
- 5 cups of chicken or fish or vegetable stock
- 1 tbsp extra virgin olive oil
- Dash of sea salt
- Dash of pepper

Directions:

1. Sauté the vegetables (not the kale or arugula just yet however), in a stock pot, on low heat for about 2 minutes so that they are still tender and still crunchy, but not cooked quite yet.
2. Add the salt and pepper.

3. Clean and chop the shrimp into bite-sized pieces that would be comfortable eating in a soup.
4. Then, add the shrimp to the potand sauté for 10 more minutes on medium-low heat.
5. Make sure the shrimp is cooked thoroughly and is not translucent.
6. When the shrimp seems to be cooked through, add the stock to the pot and cook on medium for about 20 more minutes.
7. Remove from heat and cool before serving.

Nutrition:

Energy (calories): 640 kcal; Protein: 40.05 g; Fat: 16.72 g; Carbohydrates: 85.47 g

Creamy Chicken Soup

Preparation Time: 5 minutes

Cooking Time: 30 minutes

Servings: 3

Ingredients:

- 4 chicken breasts
- 1 carrot, chopped
- 1 cup zucchini, peeled and chopped
- 2 cups cauliflower, broken into florets
- 1 celery rib, chopped
- 1 small onion, chopped
- 5 cups water
- ½ tsp salt
- Black pepper, to taste

Directions:

1. Place chicken breasts, onion, carrot, celery, cauliflower and zucchini in a deep soup pot.
2. Add in salt, black pepper and 5 cups of water.

3. Stir and bring to a boil.
4. Simmer for 30 minutes then remove chicken from the pot and let it cool slightly.
5. Blend soup until completely smooth.
6. Shred or dice the chicken meat, return it back to the pot, stirand serve.

Nutrition:

Energy (calories): 707 kcal; Protein: 82.77 g; Fat: 36.11 g; Carbohydrates: 8.79 g

Broccoli and Chicken Soup

Preparation Time: 5 minutes

Cooking Time: 30 minutes

Servings: 3

Ingredients:

- 4 boneless chicken thighs, diced
- 1 small carrot, chopped
- 1 broccoli head, broken into florets
- 1 garlic clove, chopped
- 1 small onion, chopped
- 4 cups water
- 3 tbsp extra virgin olive oil
- ½ tsp salt
- Black pepper, to taste

Directions:

1. In a deep soup pot, heat olive oil and gently sauté broccoli for 2-3 minutes, stirring occasionally.
2. Add in onion, carrot, chicken and cook, stirring, for 2-3 minutes.
3. Stir in salt, black pepper and water.
4. Bring to a boil.
5. Simmer for 30 minutes then remove from heat and set aside to cool.
6. In a blender or food processor, blend soup until completely smooth.

Nutrition:

Energy (calories): 641 kcal; Protein: 43.04 g; Fat: 48.81 g; Carbohydrates: 4.75 g

Warm Chicken and Avocado Soup

Preparation Time: 5 minutes

Cooking Time: 30 minutes

Servings: 3

Ingredients:

- 2 ripe avocados, peeled and chopped
- 1 cooked chicken breast, shredded
- 1 garlic clove, chopped
- 3 cups chicken broth
- Salt and black pepper, to taste
- Fresh coriander leaves, finely cut, to serve
- ½ cup sour cream, to serve

Directions:

1. Combine avocados, garlic and chicken broth in a blender.
2. Process until smooth and transfer to a saucepan.
3. Add in chicken and cook, stirring, over medium heat until the mixture is hot.
4. Serve topped with sour cream and finely cut coriander leaves

Nutrition:

Energy (calories): 535 kcal; Protein: 43.62 g; Fat: 10.48 g; Carbohydrates: 52.27 g

Healthy Chicken and Oat Soup

Preparation Time: 5 minutes

Cooking Time: 40 minutes

Servings: 3

Ingredients:

- 3 chicken breasts, diced
- 1 small onion, chopped
- 3 garlic cloves
- ½ cup quick-cooking oats
- 1 large carrot, chopped
- 1 red bell pepper, chopped
- 1 celery rib, chopped
- 1 tomato, diced
- 5 cups water
- 1 bay leaf
- 1 tsp salt
- ½ cup fresh parsley leaves, finely cut
- Black pepper, to taste

Directions:

1. Place the chicken, bay leaf, celery, carrot, onion, red pepper, tomato and salt into a soup pot.
2. Add in water and bring to the boil then reduce heat and simmer for 30 minutes.
3. Discard the bay leaf, season with salt and pepper, add in the oats and parsley, simmer for 5 more minutes and serve.

Nutrition:

Energy (calories): 573 kcal; Protein: 63.3 g; Fat: 27.8 g; Carbohydrates: 14.7 g

Asparagus and Chicken Soup

Preparation Time: 5 minutes

Cooking Time: 30 minutes

Servings: 3

Ingredients:

- 2 chicken breast fillets, cooked and diced
- 2-3 leeks, finely cut
- 1 bunch asparagus, trimmed and cut
- 4 cups chicken broth
- 2 tbsp extra virgin olive oil

- ½ cup fresh parsley, finely chopped
- Salt and black pepper, to taste
- Lemon juice, to serve

Directions:

1. Heat the olive oil in a large soup pot.
2. Add in the leeks and gently sauté, stirring, for 2-3 minutes.
3. Add chicken broth, the diced chickenand bring to a boil.
4. Reduce heat and simmer for 15 minutes.
5. Add in asparagus, parsley, salt and black pepperand cook for 5 minutes more.
6. Serve with lemon juice.

Nutrition:

Energy (calories): 623 kcal; Protein: 23.63 g; Fat: 5.48 g; Carbohydrates: 45.27 g

Fish and Quinoa Soup

Preparation Time: 5 minutes

Cooking Time: 40 minutes

Servings: 3

Ingredients:

- 1lb cod fillets, cubed
- 1 onion, chopped
- 3 tomatoes, chopped
- ½ cup quinoa, rinsed
- 1 red pepper, chopped
- 1 carrot, chopped
- ½ cup black olives, pitted and sliced
- 1 garlic clove, crushed
- 3 tbsp extra virgin olive oil
- A pinch of cayenne pepper
- 1 bay leaf
- 1 tsp dried thyme
- 1 tsp dried dill

- ½ tsp pepper
- ½ cup white wine
- 4 cups water
- Salt and black pepper, to taste
- ½ cup fresh parsley, finely cut

Directions:

1. Heat the olive oil over medium heat and sauté the onion, red pepper, garlic and carrot until tender.
2. Stir in the cayenne pepper, bay leaf, herbs, salt and pepper.
3. Add the white wine, water, quinoa and tomatoes and bring to a boil.
4. Reduce heat, coverand cook for 10 minutes.
5. Stir in olives and the fish and cook for another 10 minutes.
6. Stir in parsley and serve hot.

Nutrition:

Energy (calories): 673 kcal; Protein: 42.14 g; Fat: 35.63 g; Carbohydrates: 48.73 g

Bean Stew

Preparation Time: 5 minutes

Cooking Time: 35 minutes

Servings: 3

Ingredients:

- 50g of kale, chopped roughly
- ½ bird's eye chili, chopped finely (optional)
- 40g of buckwheat
- 50g of red onion, chopped finely
- 1 garlic clove, chopped finely
- 1 tbsp of roughly chopped parsley
- 200ml vegetable stock
- 1 tsp of herbes de provence
- 200g of tinned mixed beans

- 1 tsp of tomato purée
- 1 x 400g tin of chopped Italian tomatoes
- 30g celery, trimmed and chopped finely
- 1 tbsp of extra virgin olive oil
- 30g of carrot, peeled and chopped finely

Directions:

1. Heat the oil in a medium sized saucepan placed over medium low heat.
2. Add in the onion, celery, chili, carrot, garlic and herbs (if using) until the onions are soft enough but not coloured.
3. Add the stock, tomato puréeand tomatoes and bring to a boil.
4. Put in the beans and allow for 30 minutes simmering.
5. Add the kales and cook for 5-10 minutes or until the kale is tenderand then add in parsley.
6. As it cools, cook the buckwheat as per the directions on the packet.
7. Drain the buckwheat and serve with the cooked stew.

Nutrition:

Energy (calories): 375 kcal; Protein: 49.82 g; Fat: 13.48 g; Carbohydrates: 33.27 g

Pork with Pak Choi

Preparation Time: 5 minutes

Cooking Time: 40 minutes

Servings: 3

Ingredients:

- 100g of shiitake mushrooms, sliced
- 1 tbsp of corn flour
- 200g pak choi or choi sum-cut into thin slices
- 125ml of chicken stock
- 1 tbsp of tomato purée

- 1 tsp of brown sugar
- 1 clove garlic, peeled and crushed
- 1 shallot, peeled and sliced
- 100g of bean sprouts
- 1 tbsp of water
- 400g of pork mince (10% fat)
- 1 thumb (5cm) fresh ginger -peeled and grated
- 400g of firm tofu, cut into large cubes
- 1 tbsp of rice wine
- 1 tbsp of soy sauce
- A large handful (20g) of parsley, chopped
- 1 tbsp of rapeseed oil

Directions:

1. Place the tofu on kitchen paper, cover it with kitchen paperand then set it aside.
2. In a small bowl, mix water and corn flour and remove the lumps.
3. Add in rice wine, brown sugar, chicken stock, tomato pureeand soy sauce.
4. Also, add in the crushed ginger and garlic them mix.
5. Place a large frying pan or wok on high heat and add oil to it.
6. Add the mushrooms and stir-fry for 2 to 3 minutes until cooked and glossy.
7. Using a slotted spoon, remove the mushrooms from the pan and let them rest.
8. Add tofu to the pan, fry it until it is brown on all sides, remove it with a slotted spoon when done and set aside.
9. Add the pak choi to your pan or wokand stir-fry for about 2 minutes and, then add the mince.
10. Cook it until it cooks through and then add the sauce.
11. Reduce the heat a notch and allow the sauce to bubble around the meat for 1-2 minutes.
12. Add the tofu, beansproutsand mush-rooms to the pan and warm them all through.
13. Remove it from the heat and mix in parsley then serve right away.

Nutrition:

Energy (calories): 586 kcal; Protein: 58.47 g; Fat: 32.52 g; Carbohydrates: 19.69 g

Desserts and Snacks Recipes

Once you get through the first week (and I guarantee you it will be a breeze!) you can have one or max. 2 snacks a day if you need to eat something between meals. You can choose to eat an apple or a couple of walnuts. But if you want to satisfy your gourmand side and not just curb your hunger, why don't you try some of these fantastic recipes for snacks or "bites". They can all be prepared in advance and eaten when needed. They also make for fantastic appetizers for your occasional guests. I have included both savory and sweet snacks.

Crunchy potato bites

Preparation time: 10 minutes

Cooking time: 20 minutes

Servings: 2

Ingredients:

- 1 potato, sliced
- 2 bacon slices, already cooked and crumbled
- 1 small avocado, pitted and cubed
- 1 tbsp of extra virgin olive oil

Directions:

1. Spread potato slices on a lined baking sheet.
2. Toss around with the extra virgin olive oil.
3. Insert in the oven at 350 degrees F.
4. Bake for 20 minutes.
5. Arrange on a platter.
6. Top each slice with avocado and crumbled bacon.
7. Serve as a snack.

Dates in a parma ham blanket

Preparation time: 10 minutes

Cooking time: 20 minutes

Servings: 2

Ingredients:

- 12 Medjool dates
- 2 slices of Parma ham, cut into strips

Directions:

1. Wrap each date with a strip of Parma ham. Can be served hot or cold.

Mung beans snack salad

Preparation time: 10 minutes

Cooking time: 20 minutes

Servings: 2

Ingredients:

- 2 cups tomatoes, chopped
- 2 cups cucumber, chopped
- 3 cups mixed greens
- 2 cups mung beans, sprouted
- 2 cups clover sprouts

For the salad dressing:

- 1 tablespoon cumin, ground
- 1 cup dill, chopped
- 4 tablespoons lemon juice
- 1 avocado, pitted, peeled and roughly chopped
- 1 cucumber, roughly chopped

Directions:

1. In a salad bowl.
2. Mix tomatoes with 2 cups cucumber, greens, clover and mung sprouts.
3. In your blender, mix cumin with dill, lemon juice, 1 cucumberand avocado.
4. Blend really well
5. Add the blended cream to your salad, toss welland serve as a snack.

Sprouts and apples snack salad

Preparation time: 10 minutes

Cooking time: 20 minutes

Servings: 2

Ingredients:

- 1 pound Brussels sprouts, shredded
- 1 cup walnuts, chopped
- 1 apple, cored and cubed
- 1 red onion, chopped

For the salad dressing:

- 3 tablespoons red vinegar
- 1 tablespoon mustard
- ½ cup olive oil
- 1 garlic clove, minced
- Black pepper to the taste

Directions:

1. In a salad bowl, mix sprouts with apple, onion and walnuts.

2. In another bowl, mix vinegar with mustard, oil, garlic and pepper and whisk really well.
3. Add the dressing to your salad, toss well and serve as a snack.

Moroccan snack salad

Preparation time: 10 minutes

Cooking time: 20 minutes

Servings: 2

Ingredients:

- 1 bunch radishes, sliced
- 3 cups leeks, chopped
- 1 and ½ cups olives, pitted and sliced
- A pinch of turmeric powder
- Black pepper to the taste
- 2 tablespoons olive oil
- 1 cup cilantro, chopped

Directions:

1. In a bowl, mix radishes with leeks, olives and cilantro.
2. Add black pepper, oil and turmeric, toss to coat and serve as a snack.

Celery snack salad

Preparation time: 10 minutes

Cooking time: 20 minutes

Servings: 2

Ingredients:

- ½ cup raisins
- 4 cups celery, sliced
- ¼ cup parsley, chopped
- ½ cup walnuts, chopped
- Juice of ½ lemon
- 2 tablespoons olive oil
- Salt and black pepper to the taste

Lara Burns

Directions:

1. In a salad bowl, mix celery with raisins, walnuts, parsley, lemon juice, oiland black pepper and toss.
2. Divide into small cups and serve as a snack.

Dill and bell peppers snack bowl

Preparation time: 10 minutes

Cooking time: 20 minutes

Servings: 2

Ingredients:

- 2 tablespoons dill, chopped
- 1 yellow onion, chopped
- 1 pound multicolored bell peppers, cut into halves, seeded and cut into thin strips
- 3 tablespoons extra virgin olive oil
- 2 and ½ tablespoons white vinegar
- Black pepper to the taste

Directions:

1. In a salad bowl, mix bell peppers with onion, dill, pepper, oiland vinegar and toss to coat.
2. Divide into small bowls and serve as a snack.

Spicy pumpkin seeds bowl

Preparation time: 10 minutes

Cooking time: 20 minutes

Servings: 2

Ingredients:

- ½ tablespoon chili powder
- ½ teaspoon cayenne pepper
- 2 cups pumpkin seeds

- 2 teaspoons lime juice

Directions:

1. Spread pumpkin seeds on a lined baking sheet.
2. Add lime juice, cayenne and chili powderand toss well.
3. Put it in the oven and roast at 275 degrees F for 20 minutes.
4. Divide into small bowls and serve as a snack.

Apple and pecan bowls

Preparation time: 10 minutes

Cooking time: 20 minutes

Servings: 2

Ingredients: 4 portions

- 4 big apples, cored, peeled and cubed
- 2 teaspoons lemon juice
- ¼ cup pecans, chopped

Directions:

1. In a bowl, mix apples with lemon juiceand pecans and toss.
2. Divide into small bowls and serve as a snack.

Zucchini bowls

Preparation time: 10 minutes

Cooking time: 20 minutes

Servings: 2

Ingredients:

- Cooking spray
- ½ cup dill, chopped
- 1 egg
- ½ cup whole wheat flour
- Black pepper to the taste

- 1 yellow onion, chopped
- 2 garlic cloves, minced
- 3 zucchinis, grated

Directions:

1. In a bowl, mix zucchinis with garlic, onion, flour, pepper, eggand dill and stir well.
2. Shape the mix into 12 portions with the help of small bowls and arrange them on a lined baking sheet.
3. Grease them with some cooking spray and bake at 400 degrees F for 20 minutes, flipping them halfway.
4. Serve at room temperature as snacks.

Cheesy mushrooms

Preparation time: 10 minutes

Cooking time: 20 minutes

Servings: 2

Ingredients:

- 20 white mushroom caps
- 1 garlic clove, minced
- 3 tablespoons parsley, chopped
- 2 yellow onions, chopped
- Black pepper to the taste
- ½ cup low-fat parmesan, grated
- ¼ cup low-fat mozzarella, grated
- A drizzle of olive oil
- 2 tablespoons non-fat yogurt

Directions:

1. Heat up a pan with some oil over medium heat, add garlic and onion, stir, cook for 10 minutes and transfer to a bowl.
2. Add black pepper, garlic, parsley, mozzarella, parmesan and yogurt, stir well, stuff the mushroom caps with the mix.

3. Arrange them on a lined baking sheet and bake in the oven at 400 degrees F for 20 minutes.
4. Serve them as an appetizer.

Shrimp muffins

Preparation time: 10 minutes

Cooking time: 20 minutes

Servings: 2

Ingredients: 6 portions

- 1 spaghetti squash, peeled and halved
- 2 tablespoons avocado mayonnaise
- 1 cup low-fat mozzarella cheese, shredded
- 8 ounces shrimp, peeled, cooked and chopped
- 1 and ½ cups almond flour
- 1 teaspoon parsley, dried
- 1 garlic clove, minced
- Black pepper to the taste
- Cooking spray

Directions:

1. Arrange the squash on a lined baking sheet.
2. Insert in the oven at 375 degrees F and bake for 30 minutes.
3. Scrape squash flesh into a bowl and add pepper, parsley flakes, flour, shrimp, mayoand mozzarella and stir well.
4. Divide this mix into a muffin tray greased with cooking spray.
5. Bake in the oven at 375 degrees F for 15 minutes.
6. Serve them cold as a snack.

Mozzarella cauliflower bars

Preparation time: 10 minutes

227

Cooking time: 20 minutes

Servings: 2

Ingredients: 12 portions

- 1 big cauliflower head, riced
- ½ cup low-fat mozzarella cheese, shredded
- ¼ cup egg whites
- 1 teaspoon Italian seasoning
- Black pepper to the taste

Directions:

1. Spread the riced cauliflower on a lined baking sheet and cook in the oven at 375 degrees F for 20 minutes.
2. Transfer to a bowl, add black pepper, cheese, seasoning and egg whites.
3. Stir well, spread into a rectangle pan and press well on the bottom.
4. Introduce in the oven at 375 degrees F and bake for 20 minutes.
5. Let it cool and cut into 12 bars
6. Serve at room temperature as a snack.

Cinnamon apple chips

Preparation time: 10 minutes

Cooking time: 20 minutes

Servings: 2

Ingredients: 4 portions

- Cooking spray
- 2 teaspoons cinnamon powder
- 2 apples, cored and thinly sliced

Directions:

1. Arrange apple slices on a lined baking sheet, spray them with cooking oiland sprinkle cinnamon on it.
2. Put it in the oven and bake at 300 degrees F for 2 hours.

3. Divide into bowls and serve as a snack.

Vegetable and nuts bread loaf

Preparation time: 10 minutes

Cooking time: 20 minutes

Servings: 2

Ingredients: 1 loaf

- 175g (6oz) mushrooms, finely chopped
- 100g (3½ oz) haricot beans
- 100g (3½ oz) walnuts, finely chopped
- 100g (3½ oz) peanuts, finely chopped
- 1 carrot, finely chopped
- 3 sticks celery, finely chopped
- 1 bird's-eye chilli, finely chopped
- 1 red onion, finely chopped
- 1 egg, beaten
- 2 cloves of garlic, chopped
- 2 tablespoons olive oil
- 2 teaspoons turmeric powder
- 2 tablespoons soy sauce
- 4 tablespoons fresh parsley, chopped
- 100mls (3½ fl oz) water
- 60mls (2fl oz) red wine

Directions:

1. Heat the oil in a pan and add the garlic, chili, carrot, celery, onion, mushrooms and turmeric.
2. Cook for 5 minutes.
3. Place the haricot beans in a bowl and stir in the nuts, vegetables, soy sauce, egg, parsley, red wine and water.
4. Grease and line a large loaf tin with greaseproof paper.
5. Let it stand for 10 minutes then turn onto a serving plate.

Mushroom and Tofu Scramble

Preparation time: 10 minutes

Cooking time: 20 minutes

Servings: 2

Ingredients:

- 7 ounces of extra firm tofu
- 2 teaspoon turmeric powder
- 1 teaspoon black pepper
- ounce of kale, roughly chopped
- 2 teaspoons extra virgin olive oil
- ounce of red onion, thinly sliced
- 1 Thai chili, thinly sliced
- 100g mushrooms, thinly sliced
- 4 tablespoons parsley, finely chopped

Directions:

1. Wrap the tofu in paper towels and place something heavy on top to help it drain.
2. Mix the turmeric with a little water until you achieve a light paste.
3. Steam the kale for 2 to 3 minutes.
4. Heat the olive oil in a frying pan over medium heat until hot but not smoking; add the onion, chili and mushrooms and fry for 2 to 3 minutes until they have started to brown and soften.
5. Crumble the tofu into bite-size pieces and add to the pan; pour the turmeric paste over the tofu and mix thoroughly.
6. Add the black pepper and stir.
7. Cook over medium heat for 2 to 3 minutes so the spices are cooked through, and the tofu has started to brown.
8. Add the kale and continue to cook over medium heat for another minute.
9. Finally, add the parsley, mix well and serve.

Nutrition:

123 calories

Apple Pancakes with Blackcurrant Compote

Preparation time: 10 minutes

Cooking time: 20 minutes

Servings: 2

Ingredients:

- 4 ounce of porridge oats
- ounce of plain flour
- 1 tablespoon caster sugar
- ½ teaspoon baking powder
- 1 large green apple, peeled, cored, and cut into small pieces
- 150ml semi-skimmed milk
- I large egg white
- 1 teaspoon light olive oil.
- For the compote:
- an ounce of blackcurrants washed and stalked removed.
- 1 tablespoon caster sugar
- 2 tablespoon water.

Directions:

1. Make the compote first. Place the blackcurrants, sugar and water in a small pan. Bring to a simmer and cook for 10-15 minutes.
2. Place the Oats, flour, baking powder and caster sugar in a large bowl and mix properly.
3. Stir the apple into the powder mixture and then whisk in the milk a little at a time until you have a smooth mixture.
4. Whisk the egg white to a stiff peak and then fold into the pancake batter.
5. Heat ½ teaspoon olive oil in a non-stick frying pan on medium heat and pour ½ of the batter. Reduce heat and allow the

pancake to cook properly, flip to the other side with a spatula. Cook both sides until golden brown. Remove and repeat to make 2 pancakes.

6. Serve the pancakes with the blackcurrant compote drizzled over.

Nutrition:

123 calories

Sirtfood Mushroom Scramble Eggs

Preparation time: 10 minutes

Cooking time: 20 minutes

Servings: 1

Ingredients:

- 2 medium eggs
- I teaspoon turmeric
- 1 ounce of kale, roughly chopped
- 1 teaspoon extra virgin olive oil
- 1/2 chili, thinly sliced
- 0.5 ounce of red onions
- Parsley, thinly chopped
- A handful of button mushrooms, thinly sliced

Directions:

1. Steam the kale for 2-3 minutes.
2. Mix the turmeric powder with water to form a light paste.
3. Break into a bowl and whisk, add the turmeric paste, parsley and mix properly.
4. Heat the olive oil in a non-stick frying pan over medium heat and fry the onion, chili and mushroom until they have started to brown and soften.
5. Add the steamed kale to the mixture in the frying pan and stir.
6. Pour the egg mixture into the frying pan and stir.

7. Reduce the heat and allow the egg to cook and stir.

Nutrition:

Calories 156

Protein 54.

Matcha Green Juice

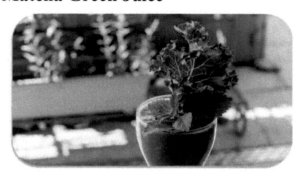

Preparation time: 10 minutes

Cooking time: 0 minutes

Total time: 10 minutes

Servings: 2

Ingredients:

- 5 ounces fresh kale
- 2 ounces fresh arugula
- ¼ cup fresh parsley
- 4 celery stalks
- 1 green apple, cored and chopped
- 1 (1-inch) piece fresh ginger, peeled
- 1 lemon, peeled
- ½ teaspoon matcha green tea

Directions:

1. Add all ingredients into a juicer
2. and extract the juice according to the manufacturer's method.
3. Pour into 2 glasses and serve immediately.

Nutrition:

Calories 113

Celery Juice

Preparation time: 10 minutes

Cooking time: 0 minutes

Servings: 2

Ingredients:

- 8 celery stalks with leaves
- 2 tablespoons fresh ginger, peeled
- 1 lemon, peeled
- ½ cup of filtered water
- Pinch of salt

Instructions

1. Place all the ingredients in a blender and pulse until well combined.
2. Through a fine mesh strainer, strain the juice and transfer into 2 glasses.
3. Serve immediately.

Nutrition:

Calories 32

Kale & Orange Juice

Preparation time: 10 minutes

Cooking time: 0 minutes

Servings: 2

Ingredients:

- 5 large oranges, peeled
- 2 bunches fresh kale

Directions:

1. Add all ingredients into a juicer
2. And extract the juice according to the manufacturer's method.
3. Pour into 2 glasses and serve immediately.

Nutrition:

Calories 315

Cucumber Juice

Preparation time: 10 minutes

Cooking time: 0 minutes

Servings: 2

Ingredients:

- 3 large apples, cored and sliced
- 2 large cucumbers, sliced
- 4 celery stalks
- 1 (1-inch) piece fresh ginger, peeled
- 1 lemon, peeled

Directions:

1. Add all ingredients into a juicer
2. And extract the juice according to the manufacturer's method.
3. Pour into 2 glasses and serve immediately.

Nutrition:

Calories 230.

Fluffy Blueberry Pancakes

Preparation time: 5 minutes

Cooking time: 15 minutes

Servings: 2

Ingredients:

- 1 egg
- 2 oz. self-raising flour
- 1 oz. buckwheat flour
- 1/3 cup skimmed milk
- 1 cup blueberries
- 2 tsp honey

Directions:

1. Mix the flours in a bowl, add the yolk and a bit of mix in a very thick batter. Keep adding the milk bit by bit to avoid lumps.
2. In another bowl, beat the egg white until stiff and then mix it carefully to the batter.
3. Put enough batter to make a 5-inch round pancake to cook 2 minutes per side until done. Repeat until all the pancakes are ready.
4. Put 1 tsp. Honey and ½ cup blueberries on top of each serving.

Nutrition:

Calories: 272, Fat: 4.3g, Carbohydrate: 26.8g, Protein: 23.6g

Banana Strawberry Smoothie

Preparation time: 5 minutes

Servings: 1

Ingredients:

- 1 cup strawberries
- ½ banana
- ½ cup almond milk, unsweetened
- ½ tsp cocoa powder
- 3 cubes ice (optional)

Directions:

1. Blend all ingredients together and serve immediately.

Nutrition: Calories: 92kcal, Fat: 1.3g, Carbohydrate: 12.8g, Protein: 3.6g

Vanilla Parfait with Berries

Preparation time: 5 minutes

Cooking time: 0 minutes

Servings: 1

Ingredients:

- 4 oz. Greek yogurt
- 1 tsp honey or maple syrup
- 1 cup mixed berries, frozen is perfect
- 1 tbsp. buckwheat granola
- ½ tsp Vanilla extract

Directions:

1. Mix yogurt, vanilla extract, and honey. Alternate yogurt and berries in a jar and top with granola.
2. Frozen berries are perfect if the parfait is made in advance because they release their juices in the yogurt.

Nutrition: Calories: 318, Fat: 5.4g, Carbohydrate: 22.8g, Protein: 21.9g

Blueberry Smoothie

Preparation time: 5 minutes

Servings: 1

Ingredients:

- 1 cup blueberries
- ½ banana
- ½ cup orange juice
- 3 cubes ice (optional)

Directions:

1. Blend all ingredients together and serve immediately.

Nutrition: Calories: 87, Fat: 1.1g, Carbohydrate: 11.8g, Protein: 1.6g

Overnight Oats with Strawberries and Chocolate

Preparation time: 5 minutes + 8h

Cooking time: 0 minutes

Servings: 2

Ingredients:

- 2 oz. rolled oats
- 4 oz. almond milk, unsweetened
- 2 tbsp. plain yogurt
- 1 cup strawberries
- 1 tsp honey
- 1 square 85% chocolate

Directions:

1. Mix the oats and the milk and leave overnight.
2. In the morning, top the jar with yogurt, honey, strawberries, and chocolate cut into small pieces.
3. It can be prepared in advance and left up to 3 days in the fridge.

Nutrition:

Calories: 258, Fat: 3.3g, Carbohydrate: 29.8g, Protein: 13.6g

Chocolate Mousse

Preparation time: 5 minutes

Servings: 1

Ingredients:

- ½ avocado
- 1 tsp cocoa powder
- 1 tsp honey

Directions:

1. Blend all ingredients together and serve immediately.

Nutrition: Calories: 87, Fat: 1.1g, Carbohydrate: 11.8g, Protein: 1.6g

Banana Vanilla Pancake

Preparation time: 10 minutes

Cooking time: 15 minutes

Servings: 2

Ingredients:

- 1 Egg
- 1 Egg White
- 1 Banana
- 2 tsp honey
- 1 cup Rolled Oats
- ¼ tsp Baking Powder
- A pinch of salt
- 1 tsp Vanilla extract
- ½ cup almond milk, unsweetened

Directions:

1. Put half banana, eggs, oats, vanilla, baking powder, salt and almond milk in a blender and blend until smooth.
2. Heat a skillet and, when hot but batter in to form pancakes.
3. Top with honey and the other half banana.

Nutrition: Calories: 232, Fat: 5.3g, Carbohydrate: 22.8g, Protein: 18.6g

Arugula Salad with Turkey and Italian Dressing

Preparation time: 5 minutes

Cooking time: 30 minutes

Servings: 2

Ingredients:

- 8oz. turkey breast
- 1 cup arugula
- 1 cup lettuce
- 2 tsp. Dijon mustard

- 1 tbsp. cumin
- 1/2 cup celery, finely diced
- 2 tsp. oregano
- 1/4 cup scallions, sliced
- 2 tsp. extra virgin olive oil
- Salt and pepper to taste

Directions:

1. Grill the turkey and shred it. Set aside.
2. Mix lettuce and arugula on a plate. Evenly distribute shredded turkey, celery, and scallions.
3. In a small bowl mix all dressing ingredients mustard, oil, lemon juice, oregano, salt and pepper and pour it over the salad just before serving.

Nutrition: Calories: 165 kcal, Fat: 2.9g, Carbohydrate: 13.6g, Protein: 26.1g

Lemon Ginger Shrimp Salad

Preparation time: 15 minutes

Cooking time: 5 minutes

Servings: 2

Ingredients:

- 1 cup chicory leaves
- ½ cup arugula
- ½ cup baby spinach
- 2 tsp. of extra virgin olive oil
- 6 walnuts, chopped
- 1 avocado-peeled, stoned and sliced
- Juice of ½ lemon
- 8 oz. shrimps
- 1 pinch chili

Directions:

1. Mix chicory, baby spinach, and arugula and put them on a large plate.
2. Heat a skillet on medium-high temperature, put 1 tbsp. oil and cook shrimps

with garlic, chili, salt, and pepper until they are not transparent anymore (5 minutes)
3. Blend avocado with oil, lemon juice with a pinch of salt and pepper and distribute the dressing on top.
4. Chop the walnuts, put them on the plate as last ingredient and serve.

Nutrition: Calories: 353, Fat: 4.8g, Carbohydrate: 28.1g, Protein: 28.3g

Asian Beef Salad

Preparation time: 15 minutes

Cooking time: 8 minutes

Servings: 2

Ingredients:

- 3 tsp. extra virgin olive oil
- 8 0z. sirloin steaks
- ½ red onion, finely sliced
- ½ cucumber, sliced
- ½ cup cherry tomatoes halved
- 2 cups lettuce
- 1 handful parsley
- 1 tbsp. soy sauce
- ½ bird's eye chili
- 3 tbsp. lemon juice

Directions:

1. Crush the garlic, mix it with finely sliced chili and parsley, 2 tsp olive oil and soy sauce. This will be dressing.
2. Prepare the salad in a bowl placing lettuce on the bottom, then onion, cherry tomatoes and cucumber.
3. Heat a skillet until very hot. Brush the steaks with remaining oil, season them with salt and pepper and cook them to your taste. Transfer the steaks onto a

cutting board for 5 minutes before slicing.

4. Drizzle the dressing on the salad and mix well. Place steak slices on top and serve.

Nutrition: Calories 262, Total Fat 12 g, Total Carbs 15.2 g Protein 25.2 g

Avocado Mayo Medley

Preparation time: 5 minutes

Cooking time: 0 minutes

Servings: 3

Ingredients:

- 1 medium avocado, cut into chunks
- ½ teaspoon ground cayenne pepper
- 2 tablespoons fresh cilantro
- ¼ cup olive oil
- ½ cup mayo, low fat and low sodium

Directions:

1. Take a food processor and add avocado, cayenne pepper, lime juice, salt and cilantro.
2. Mix until smooth.
3. Slowly incorporate olive oil, add 1 tablespoon at a time and keep processing between additions.
4. Store and use as needed!

Nutrition:

- Calories: 231
- Fat: 20g
- Carbohydrates: 5g
- Protein: 3g

Amazing Garlic Aioli

Preparation time: 5 minutes

Cooking time: 0 minutes

Servings: 3

Ingredients:

- ½ cup mayonnaise, low fat and low sodium
- 2 garlic cloves, minced
- Juice of 1 lemon
- 1 tablespoon fresh-flat leaf Italian parsley, chopped
- 1 teaspoon chives, chopped
- Salt and pepper to taste

Directions:

1. Add mayonnaise, garlic, parsley, lemon juice, chives and season with salt and pepper.
2. Blend until combined well.
3. Pour into refrigerator and chill for 30 minutes.
4. Serve and use as needed!

Nutrition:

Calories: 813

Fat: 88g

Carbohydrates: 9g

Protein: 2g

Easy Seed Crackers

Preparation time: 10 minutes

Cooking Time: 60 minutes

Ingredients:

- 1 cup boiling water
- 1/3 cup chia seeds
- 1/3 cup sesame seeds
- 1/3 cup pumpkin seeds
- 1/3 cup Flaxseeds
- 1/3 cup sunflower seeds
- 1 tablespoon Psyllium powder
- 1 cup almond flour

235

- 1 teaspoon salt
- ¼ cup coconut oil, melted

Directions:

1. Preheat your oven to 300 degrees F.
2. Line a cookie sheet with parchment paper and keep it on the side.
3. Add listed ingredients (except coconut oil and water) to food processor and pulse until ground.
4. Transfer to a large mixing bowl and pour melted coconut oil and boiling water, mix.
5. Transfer mix to prepared sheet and spread into a thin layer.
6. Cut dough into crackers and bake for 60 minutes.
7. Cool and serve.
8. Enjoy!

Nutrition:

- Total Carbs: 10.6g
- Fiber: 3g
- Protein: 5g
- Fat: 14.6g

Hearty Almond Crackers

Preparation time: 10 minutes

Cooking Time: 20 minutes

Ingredients:

- 1 cup almond flour
- ¼ teaspoon baking soda
- 1/8 teaspoon black pepper
- 3 tablespoons sesame seeds
- 1 egg, beaten
- Salt and pepper to taste

Directions:

1. Preheat your oven to 350 degrees F.

2. Line two baking sheets with parchment paper and keep them on the side.
3. Divide dough into two balls.
4. Roll out the dough between two pieces of parchment paper.
5. Cut into crackers and transfer them to prepared baking sheet.
6. Bake for 15-20 minutes.
7. Repeat until all the dough has been used up.
8. Leave crackers to cool and serve.
9. Enjoy!

Nutrition:

Total Carbs: 8g

Fiber: 2g

Protein: 9g

Fat: 28g

Black Bean Salsa

Preparation time: 5 minutes

Cooking time: 0 minutes

Servings: 3

Ingredients:

- 1 tablespoon coconut aminos
- ½ teaspoon cumin, ground
- 1 cup canned black beans, no salt
- 1 cup salsa
- 6 cups romaine lettuce, torn
- ½ cup avocado, peeled, pitted and cubed

Directions:

1. Take a bowl and add beans, alongside other ingredients.
2. Toss well and serve.
3. Enjoy!

Nutrition:

Calories: 181

Fat: 5g

Carbohydrates: 14g

Protein: 7g

Corn Spread

Preparation time: 5 minutes

Cooking time: 0 minutes

Servings: 3

Ingredients:

- 30 ounce canned corn, drained
- 2 green onions, chopped
- ½ cup coconut cream
- 1 jalapeno, chopped
- ½ teaspoon chili powder

Directions:

1. Take a pan and add corn, green onions, jalapeno, chili powder, stir well.
2. Bring to a simmer over medium heat and cook for 10 minutes.
3. Let it chill and add coconut cream.
4. Stir well.
5. Serve and enjoy!

Nutrition:

Calories: 192

Fat: 5g

Carbohydrates: 11g

Protein: 8g

Moroccan Leeks Snack

Preparation time: 5 minutes

Cooking time: 0 minutes

Servings: 3

Ingredients:

- 1 bunch radish, sliced
- 3 cups leeks, chopped
- 1 ½ cups olives, pitted and sliced
- Pinch turmeric powder
- 2 tablespoons essential olive oil
- 1 cup cilantro, chopped

Directions:

1. Take a bowl and mix in radishes, leeks, olives and cilantro.
2. Mix well.
3. Season with pepper, oil, turmeric and toss well.
4. Serve and enjoy!

Nutrition:

Calories: 120

Fat: 1g

Carbohydrates: 1g

Protein: 6g

The Bell Pepper Fiesta

Preparation time: 5 minutes

Cooking time: 0 minutes

Servings: 3

Ingredients:

- 2 tablespoons dill, chopped
- 1 yellow onion, chopped
- 1 pound multicolored peppers, cut, halved, seeded and cut into thin strips
- 3 tablespoons organic olive oil
- 2 ½ tablespoons white wine vinegar
- Black pepper to taste

Directions:

1. Take a bowl and mix in sweet pepper, onion, dill, pepper, oil, vinegar and toss well.
2. Divide between bowls and serve.
3. Enjoy!

Nutrition:

Calories: 120

Fat: 3g

Carbohydrates: 1g

Protein: 6g

Spiced Up Pumpkin Seeds Bowls

Preparation time: 5 minutes

Cooking time: 30 minutes

Servings: 3

Ingredients:

- ½ tablespoon chili powder
- ½ teaspoon cayenne
- 2 cups pumpkin seeds
- 2 teaspoons lime juice

Directions:

1. Spread pumpkin seeds over lined baking sheet, add lime juice, cayenne and chili powder.
2. Toss well.
3. Preheat your oven to 275 degrees F.
4. Roast in your oven for 20 minutes and transfer to small bowls.
5. Serve and enjoy!

Nutrition:

- Calories: 170
- Fat: 3g
- Carbohydrates: 10g
- Protein: 6g

Cauliflower Bars

Preparation time: 5 minutes

Cooking time: 30 minutes

Servings: 3

Ingredients:

- 1 cauliflower head, riced
- 12 cup low-fat mozzarella cheese, shredded
- ¼ cup egg whites
- 1 teaspoon Italian dressing, low fat
- Pepper to taste

Directions:

1. Spread cauliflower rice over lined baking sheet.
2. Preheat your oven to 375 degrees F.
3. Roast for 20 minutes.
4. Transfer to bowl and spread pepper, cheese, seasoning, egg whites.
5. And stir well.
6. Spread in a rectangular pan and press.
7. Transfer to oven and cook for 20 minutes more.
8. Serve and enjoy!

Nutrition:

Calories: 140

Fat: 2g

Carbohydrates: 6g

Protein: 6g

Green Juice Recipe

Preparation time: 10 Minutes

Cooking Time: 0 Minutes

Servings 2

Ingredients:

- 1 large handful of rockets
- Two large handfuls of kale
- ½ medium green apple
- Juice of ½ lemon
- ½ level teaspoon of matcha

Directions:

1. Mix the greens well and juice them to get about 50 ml of juice.
2. Juice the apple and the celeryand then peel the lemon and juice it by hand.
3. Pour a little of the juice in a glass, add matcha powderand then stir vigorously. Once it has dissolved, pour it back on the juiceand stir it in. Add some water if the blend is a little too strong for you and serve.

Nutrition: calories 302, fat 8.5, fiber 9.8, carbs 21.8, protein 11.3

Matcha Green Tea Smoothie

Preparation time: 10 Minutes

Cooking Time: 0 Minutes

Servings 2

Ingredients:

- 2 bananas
- 2 tsp Matcha green tea powder
- 1/2 tsp vanilla bean paste or scraped from a vanilla bean pod
- 1 ½ cups milk
- 4-5 ice cubes
- 2 tsp honey

Directions:

1. Add all ingredients except the Matcha to a blender. Blend until smooth. Sprinkle in the Matcha tea powder, stir well or blend a few seconds more or add cooled green tea).

Nutrition: calories 238, fat 9, fiber 5.6, carbs 14.4, protein 8.4

Fruity Granola Bars

Preparation time: 5 minutes

Cooking time: 30 minutes

Servings: 3

Ingredients:

- ¾ cup packed brown sugar
- ½ cup honey
- ¼ cup water
- 1 teaspoon salt
- ½ cup cocoa butter
- 3 cups rolled oats
- 1 cup walnuts, chopped
- 1 cup ground buckwheat
- ¼ cup sesame seeds
- ½ cup dried strawberries or mixed fruits
- ½ cup raisins
- ½ cup Medjool dates, chopped

Directions:

1. In a large pan, combine sugar, cocoa butter, honey, water and salt. Bring to a simmer and cook for 5 minutes.
2. Score deeply into bars roughly 2" wide by 4" tall.
3. Allow to cool for 30 minutes before breaking or cutting along score lines. Store in an airtight container.

Nutrition: calories 188, fat 12.8, fiber 9.2, carbs 22.2, protein 16.8

Cardamom Granola Bars

Preparation time: 5 minutes

Cooking time: 30 minutes

Servings: 3

Ingredients:

- 2 cups rolled oats
- ½ cup raisins
- ½ cup walnuts, chopped and toasted
- 1 ½ teaspoons ground cardamom
- 6 tablespoons cocoa butter
- 1/3 cup packed brown sugar
- 3 tablespoons honey
- Coconut oil, for greasing pan

Directions:

1. Preheat oven to 350 degrees F.
2. Line a 9-inch square pan with foil, extending the foil over the sides. Grease the foil with coconut oil.
3. Mix the oats, raisins, walnuts and cardamom in a large bowl.
4. Heat the cocoa butter, brown sugar and honey in a saucepan until the butter melts and begins to bubble.
5. Bake for 30 minutes or until the top is golden brown.
6. Allow to cool for 30 minutes. Using the foil, lift the granola out of the pan and place on cutting board.
7. Cut into 18 bars.

Nutrition: calories 232, fat 5.5, fiber 7.5, carbs 20.9, protein 16.8

Coconut Brownie Bites

Preparation time: 5 minutes

Cooking time: 40 minutes

Servings: 3

Ingredients:

- ¼ cup unsweetened cocoa powder
- ¼ cup unsweetened desiccated or shredded coconut

Directions:

1. Place everything in a food processor and blend until well combined.
2. Roll into 1" balls.
3. Roll balls in coconut until well-covered and place on wax paper lined baking sheet.
4. Freeze for 30 minutes or refrigerate for up to 2 hours.

Nutrition: calories 282, fat 11.5, fiber 5.5, carbs 17.9, protein 14.8

Kale & Fruit Juice

Preparation Time: 10 minutes

Cooking Time: 10 minutes

Servings: 2

Ingredients:

- 2 large green apples, cored and sliced
- Large pears, cored and sliced
- 3 cups fresh kale leaves
- 3 celery stalks
- 1 lemon, peeled

Directions:

1. Add all ingredients into a juicer
2. and extract the juice according to the manufacturer's method.
3. Pour into 2 glasses and serve immediately.

Nutrition:

Calories 293, Fat 0.8 g, Carbs 74.6 g, Protein 4.6 g, Sodium 69 mg

Kale, Carrot, & Grapefruit Juice

Preparation Time: 10 minutes

Cooking Time: 10 minutes

Servings: 2

Ingredients:

- 3 cups fresh kale
- 2 large Granny Smith apples, cored and sliced
- 2 medium carrots, peeled and chopped
- 2 medium grapefruit, peeled
- 1 teaspoon fresh lemon juice

Directions:

1. Add all ingredients into a juicer.
2. and extract the juice according to the manufacturer's method.
3. Pour into 2 glasses and serve immediately.

Nutrition: Calories 232 g, Fat 0.6g, Carbs 57.7g, Protein 4.9g, Sodium 88mg

Buckwheat Granola

Preparation Time: 15 minutes

Cooking Time: 30 minutes

Servings: 10

Ingredients:

- 2 cups raw buckwheat groats
- ¾ cup pumpkin seeds
- ¾ cup almonds, chopped
- 1 cup unsweetened coconut flakes
- 1 teaspoon ground cinnamon
- 1 teaspoon ground ginger
- 1 ripe banana, peeled
- 2 tablespoons maple syrup
- 2 tablespoons olive oil

Directions:

1. Preheat your oven to 350°F. In a bowl, place the buckwheat groats, coconut flakes, pumpkin seeds, almonds and spices and mix well.
2. In another bowl, add the banana and with a fork, mash well.
3. Add to the buckwheat mixture maple syrup and oil and mix until well combined.
4. Transfer the mixture onto the prepared baking sheet and spread in an even layer. Bake for about 25–30 minutes, stirring once halfway through.
5. Remove the baking sheet from oven and set aside to cool.

Nutrition: Calories 252, Fat 14.3 g, Carbs 27.6 g,

Apple Pancakes

Preparation Time: 15 minutes

Cooking Time: 24 minutes

Servings: 6

Ingredients:

- ½ cup buckwheat flour
- 2 tablespoons coconut sugar
- 1 teaspoon baking powder
- ½ teaspoon ground cinnamon
- 1/3 cup unsweetened almond milk
- 1 egg, beaten lightly
- 2 granny smith apples, peeled, coredand grated

Directions:

1. In a bowl, place the flour, coconut sugarand cinnamonand mix well.
2. In another bowl, place the almond milk and egg and beat until well combined.
3. Now, place the flour mixture and mix until well combined.
4. Fold in the grated apples.
5. Heat a lightly greased non-stick wok over medium-high heat.

6. Add desired amount of mixture and with a spoon, spread into an even layer.
7. Cook for 1–2 minutes on each side.
8. Repeat with the remaining mixture.
9. Serve warm with the drizzling of honey.

Nutrition: Calories 93, Fat 21g, Carbs 22g, Protein 25g, Sodium 23mg

Matcha Pancakes

Preparation Time: 15 minutes

Cooking Time: 24 minutes

Servings: 6

Ingredients:

- 2 tablespoons flax meal
- 5 tablespoons warm water
- 1 cup spelt flour
- 1 cup buckwheat flour
- 1 tablespoon matcha powder
- 1 tablespoon baking powder
- Pinch of salt
- ¾ cup unsweetened almond milk
- 1 tablespoon olive oil
- 1/3 cup raw honey

Directions:

1. In a bowl, add the flax meal and warm water and mix well. Set aside for about 5 minutes.
2. In another bowl, place the flours, matcha powder, baking powder and salt and mix well.
3. In the bowl of flax meal mixture, place the almond milk, oil and vanilla extract and beat until well combined.
4. Now, place the flour mixture and mix until a smooth textured mixture is formed.

5. Heat a lightly greased non-stick wok over medium-high heat.
6. Add desired amount of mixture and with a spoon, spread into an even layer.
7. Cook for about 2–3 minutes.
8. Carefully, flip the side and cook for about 1 minute.
9. Repeat with the remaining mixture.
10. Serve warm with the drizzling of honey.

Nutrition: Calories 232, Fat 4.6g, Carbs 46.3 g

Smoked Salmon & Kale Scramble

Preparation Time: 10 minutes

Cooking Time: 9 minutes

Servings: 3

Ingredients:

- 2 cups fresh kale, tough ribs removed and chopped finely
- 1 tablespoon coconut oil
- Ground black pepper, to taste
- ½ cup smoked salmon, crumbled
- 4 eggs, beaten

Directions:

1. In a wok, melt the coconut oil over high heat and cook the kale with black pepper for about 3–4 minutes.
2. Stir in the smoked salmon and reduce the heat to medium.
3. Add the eggs and cook for about 3–4 minutes, stirring frequently.
4. Serve immediately.

Nutrition: Calories 257, Fat 17g, Carbs 7.7g, Protein 19.3 g, Sodium 419 mg

Kale & Mushroom Frittata

Preparation Time: 15 minutes

Cooking Time: 30 minutes

Servings: 5

Ingredients:

- 8 eggs
- ½ cup unsweetened almond milk
- Salt and ground black pepper, to taste
- 1 tablespoon olive oil
- 1 onion, chopped
- 1 garlic clove, minced
- 1 cup fresh mushrooms, chopped
- 1½ cups fresh kale, tough ribs removed and chopped

Directions:

1. Preheat oven to 350°F.
2. In a large bowl, place the eggs, coconut milk, salt and black pepper.
3. and beat well. Set aside.
4. In a large ovenproof wok, heat the oil over medium heat.
5. and sauté the onion and garlic for about 3–4 minutes.
6. Add the squash, kale, bell pepper, salt and black pepper.
7. and cook for about 8–10 minutes.
8. Stir in the mushrooms and cook for about 3–4 minutes.
9. Add the kale and cook for about 5 minutes.
10. Place the egg mixture on top evenly.
11. and cook for about 4 minutes, without stirring.
12. Transfer the wok in the oven.
13. and bake for about 12–15 minutes or until desired doneness.
14. Remove from the oven.
15. and place the frittata side for about 3–5 minutes before serving.
16. Cut into desired sized wedges and serve.

Sirtfood Diet Cookbook

Nutrition: Calories 151, Fat 10.2g, Protein 10.3g, Sodium 156 mg

Kale, Apple, & Cranberry Salad

Preparation Time: 15 minutes

Cooking Time: 15 minutes

Servings: 4

Ingredients:

- 6 cups fresh baby kale
- 3 large apples, cored and sliced
- ¼ cup unsweetened dried cranberries
- ¼ cup almonds, sliced
- 2 tablespoons extra-virgin olive oil
- 1 tablespoon raw honey
- Salt and ground black pepper, to taste

Directions:

1. In a salad bowl, place all the ingredients and toss to coat well.
2. Serve immediately.

Nutrition: Calories 253. Fat 10.3g, Carbs 40.7g, Protein 4.7 g, Sodium 84mg

Arugula, Strawberry, & Orange Salad

Preparation Time: 15 minutes

Cooking Time: 15 minutes

Servings: 4

Ingredients:

- Salad
- 6 cups fresh baby arugula
- 1½ cups fresh strawberries, hulled and sliced
- 2 oranges, peeled and segmented
- Dressing
- 2 tablespoons fresh lemon juice

243

- 1 tablespoon raw honey
- 2 teaspoons extra-virgin olive oil
- 1 teaspoon Dijon mustard
- Salt and ground black pepper, to taste

Directions:

1. For salad: in a salad bowl, place all ingredients and mix.
2. For dressing: place all ingredients in another bowl and beat until well combined.
3. Place dressing on top of salad and toss to coat well.
4. Serve immediately.

Nutrition: Calories 107, Fat 2.9g, Carbs 20.6g,

Protein 2.1g, Sodium 63 mg

Beef & Kale Salad

Preparation Time: 15 minutes

Cooking Time: 8 minutes

Servings: 2

Ingredients:

- For Steak
- 2 teaspoons olive oil
- 2 (4-ounce) strip steaks
- Salt and ground black pepper, to taste
- Salad
- ¼ cup carrot, peeled and shredded
- ¼ cup cucumber, peeled, seededand sliced
- ¼ cup radish, sliced
- ¼ cup cherry tomatoes, halved
- 3 cups fresh kale, tough ribs removed and chopped
- For Dressing
- 1 tablespoon extra-virgin olive oil
- 1 tablespoon fresh lemon juice
- Salt and ground black pepper, to taste

Directions:

1. For steak: in a large heavy-bottomed wok.
2. Heat the oil over high heat.
3. Cook the steaks with salt and black pepper for about 3–4 minutes per side.
4. Transfer the steaks onto a cutting board for about 5 minutes before slicing.
5. For salad: place all ingredients in a salad bowl and mix.
6. For dressing: place all ingredients in another bowl and beat until well combined.
7. Cut the steaks into desired sized slices against the grain.
8. Place the salad onto each serving plate.
9. Top each plate with steak slices.
10. Drizzle with dressing and serve.

Nutrition: Calories 262, Fat 12g, Protein 25.2g, Sodium 506 mg

Salmon Burgers

Preparation Time: 20 minutes

Cooking Time: 15 minutes

Servings: 5

Ingredients:

- For Burgers
- 1 teaspoon olive oil
- 1 cup fresh kale, tough ribs removed and chopped
- 1/3 cup shallots, chopped finely
- Salt and ground black pepper, to taste
- 16 ounces skinless salmon fillets
- ¾ cup cooked quinoa
- 2 tablespoons Dijon mustard
- 1 large egg, beaten
- For Salad
- 2½ tablespoons olive oil

244

- 2½ tablespoons red wine vinegar
- Salt and ground black pepper, to taste
- 8 cups fresh baby arugula
- 2 cups cherry tomatoes, halved

Directions:

1. For burgers: in a large non-stick wok, heat the oil over medium heat and sauté the kale, shallots, salt and black pepper for about 4–5 minutes.
2. Remove from heat and transfer the kale mixture into a large bowl.
3. Set aside to cool slightly.
4. With a knife, chop 4 ounces of salmon and transfer into the bowl of kale mixture.
5. In a food processor, add the remaining salmon and pulse until finely chopped.
6. Transfer the finely chopped salmon into the bowl of kale mixture.
7. Then, add remaining ingredients and stir until fully combined.
8. Make 5 equal-sized patties from the mixture.
9. Heat a lightly greased large non-stick wok over medium heat and cook the patties for about 4–5 minutes per side.
10. For dressing: in a glass bowl, add the oil, vinegar, shallots, salt and black pepperand beat until well combined.
11. Add arugula and tomatoes and toss to coat well.
12. Divide the salad onto on serving plates and top each with 1 patty.
13. Serve immediately.

Nutrition: Calories 329, Fat 15.8g, Carbs 24g, Protein 24.9g, Sodium 177 mg

Chicken with Broccoli & Mushrooms

Preparation Time: 15 minutes

Cooking Time: 25 minutes

Servings: 6

Ingredients:

- 3 tablespoons olive oil
- 1-pound skinless, boneless chicken breast, cubed
- 1 medium onion, chopped
- 6 garlic cloves, minced
- 2 cups fresh mushrooms, sliced
- 16 ounces small broccoli florets
- ¼ cup water
- Salt and ground black pepper, to taste

Directions:

1. Heat the oil in a large wok over medium heat and cook the chicken cubes for about 4–5 minutes.
2. With a slotted spoon, transfer the chicken cubes onto a plate.
3. In the same wok, add the onion and sauté for about 4–5 minutes.
4. Add the mushrooms and cook for about 4–5 minutes.
5. Stir in the cooked chicken, broccoli and water and cook (covered) for about 8–10 minutes, stirring occasionally.
6. Stir in salt and black pepper and remove from heat.
7. Serve hot.

Nutrition: Calories 197, Fat 10.1 g, Carbs 8.5g; Protein20.1g, Sodium 82mg

Lemon Ricotta Cookies with Lemon Glaze

Preparation Time: 10 Minutes

Cooking Time: 15 Minutes

Servings: 10

Ingredients:

- 2 ½ cups all-purpose flour

Lara Burns

- 1 tsp. baking powder
- 1 tsp. salt
- 1 tbsp. unsalted butter softened
- 2 cups of sugar
- 2 eggs
- 1 teaspoon (15-ounces) container whole-milk ricotta cheese
- 3 tbsp. lemon juice
- zest of one lemon

Glaze:

- 11/2 cups powdered sugar
- 3 tbsp. lemon juice
- zest of one lemon

Directions:

1. Preheat the oven to 375 degrees f.
2. Prepare a medium bowl; combine the flour, baking powder and salt. Set-aside.
3. From the big bowl, blend the butter and the sugar. With an electric mixer, beat the sugar and butter until light and fluffy, about three minutes. Then add eggs one at a time, beating until incorporated.
4. Insert the ricotta cheese, lemon juice and lemon zest. Beat to blend. Stir in the dry ingredients.
5. Line two baking sheets with parchment paper. Spoon the dough (approximately 2 tablespoons of each cookie) on the prepared baking sheets.
6. Then bake for 15 minutes or until slightly golden at the borders. Remove from the oven and allow the cookies to remain on the baking sheet for about 20 minutes.
7. For Glaze: combine the powdered sugar, lemon juice and lemon zest in a small bowl and then stir until smooth. Spoon approximately 1/2-tsp on each

cookie and use of the back of the spoon to disperse lightly. Allow glaze to harden for approximately two hours. Pack the biscuits in a decorative jar.

Nutrition:

Calories: 360 Cal

Fat: 2.5 g

Carbs: 82.3 g

Fiber: 0.9 g

Protein: 4.5 g

Dark Chocolate Pretzel Cookies

Preparation Time: 20 Minutes

Cooking Time: 25 Minutes

Servings: 4

Ingredients:

- 1 cup yogurt
- 1/2 tsp. baking soda
- 1/4 teaspoon of salt
- 1/4 tsp. cinnamon
- 4 tbsp. butter (softened/0
- 1/3 cup brown sugar
- 1 egg
- 1/2 tsp. vanilla
- 1/2 cup dark chocolate chips
- 1/2 cup pretzels, chopped

Directions:

1. Preheat the oven to 350 degrees.
2. First, whisk together the butter, sugar, vanilla and egg in a medium mixing bowl.
3. In a separate bowl, place and stir together the salt, baking soda and flour.

4. Stir the bread mixture in, using all the wet components, along with the chocolate chips and pretzels until just blended.
5. Drop a large spoonful of dough on a baking sheet (unlined).
6. Bake for 15-17 minutes, or until the bottoms are somewhat all crispy.
7. Allow cooling on a wire rack.

Nutrition:

Calories: 392 Cal

Fat: 18.2 g

Carbs: 50.2 g

Fiber: 1 g

Protein: 9.1 g

Mascarpone Cheesecake with Almond Crust

Preparation Time: 5 Minutes

Cooking Time: 10 Minutes

Servings: 4

Ingredients:

Crust:

- 1/2 cup slivered almonds
- 8 tsp. -- or 2/3 cup graham cracker crumbs
- 2 tbsp. sugar
- 1 tbsp. salted butter melted

Filling:

- 1 (8-ounces) packages cream cheese, room temperature
- 1 (8-ounces) container mascarpone cheese, room temperature
- 3/4 cup sugar
- 1 tsp. fresh lemon juice (I needed to use imitation lemon-juice)

- 1 tsp. vanilla extract
- 2 large eggs, room temperature

Directions:

For the crust:

1. First, preheat oven to 350 degrees F. You will need a 9-inch pan (I had a throw off). Finely grind the almonds, cracker crumbs sugar in a food processor (I used my Magical Bullet). Then add the butter and process until moist crumbs form.
2. Press the almond mixture on the base of the prepared pan (maybe not on the edges of the pan). Bake the crust until its set and start to brown, about 1-2 minutes. Cool. Reduce the oven temperature to 325 degrees F.
3. For your filling: with an electric mixer, beat the cream cheese, mascarpone cheese and sugar in a large bowl until smooth, occasionally scraping down the sides of the jar using a rubber spatula. Beat in the lemon juice and vanilla. Add the eggs one at a time and beat until combined after each addition.
4. Pour the cheese mixture on the crust from the pan. Put the pan into a big skillet or Pyrex dish pour enough hot water to the roasting pan to come halfway up the sides of one's skillet. Bake until the middle of the filling moves slightly when the pan is gently shaken, about 1 hour (the dessert will get hard when it's cold). Transfer the cake to a stand; cool for 1 hour. Refrigerate until the cheesecake is cold, at least eight hours.
5. Topping: squeeze just a small thick cream in the microwave using a chopped Lindt dark chocolate - afterward, get a Ziplock baggie and cut out a hole at the corner, then pour the

melted chocolate into the baggie and used this to decorate the cake!

Nutrition:

Calories: 550 Cal

Fat: 40.7 g

Carbs: 36.9 g

Fiber: 3.5 g

Protein: 11.5 g

Home-made Ice Cream Drumsticks

Preparation Time: 20 Minutes

Cooking Time: 0 Minutes

Servings: 4

Ingredients:

- Vanilla ice cream
- Two Lindt hazelnut chunks
- Magical shell - out chocolate
- Sugar levels
- Nuts (I mixed crushed peppers and un-salted peanuts)
- Parchment paper

Directions:

1. Soften ice cream and mixing topping - I had two sliced Lindt hazelnut balls.
2. Fill underside of Magic shell with sugar and nuts and top with ice-cream.
3. Wrap parchment paper round cone and then fill cone over about 1.5 inches across the cap of the cone (the paper can help to carry its shape).
4. Sprinkle with magical nuts and shells.
5. Freeze for about 20 minutes before the ice cream is eaten.

Nutrition:

Calories: 419 Cal

Fat: 18.6 g

Carbs: 63.6 g

Fiber: 2.9 g

Protein: 5 g

Peach and Blueberry Pie

Preparation Time: 10 Minutes

Cooking Time: 40 Minutes

Servings: 16

Ingredients:

- 1 box of noodle dough
- Filling:
- 5 peaches, peeled and chopped (I used roasted peaches)
- 3 cups strawberries
- 3/4 cup sugar
- 1/4 cup bread
- Juice of 1/2 lemon
- 1 egg yolk, beaten

Directions:

1. Preheat oven to 400 degrees.
2. Place dough to a 9-inch pie plate
3. In a big bowl, combine tomatoes, sugar, bread and lemon juice, then toss to combine. Pour into the pie plate, mounding at the center.
4. Simply take some bread and then cut into bits, then put a pie shirt and put the dough in addition to pressing on edges.
5. Brush crust with egg wash then sprinkles with sugar.
6. Set onto a parchment paper-lined baking sheet.
7. Bake at 400 for about 20 minutes, until crust is browned at borders.
8. Turn oven down to 350, bake for another 40 minutes.
9. Remove and let sit at least 30 minutes.

10. Have with vanilla ice-cream.

Nutrition:

Calories: 80 Cal

Fat: 1.1 g

Carbs: 17.8 g

Fiber: 1.3 g

Protein: 1.1 g

Pear, Cranberry and Chocolate Crisp

Preparation Time: 15 Minutes

Cooking Time: 10 Minutes

Servings: 10

Ingredients:

- 1/2 cup flour
- 1/2 cup brown sugar
- 1 tsp. cinnamon
- 1/8 tsp. salt
- 3/4 cup yogurt
- 1/4 cup sliced peppers
- 1/3 cup butter, melted
- 1 teaspoon vanilla

Filling:

- 1 tbsp. brown sugar
- 1/4 cup dried cranberries
- 1 teaspoon of lemon juice
- Two handfuls of milk chocolate chips

Directions:

1. Preheat oven to 375.
2. Spray a casserole dish with a butter spray.
3. Put all of the topping ingredients: flour, sugar, cinnamon, salt, nuts, etc.
4. Butter a bowl and then mix. Set aside.
5. In a large bowl, combine the sugar, lemon juice, pears and cranberries.

6. Once is fully blended, move to the prepared baking dish.
7. Spread the topping evenly over the fruit.
8. Bake for about half an hour.
9. Disperse chocolate chips out at the top.
10. Cook for another 10 minutes.
11. Have with ice cream.

Nutrition:

Calories: 128 Cal

Fat: 6.6 g

Carbs: 15 g

Fiber: 0.7 g

Protein: 2 g

Crunchy Chocolate Chip Coconut Macadamia Nut Cookies

Preparation Time: 10 Minutes

Cooking Time: 10 Minutes

Servings: 10

Ingredients:

- 1 cup yogurt
- 1 cup yogurt
- 1/2 tsp. baking soda
- 1/2 tsp. salt
- 1 tbsp. of butter, softened
- 1 cup firmly packed brown sugar
- 1/2 cup sugar
- 1 large egg
- 1/2 cup semi-sweet chocolate chips
- 1/2 cup sweetened flaked coconut
- 1/2 cup coarsely chopped dry-roasted macadamia nuts
- 1/2 cup raisins

Directions:

1. Preheat the oven to 325°f.

2. In a little bowl, whisk together the flour, oats and baking soda and salt, then place aside.
3. In your mixer bowl, mix the butter/sugar/egg mix.
4. Mix in the flour/oats mix until just combined and stir into the chocolate chips, raisins, nuts and coconut.
5. Place outsized bits on a parchment-lined cookie sheet.
6. Bake for 1-3 minutes before biscuits are only barely golden brown.
7. Remove from the oven and then leave the cookie sheets to cool at least 10 minutes.

Nutrition:

Calories: 243 Cal

Fat: 12.6 g

Carbs: 30.3 g

Fiber: 1.5 g

Protein: 4.4 g

Ultimate Chocolate Chip Cookie N' Oreo Fudge Brownie Bar

Preparation Time: 15 Minutes

Cooking Time: 60 Minutes

Servings: 10

Ingredients:

- 1 cup (2 sticks) butter, softened
- 1 cup granulated sugar
- 3/4 cup light brown sugar
- 2 large eggs
- 1 tablespoon pure vanilla extract
- 2 ½ cups all-purpose flour
- 1 tsp. baking soda
- 1 tsp. lemon
- 2 cups (12 oz.) milk chocolate chips

- 1 package double-stuffed Oreo
- 1 family-size (9×1 3) brownie mixture
- 1/4 cup hot fudge topping

Directions:

1. Preheat oven to 350 degrees F.
2. First, cream the butter and sugars in a bowl using an electric mixer at medium speed for 35 minutes.
3. Add the vanilla and eggs and mix well to combine thoroughly. In a separate bowl, whisk together the salt, flour and baking soda then slowly incorporate it in the mixer until everything is combined.
4. Stir in chocolate chips.
5. Spread the cookie dough at the bottom of a 9×1-3 baking dish that is wrapped with wax paper and then coated with cooking spray.
6. Shirt with a coating of Oreos. Mix brownie mix, adding an optional 1/4 cup of hot fudge directly into the mixture.
7. Stir the brownie batter within the cookie-dough and Oreos.
8. Cover with a foil and bake it at 350 degrees F for 30 minutes.
9. Remove foil and continue baking for another 15 25 minutes.
10. Let cool before cutting on brownies. They may be gooey while warm but will also set up perfectly once chilled.

Nutrition:

Calories: 490 Cal

Fat: 21.9 g

Carbs: 69 g

Fiber: 1.5 g

Protein: 5.5 g

Radish green pesto

Preparation Time: 15 Minutes

Cooking Time: 60 Minutes

Servings: 10

Ingredients:

- 2 handfuls
- fresh radish leaf (from 1–2 bunch of radishes in organic quality)
- 1 garlic
- 30 g pine nuts (2 tbsp)
- 30 g parmesan (1 piece; 30% fat in dry matter)
- 100 ml olive oil
- salt
- pepper
- 1 tsp lemon juice

Directions:

1. Wash the radish leaves and shake them dry. Peel and chop the garlic.
2. Roast pine nuts in a hot pan without fat over medium heat for 3 minutes. Grate the Parmesan finely.
3. Puree the radish leaves, garlic, pine nuts and the oil with a hand blender. Mix in the Parmesan. Season with salt, pepper and lemon juice.

Watercress smoothie

Preparation Time: 15 Minutes

Cooking Time: 60 Minutes

Servings: 10

Ingredients:

- 150 g watercress
- 1 small onion
- ½ cucumber
- 1 tbsp lemon juice
- 200 ml mineral water
- salt
- pepper
- 4 tbsp crushed ice

Directions:

1. Wash and spin dry watercress; put some sheets aside for the garnish.
2. Peel the onion and cut it into small cubes. Wash the cucumber half, halve lengthways and cut the pulp into tiny cubes; Set aside 4 tablespoons of cucumber cubes.
3. Puree the remaining cucumber cubes with cress, onion cubes, lemon juice, mineral water and ice in a blender.
4. Season the smoothie with salt and pepper, pour into 2 glasses and sprinkle with cucumber cubes and cress leaves.

Melon and spinach juice with cinnamon

Preparation Time: 15 Minutes

Cooking Time: 60 Minutes

Servings: 10

Ingredients:

- 350 g small honeydew melon (0.5 small honeydew melons)
- 250 g young tender spinach leaves
- 1 PC cinnamon stick (approx. 1 cm)
- nutmeg

Directions:

1. Core the melon with a teaspoon. First cut the melon into wedges, then cut the pulp from the skin and roughly dice.
2. Clean the spinach and wash thoroughly in a bowl of water. Renew the water several times until it remains clear.

251

3. Using a small sharp knife, scrape thin strips off the cinnamon stick.
4. Squeeze the spinach lightly; Put back a leaflet and a small stem for the garnish as you like. Juice the rest with the melon in a juicer and pour it into a glass with ice cubes. Rub a little nutmeg over it, garnish with cinnamon and possibly with the spinach set aside and enjoy immediately.

Christmas cocktail - vegan eggnog

Ingredients:

- 1 cup cashew nuts
- 1 cup soy or almond milk
- 2-3 glasses of water
- about 5 pieces of dates (more if you like sweeter drinks)
- 2-3 scoops of brandy or whiskey
- 1 tablespoon lemon juice (optional, to taste)
- 1-2 teaspoons cinnamon
- ½ teaspoons ground anise
- ½ teaspoons ground ginger
- 2 pinches nutmeg
- pinch of salt
- Process

Directions:

1. Pour dates and cashews with boiling water and leave to soak for 20 minutes. Transfer the remaining ingredients to the blender dish and finally add the drained nuts and dates.
2. Mix thoroughly in a high-speed blender for a few minutes, until a thick and creamy cocktail without lumps is formed. If your blender can't do it, mix the cashews with water first and strain them with gauze.

3. Season the cocktail with more lemon juice and salt to taste and if you prefer sweeter drinks, add 2-3 pieces of dates. Serve it chilled with a pinch of cinnamon.

Orange and mandarin liqueur

Preparation Time: 15 Minutes

Cooking Time: 60 Minutes

Servings: 10

Ingredients:

- 2 large oranges
- 2 tangerines
- 1 small lemon
- 300 g white sugar candy
- 1 stick of vanilla
- 50 ml of orange juice
- 250 ml double grain

Directions:

1. Put the sugar candy in a bottle or a screw-top jar.
2. Pour the citrus into small pieces and remove the skin.
3. Pour in the orange juice.
4. Add the vanilla stick.
5. Baste with the double grain
6. Fill up to the top of the bottle if desired.
7. Close the bottle.
8. Shake daily until the sugar candy has dissolved.
9. After 2 - 3 weeks pour the liqueur through a sieve.
10. Pour it back into the bottle.

Cucumber-apple-banana shake

Preparation Time: 15 Minutes

Cooking Time: 60 Minutes

Servings: 10

Ingredients:

- 1 lemon
- 1 banana
- 4th sour apples (e.g. granny smith)
- 1 bunch parsley
- ½ cucumber
- mineral water to fill up
- 10 dice ice cubes

Directions:

1. Halve the lemon and squeeze out the juice. Peel and dice the banana. Clean, wash, quarter the apples, remove the core, dice the pulp. Mix the apples with the banana cubes and lemon juice.
2. Wash parsley, shake dry and chop. Clean, peel and halve the cucumber, coreand cut into bite-size pieces. Put 3 pieces of cucumber on 4 wooden skewers.
3. Puree the remaining pieces of cucumber with fruit, parsley and ice in a blender. Spread over 4 glasses, fill up with mineral water to the desired consistency and garnish with 1 cucumber skewer each.

Kefir avocado shake with herbs

Preparation Time: 15 Minutes

Cooking Time: 60 Minutes

Servings: 10

Ingredients:

- 2 stems dill
- 2 stems parsley
- straws of chives
- 1 avocado
- 1 tsp honey
- 1 splash lime juice
- 4 ice cubes
- 300 ml kefir chilled
- salt
- 1 pinch wasabi powder

Directions:

1. Spray the herbs, pat dry, pluck and cut roughly except for a few dill tips for the garnish.
2. Peel, halve, core and cut the avocado into pieces. Puree with the herbs, honey, lime juice, ice cubes and kefir in a blender until creamy.
3. Season the smoothie with salt and wasabi and pour into glasses. Serve garnished with dill tips.

Mandarin liqueur

Preparation Time: 15 Minutes

Cooking Time: 60 Minutes

Servings: 10

Ingredients:

- 2 large oranges
- 2 tangerines
- 1 small lemon
- 300 g white sugar candy
- 1 stick of vanilla
- 50 ml of orange juice
- 250 ml double grain

Directions:

1. Put the sugar candy in a bottle or a screw-top jar.
2. Pour the citrus into small pieces and remove the skin.
3. Pour in the orange juice.
4. Add the vanilla stick.

5. Baste with the double grain and fill up to the top of the bottle if desired.
6. Close the bottle.
7. Shake daily until the sugar candy has dissolved.
8. After 2 - 3 weeks pour the liqueur through a sieve and pour it back into the bottle.

Pear and lime marmalade

Ingredients: for 1.5 l jam

- 3-4 untreated limes
- 1 kg ripe pears
- 500 g jam sugar 2: 1

Preparation

1. Wash 2 limes and grate dry.
2. Peel the peels thinly with the zest ripper.
3. Then cut all limes in half and squeeze them out. Measure out 100 ml of lime juice.
4. Wash and peel the pears, remove the core and then quarter them. Weigh 900 g of pulp.
5. Then puree the pears together with the lime juice.
6. Now put the pear puree together with the lime peels and the jellied sugar in a saucepan.
7. Bring all ingredients to the boil together.
8. Simmer for 4 minutes, stirring, taking care not to burn anything.
9. Make a gelation test with a small blob on a cold saucer. If this becomes solid in a short time, the jam is ready Remove any foam that may have formed with a spade, but you can also simply stir it in.
10. Then pour the hot mass into hot rinsed jars, close and let stand upside down.

Healthy green shot

Preparation Time: 15 Minutes

Cooking Time: 60 Minutes

Servings: 10

Ingredients:

- 2 pears
- 3 green apples (e.g. granny smith)
- 3 sticks celery
- 60 g organic ginger
- 1 bunch parsley (20 g)
- 3 kiwi fruit
- 2 limes
- 1 tsp turmeric

Directions:

1. Wash pears, apples, celery, ginger and parsley and cut into pieces. Halve the kiwi fruit and remove the pulp with a spoon. Halve limes and squeeze out juice.
2. Put the pears, apples, kiwi, celery, ginger and parsley in the juicer and squeeze out the juice.
3. Mix freshly squeezed juice with the lime juice and season with turmeric. Serve the mixture as shots immediately or freeze it in portions.

Spinach kiwi smoothie bowl

Preparation Time: 15 Minutes

Cooking Time: 60 Minutes

Servings: 10

Ingredients:

- 1 green apple
- 2 kiwi fruit
- 300 g bananas (2 bananas)
- 100 g baby spinach

- 1 lemon
- 6 g chia seeds (2 tsp)
- 20 g grated coconut (2 tbsp)

Directions:

1. Clean, wash, core and chop the apple. Peel and cut the kiwis and bananas and put half aside. Wash the spinach and put some leaves aside. Halve the lemon and squeeze out the juice.
2. Put half of the fruit, spinach and lemon juice in a blender and mash finely. Divide the smoothie into 4 bowls.
3. Put the remaining pieces of fruit as a topping on the smoothie bowls. Sprinkle with chia seeds and grated coconut and serve with the remaining spinach leaves.

Avocado smoothie with basil

Preparation Time: 15 Minutes

Cooking Time: 60 Minutes

Servings: 10

Ingredients:

- 2 kiwi fruit
- 1 yellow-peeled apple
- 200 g honeydew melon meat
- 1 avocado
- 1 green chili pepper
- 20 g basil (1 handful)
- 20 g arugula (0.25 bunch)
- 1 tbsp sprouts (suitable for raw consumption)

Directions:

1. Peel and slice the kiwi fruit. Wash, quarter and core the apple and cut the quarters into slices. Cut the melon meat into pieces. Peel, core and cut avocado

into pieces. Wash the chili pepper and cut it into rings. Wash the basil and rocket and shake dry. Shower sprouts in a sieve.
2. Put all prepared ingredients in a blender and mash them finely. Add about 100 ml of cold water and serve in 4 glasses.

Gooseberry buttermilk drink

Preparation Time: 15 Minutes

Cooking Time: 60 Minutes

Servings: 10

Ingredients:

- 300 g gooseberries
- 2 bananas
- 600 ml buttermilk
- 30 g honey (2 tbsp)
- 4 small stems of mint
- ice cubes

Directions:

1. Wash and clean gooseberries and drain well. Set some berries aside for the garnish.
2. Peel and slice bananas. Puree together with gooseberries and 200 ml buttermilk. Add the remaining buttermilk and honey and mix until frothy.
3. Fill 4 glasses about halfway with ice cubes and spread the drink on them.
4. Wash the mint, shake it dry and spread it with the rest of the gooseberries on the drinks.

Blackberry and vanilla smoothie

Preparation Time: 15 Minutes

Cooking Time: 60 Minutes

Servings: 10

Ingredients:

- 500 g blackberry
- 1 vanilla bean
- 1 tsp lemon juice
- 700 ml buttermilk (ice cold)
- 80 g lean quark (4 tbsp)
- 40 g cashews
- 80 ml whipped cream

Directions:

1. Wash and drain blackberries.
2. Cut the vanilla pod lengthways, scrape out the pulp and puree creamy with blackberries, lemon juice, buttermilk, curd cheese and cashew nuts in a blender.
3. Whip the cream. Pour smoothie into 4 glasses and garnish with cream

Dijon Celery Salad

Preparation Time: 10 minutes

Cooking Time: 0 minutes

Servings: 4

Ingredients:

- 5 teaspoons stevia
- ½ cup lemon juice
- 1/3 cup dijon mustard
- 2/3 cup olive oil
- black pepper to the taste
- 2 apples, cored, peeled and cubed
- 1 bunch celery and leaves, roughly chopped
- ¾ cup walnuts, chopped

Directions:

1. In a salad bowl, mix celery and its leaves with apple pieces and walnuts.
2. Add black pepper, lemon juice, mustard, stevia and olive oil.

3. Whisk well, add to your salad, toss.
4. Divide into small cups and serve as a snack.

Nutrition:

Calories: 125 Cal

Fat: 2 g

Carbohydrates: 7 g

Protein: 7 g

Fiber: 2 g

Dill Bell Pepper Snack Bowls

Preparation Time: 10 minutes

Cooking Time: 0 minutes

Servings: 4

Ingredients:

- 2 tablespoons dill, chopped
- 1 yellow onion, chopped
- 1-pound multicolored bell peppers, cut into halves, seeded and cut into thin strips
- 3 tablespoons olive oil
- 2 and ½ tablespoons white vinegar
- Black pepper to the taste

Directions:

1. In a salad bowl, mix bell peppers with onion, dill, pepper, oil and vinegar, toss to coat, divide into small bowls and serve as a snack.

Nutrition:

Calories: 120 Cal

Fat: 3 g

Carbohydrates: 2 g

Protein: 3 g

Fiber: 3 g

Cinnamon Apple Chips

Preparation Time: 10 minutes

Cooking Time: 2 hours

Servings: 4

Ingredients:

- Cooking spray
- 2 teaspoons cinnamon powder
- 2 apples, cored and thinly sliced

Directions:

1. Arrange apple slices on a lined baking sheet, spray them with cooking oil, sprinkle cinnamon, introduce in the oven and bake at 300 degrees F for 2 hours.
2. Divide into bowls and serve as a snack.

Nutrition:

Calories: 80 Cal

Fat: 0 g

Carbohydrates: 7 g

Protein: 4 g

Fiber: 3 g

Potato Bites

Preparation Time: 10 minutes

Cooking Time: 20 minutes

Servings: 3

Ingredients:

- 1 potato, sliced
- 2 bacon slices, already cooked and crumbled
- 1 small avocado, pitted and cubed
- Cooking spray

Directions:

1. Spread potato slices on a lined baking sheet, spray with cooking oil, introduce in the oven at 350 degrees F, bake for 20 minutes, arrange on a platter, top each slice with avocado and crumbled bacon and serve as a snack.

Nutrition:

Calories: 180 Cal

Fat: 4 g

Carbohydrates: 8 g

Protein: 6 g

Fiber: 1 g

Beans Snack Salad

Preparation Time: 10 minutes

Cooking Time: 0 minutes

Servings: 6

Ingredients:

- 2 cups tomatoes, chopped
- 2 cups cucumber, chopped
- 3 cups mixed greens
- 2 cups mung beans, sprouted
- 2 cups clover sprouts
- for the salad dressing:
- 1 tablespoon cumin, ground
- 1 cup dill, chopped
- 4 tablespoons lemon juice
- 1 avocado, pitted, peeled and roughly chopped
- 1 cucumber, roughly chopped

Directions:

2. In a salad bowl.
3. Mix tomatoes with 2 cups cucumber, greens, clover and mung sprouts.
4. In your blender, mix cumin with dill, lemon juice, 1 cucumber and avocado.

5. Blend well, add this to your salad, toss well and serve as a snack.

Nutrition:

Calories: 120 Cal

Fat: 0 g

Carbohydrates: 1 g

Protein: 6 g

Fiber: 2 g

Sprouts and Apple Snack Salad

Preparation Time: 10 minutes

Cooking Time: 0 minute

Servings: 4

Ingredients:

- 1-pound brussels sprouts, shredded
- 1 cup walnuts, chopped
- 1 apple, cored and cubed
- 1 red onion, chopped
- For the salad dressing:
- 3 tablespoons red vinegar
- 1 tablespoon mustard
- 1/2 cup olive oil
- 1 garlic clove, minced
- Black pepper to the taste

Directions:

1. In a salad bowl, mix sprouts with apple, onion and walnuts.
2. In another bowl, mix vinegar with mustard, oil, garlic and pepper, whisk well, add this to your salad, toss well and serve as a snack.

Nutrition:

Calories: 120 Cal

Fat: 2 g

Carbohydrates: 8 g

Protein: 6 g

Fiber: 2 g

Moroccan Leeks Snack Salad

Preparation Time: 10 minutes

Cooking Time: 0 minutes

Servings: 4

Ingredients:

- 1 bunch radishes, sliced
- 3 cups leeks, chopped
- 1 and ½ cups olives, pitted and sliced
- A pinch of turmeric powder
- Black pepper to the taste
- 2 tablespoons olive oil
- 1 cup cilantro, chopped

Directions:

1. In a bowl, mix radishes with leeks, olives and cilantro.
2. Add black pepper, oil and turmeric, toss to coat and serve as a snack.

Nutrition:

Calories: 120 Cal

Fat: 1 g

Carbohydrates: 8 g

Protein: 6 g

Fiber: 1 g

Celery and Raisins Snack Salad

Preparation Time: 10 minutes

Cooking Time: 0 minutes

Servings: 4

Ingredients:

- ½ cup raisins
- 4 cups celery, sliced
- ¼ cup parsley, chopped
- ½ cup walnuts, chopped
- Juice of ½ lemon
- 2 tablespoons olive oil
- Salt and black pepper to the taste

Directions:

1. In a salad bowl.
2. Mix celery with raisins, walnuts, parsley, lemon juice, oil and black pepper, toss
3. Divide into small cups and serve as a snack.

Nutrition:

Calories: 120 Cal

Fat: 1 g

Carbohydrates: 6 g

Protein: 5 g

Fiber: 2 g

Dijon Celery Salad

Preparation Time: 10 minutes

Cooking Time: 0 minutes

Servings: 4

Ingredients:

- 5 teaspoons stevia
- ½ cup lemon juice
- 1/3 cup Dijon mustard
- 2/3 cup olive oil
- Black pepper to the taste
- 2 apples, cored, peeled and cubed
- 1 bunch celery and leaves, roughly chopped
- ¾ cup walnuts, chopped

Directions:

1. In a salad bowl, mix celery and its leaves with apple pieces and walnuts.
2. Add black pepper, lemon juice, mustard, stevia and olive oil, whisk well, add to your salad, toss, divide into small cups and serve as a snack.

Nutrition:

Calories: 125 Cal

Fat: 2 g

Carbohydrates: 7 g

Protein: 7 g

Fiber: 2 g

Mozzarella Bars

Preparation Time: 10 minutes

Cooking Time: 40 minutes

Servings: 12

Ingredients:

- 1 big cauliflower head, riced
- ½ cup low-fat mozzarella cheese, shredded
- ¼ cup egg whites
- 1 teaspoon Italian seasoning
- Black pepper to the taste

Directions:

1. Spread the cauliflower rice on a lined baking sheet, cook in the oven at 375 degrees F for 20 minutes.
2. Transfer to a bowl, add black pepper, cheese, seasoning and egg whites.
3. Stir well, spread into a rectangle pan and press on the bottom.
4. Introduce in the oven at 375 degrees F, bake for 20 minutes, cut into 12 bars.
5. and serve as a snack.

Nutrition:

Calories: 140 Cal

Fat: 1 g

Carbohydrates: 6 g

Protein: 6 g

Fiber: 3 g

Baby Spinach Snack

Preparation Time: 10 minutes

Cooking Time: 10 min

Servings: 3

Ingredients:

- 2 cups baby spinach, washed
- A pinch of black pepper
- ½ tablespoon olive oil
- ½ teaspoon garlic powder

Directions:

1. Spread the baby spinach on a lined baking sheet, add oil, black pepper and garlic powder, toss a bit, introduce in the oven, bake at 350 degrees F for 10 minutes, divide into bowls and serve as a snack.

Nutrition:

Calories: 125 Cal

Fat: 4 g

Carbohydrates: 4 g

Protein: 2 g

Fiber: 1 g

Italian Veggie Salsa

Preparation Time: 10 minutes

Cooking Time: 10 minutes

Servings: 4

Ingredients:

- 2 red bell peppers, cut into medium wedges
- 3 zucchinis, sliced
- ½ cup garlic, minced
- 2 tablespoons olive oil
- A pinch of black pepper
- 1 teaspoon Italian seasoning

Directions:

1. Heat a pan with the oil over medium-high heat, add bell peppers and zucchini, toss and cook for 5 minutes.
2. Add garlic, black pepper and Italian seasoning, toss, cook for 5 minutes more, divide into small cups and serve as a snack.

Nutrition:

Calories: 132 g

Fat: 3 g

Carbohydrates: 7 g

Protein: 4 g

Fiber: 3 g

Black Bean Salsa

Preparation Time: 10 minutes

Cooking Time: 0 minutes

Servings: 6

Ingredients:

- 1 tablespoon coconut amino
- ½ teaspoon cumin, ground
- 1 cup canned black beans, no-salt-added, drained and rinsed
- 1 cup salsa
- 6 cups romaine lettuce leaves, torn

- ½ cup avocado, peeled, pitted and cubed

Directions:

1. In a bowl, combine the beans with the amino, cumin, salsa, lettuce and avocado, toss, divide into small bowls and serve as a snack

Nutrition:

Calories: 181 Cal

Fat: 4 g

Carbohydrates: 14 g

Protein: 7 g

Fiber: 7 g

Pumpkin Seeds Bowls

Preparation Time: 10 minutes

Cooking Time: 20 minutes

Servings: 6

Ingredients:

- ½ tablespoon chili powder
- ½ teaspoon cayenne pepper
- 2 cups pumpkin seeds
- 2 teaspoons lime juice

Directions:

1. Spread pumpkin seeds on a lined baking sheet.
2. Add lime juice, cayenne and chili powder, toss well, introduce in the oven.
3. Roast at 275 degrees F for 20 minutes.
4. Divide into small bowls and serve as a snack.

Nutrition:

Calories: 170 Cal

Fat: 2 g

Carbohydrates: 12 g

Protein: 6 g

Fiber: 7 g

Eggplant Salsa

Preparation Time: 10 minutes

Cooking Time: 10 minutes

Servings: 4

Ingredients:

- 1 And ½ Cups Tomatoes, Chopped
- 3 Cups Eggplant, Cubed
- A Drizzle Of Olive Oil
- 2 Teaspoons Capers
- 6 Ounces Green Olives, Pitted And Sliced
- 4 Garlic Cloves, Minced
- 2 Teaspoons Balsamic Vinegar
- 1 Tablespoon Basil, Chopped
- Black Pepper To The Taste

Directions:

1. Heat A Pan With The Oil Over Medium-High Heat, Add Eggplant, Stir and Cook For 5 Minutes. Add Tomatoes, Capers, Olives, Garlic, Vinegar, Basil And Black Pepper, Toss, Cook For 5 Minutes More, Divide Into Small Cups and Serve Cold.

Nutrition:

Calories: 120 Cal

Fat: 6 g

Carbohydrates: 9 g

Protein: 7 g

Fiber: 5 g

Date Nut Bread

Preparation Time: 30 minutes

Cooking Time: 4-6 hours

Servings: 4-6

Ingredients:

- ¾ cup Medjool dates
- 1 ¼ cup All-Purpose flour
- 2 teaspoon baking powder
- ¼ teaspoon baking soda
- ½ teaspoon salt
- ½ cup sugar
- ¾ cup milk
- 1 egg, slightly beaten
- 1 tablespoon orange peel, grated
- 1 tablespoon coconut oil, melted
- ¼ cup buckwheat flour
- 1 cup walnuts, chopped

Directions:

2. Place the dates on a chopping block and sprinkle 1 tablespoon of All-Purpose flour over them. Dip a knife into the flour and chop the dates finely. Flour the knife often to keep the cut-up fruit from sticking together.
3. Sift the remaining All-Purpose flour, baking powder, baking soda, salt and sugar into a large bowl.
4. In a separate bowl, combine the milk, egg, orange peel and oil.
5. Add the buckwheat flour to the flour mixture, mix well and gently fold in the dates, along with any flour left on the cutting block and the walnuts.
6. Pour in the liquid ingredients and mix until just combined.
7. Transfer dough into a well-greased and floured baking unit. Cover and place in the slow cooker

8. Use a toothpick or small amount of twisted aluminum foil to prop the crockpot lid open a tiny fraction to allow steam to escape.
9. Cook on high for 4 to 6 hours. Cool on a rack for 10 minutes. Serve warm or cold.
10. Do NOT lift the crockpot lid while the bread is baking.

Nutrition:

Calories: 70 Cal

Fat:1 g

Carbohydrates: 15 g

Protein: 1 g

Fiber: 1 g

Strawberry Rhubarb Crisp

Preparation Time: 10 minutes

Cooking Time: 45 minutes

Servings: 6-8

Ingredients:

- 1 cup white sugar
- ½ cup buckwheat flour + 3 tablespoons
- 3 cups strawberries, sliced
- 3 cups rhubarb, diced
- ½ lemon, juiced
- 1 cup packed brown sugar
- 1 cup coconut oil, melted
- ¾ cup rolled oats
- ¼ cup buckwheat groats
- ¼ cup walnuts, chopped

Directions:

1. Preheat oven to 375 degrees F
2. In a large bowl, mix white sugar, 3 tablespoons flour, strawberries, rhubarb

and lemon juice. Place the mixture in a 9x13 inch baking dish.

3. In a separate bowl, mix ½ cup flour, brown sugar, coconut oil, oats, buckwheat groats and walnuts until crumbly. You may want to use a pastry blender for this. Crumble on top of the rhubarb and strawberry mixture.
4. Bake 45 minutes in the preheated oven, or until crisp and lightly browned.

Nutrition:

Calories: 240 Cal

Fat: 7 g

Carbohydrates: 42 g

Protein: 2 g

Fiber: 3 g

Avocado Smoothie

Preparation Time: 5 Minutes

Cooking Time: 5 Minutes

Servings: 2

Ingredients:

- 1 cup Coconut Milk, preferably full-fat
- 1 cup Ice
- 3 cups Baby Spinach
- 1 Banana, frozen & quartered
- 1/2 cup pineapple chunks, frozen
- 1/2 of 1 Avocado, smooth

Directions:

1. First, place ice, pineapple chunks, pineapple chunks, banana, avocado, baby spinach in the blender pitcher.
2. Now, press the 'extract' button.
3. Finally, transfer to a serving glass.
4. To make it more nutritious and filling, you can even add banana to it.

Nutrition:

130 calories

Tofu Smoothie

Preparation Time: 5 Minutes

Cooking Time: 5 Minutes

Servings: 2

Ingredients:

- 1 Banana, sliced & frozen
- 3/4 cup Almond Milk
- 2 tbsp. Peanut Butter
- 1/2 cup Yoghurt, plain & low-fat
- 1/2 cup Tofu, soft & silken
- 1/3 cup Dates, chopped

Directions:

1. First, place tofu, banana, dates, yogurt, peanut butter and almond milk in the blender pitcher.
2. After that, press the 'smoothie' button.
3. Finally, transfer to serving glass and enjoy it.
4. Tip: You can try adding herbs to your preference.

Nutrition:

Calories: 119 Sugar: 13

Sodium: 31 Fat: 2 Carbohydrates: 22

Fiber: 3 Protein: 5

Carrot Strawberry Smoothie

Preparation Time: 5 Minutes

Cooking Time: 5 Minutes

Servings: 2

Ingredients:

- 1/3 cup Bell Pepper, diced

- 1 cup Carrot Juice, chilled
- 1 cup Mango, diced
- 1 cup Strawberries, unsweetened & frozen

Directions:

1. To start with, place strawberries, bell pepper and mango in the blender pitcher.
2. After that, pulse it a few times.
3. Pour the carrot juice into it.
4. Finally, press the 'smoothie' button.
5. Tip: You can try adding pineapple chunks to it for enhanced flavour.

Nutrition:

70 calories

Green Smoothie

Preparation Time: 5 Minutes

Cooking Time: 5 Minutes

Servings: 3 to 4

Ingredients:

- 1/4 cup Baby Spinach
- 1/2 cup Ice
- 1/4 cup Kale
- 1/2 cup Pineapple Chunks
- 1/2 cup Coconut Water
- 1/2 cup mango, diced
- 1/2 Banana, diced

Directions:

1. Begin by placing all the ingredients needed to make the smoothie in the blender pitcher.
2. Now, press the 'extract' button.
3. Transfer the smoothie into the serving glass.

Nutrition:

Calories: 207 Carbohydrates: 33 grams Fat: 2 grams

Protein: 15 grams Sodium: 73 milligrams Sugar: 25 grams

Fiber: 5 grams Cholesterol: 4 milligrams

Yoghurt & Fruit Jam Parfait

Preparation Time: 5 Minutes

Cooking Time: 5 Minutes

Servings: 6

Ingredients:

- 3 cups Mixed Berries
- 1 tbsp. Lemon Juice
- 7/8 cup Honey
- 2 tsp. Fruit Pectin
- 1 cup Granola
- 3 cups Greek Yoghurt

Directions:

1. For making this healthy jam, you need to place the mixed berries, honey, lemon juice and pectin in the blender pitcher.
2. Pulse the mixture 3 to 4 times and then press the 'sauce/ dip' button.
3. Now, transfer the jam to a safe heat container and then place it in the refrigerator for 2 to 3 hours.
4. Once the jam is chilled, layer 1/3 cup of the Greek Yoghurt into the bottom of the parfait glass.
5. After that, spoon in a jam into it and then add the granola.
6. Serve immediately.

Tip: If you don't want to use honey, you can use 1 cup of granulated sugar.

Nutrition: 154 calories

Kiwi Smoothie

Preparation Time: 5 Minutes

Cooking Time: 5 Minutes

Servings: 3

Ingredients:

- 1/4 of 1 Avocado, ripe & pitted
- 1/4 cup Ice
- 1/4 cup Coconut Water
- 3/4 cup Kale Leaves
- 1/2 cm Ginger, fresh & peeled
- 2 Kiwis, quartered
- 1 Date pitted & halved
- 1 tsp. Lime Juice

Directions:

1. First, place ice, kale leaves, avocado, dates, kiwis, lime juice, ginger and coconut water in the blender pitcher.
2. Then, press the 'smoothie' button.
3. Finally, transfer to a serving glass and enjoy it.

Nutrition:

Calories: 268.0 Total Fat: 2.3 g Cholesterol: 40.0 mg

Sodium: 141.2 mg Total Carbs: 34.3 g Dietary Fiber: 6.0 g Protein: 27.9 g

Pineapple Kale Smoothie

Preparation Time: 5 Minutes

Cooking Time: 5 Minutes

Servings: 3

Ingredients:

- 3/4 cup Kale leaves
- 1 cup Pineapple, fresh & chopped into chunks
- 1/4 cup Ice

- 3/4 cup Coconut Water
- 1/4 of 1 Avocado, ripe & pitted
- 1/2 of 1 Lime
- 1 Date pitted & halved

Directions:

1. For making this bright, tasty smoothie, place ice, kale leaves, avocado, date, coconut water, lime and pineapple in the blender pitcher.
2. After that, press the 'smoothie' button.
3. Finally, transfer the smoothie to a serving glass and enjoy it.
4. For a richer smoothie, you can try substituting coconut water with light coconut milk.

Nutrition:

Calories: 266.3 Total Fat: 0.6 g Cholesterol: 0.0 mg

Sodium: 34.9 mg Total Carbs: 68.6 g Dietary Fiber: 8.8 g Protein: 4.0 g

Antioxidant Smoothie

Preparation Time: 5 Minutes

Cooking Time: 5 Minutes

Servings: 3

Ingredients:

- 1/2 cup Celery Stalk, halved
- 1/3 cup Watermelon, chopped into chunks
- 1/4 cup Ice
- 1/8 cup Red Cabbage, chopped
- 1/2 cup Blueberries
- 1/2 cup Pomegranate Juice
- 1/2 of 1 Apple, unpeeled & halved

Directions:

1. Begin by placing ice, red cabbage, celery stalk, apple, blueberries and watermelon in the blender pitcher.
2. Now, select the 'smoothie' button.
3. Finally, transfer the smoothie to the serving glass and enjoy it.

Nutrition:

Calories: 225.3 Total Fat: 9.1 g

Cholesterol: 10.0 mg Sodium: 135.5 mg

Total Carbs: 29.7 g

Dietary Fiber: 7.2 g

Protein: 9.1 g

Carrot Beetroot Smoothie

Preparation Time: 5 Minutes

Cooking Time: 5 Minutes

Servings: 3

Ingredients:

- 1/2 of 1 Beet, small & halved
- 3/4 cup Water
- 1/2 cup Ice
- 1 Celery Stalk
- 1/2 of 1 Lemon
- 1/2 of 1 Carrot, halved
- 1/2 cm Ginger, fresh & peeled
- 1/2 of 1 Orange, halved

Directions:

1. To start with, place ice, carrot, beet, celery stalk, lemon, ginger, orange and water in the blender pitcher.
2. Then select the 'smoothie' button.
3. Finally, transfer the smoothie to the serving glass.
4. Tip: For a more vibrant smoothie, you can try substituting coconut water with light coconut milk.

Nutrition:

Calories: 169.7 Total Fat: 1.0 g Cholesterol: 0.0 mg

Sodium: 112.3 mg Total Carbs: 38.3 g Dietary Fiber: 3.6 g Protein: 3.7 g

Black Tea Cake

Preparation Time: 10 minutes.

Cooking Time: 35 minutes.

Servings: 8

Ingredients:

- 6 tablespoons black tea powder
- 2 cups almond milk, warmed up
- 1 cup avocado oil
- 2 cups stevia
- 4 eggs
- 2 teaspoons vanilla extract
- 3 and ½ cups almond flour
- 1 teaspoon baking soda
- 3 teaspoons baking powder

Directions:

1. In a bowl, combine the almond milk with the oil, stevia and the rest of the ingredients and whisk well.
2. Pour this into a cake pan lined with parchment paper, introduce in the oven at 350ºF and bake for 35 minutes.
3. Leave the cake to cool down, slice and serve.

Nutrition:

Carbs: 6.5g.

Protein: 5.4g.

Green Tea and Vanilla Cream

Preparation Time: 2 hours.

Cooking Time: 0 minutes.

Servings: 4

Ingredients:

- 14 ounces almond milk, hot
- 2 tablespoons green tea powder
- 14 ounces heavy cream
- 3 tablespoons stevia
- 1 teaspoon vanilla extract
- 1 teaspoon gelatin powder

Directions:

1. In a bowl, combine the almond milk with the green tea powder and the rest of the ingredients, whisk well, cool down, divide into cups and keep in the fridge for 2 hours before serving.

Nutrition:

Calories: 120

Fat: 3g.

Carbs: 7g.

Protein: 4g.

120. Figs Pie

Preparation Time: 10 minutes.

Cooking Time: 1 hour.

Servings: 8

Ingredients:

- ½ cup stevia
- 6 figs, cut into quarters
- ½ teaspoon vanilla extract
- 1 cup almond flour
- 4 eggs, whisked

Directions:

1. Spread the figs on the bottom of a springform pan lined with parchment paper.

2. In a bowl, combine the other ingredients, whisk and pour over the figs.
3. Bake at 375ºF for 1 hour, flip the pie upside down when it's done and serve.

Nutrition:

Calories: 200

Fat: 4.4g.

Carbs: 7.6g.

Protein: 8g.

Cherry Cream

Preparation Time: 2 hours.

Cooking Time: 0 minutes.

Servings: 4

Ingredients:

- 2 cups cherries, pitted and chopped
- 1 cup almond milk
- ½ cup whipping cream
- 3 eggs, whisked
- 1/3 cup stevia
- 1 teaspoon lemon juice
- ½ teaspoon vanilla extract

Directions:

1. In your food processor, combine the cherries with the milk and the rest of the ingredients, pulse well, divide into cups and keep in the fridge for 2 hours before serving.

Nutrition:

Calories: 200

Fat: 4.5g.

Carbs: 5.6g.

Protein: 3.4g.

Lara Burns

Strawberries Cream

Preparation Time: 10 minutes.

Cooking Time: 20 minutes.

Servings: 4

Ingredients:

- ½ cup stevia
- 2 pounds strawberries, chopped
- 1 cup almond milk
- Zest of 1 lemon, grated
- ½ cup heavy cream
- 3 egg yolks, whisked

Directions:

2. Heat up a pan with the milk over medium-high heat, add the stevia and the rest of the ingredients, whisk well, simmer for 20 minutes, divide into cups and serve cold.

Nutrition:

Calories: 152

Fat: 4.4g.

Carbs: 5.1g.

Protein: 0.8g.

A 21 Day Sirtfood Diet Meal Plan

DAYS	BREAKFAST	LUNCH	DINNER	DESSERT
1.	Kale Scramble	King Prawn Stir-fry & Soba	Lamb Chops with Kale	Italian Veggie Salsa
2.	Buckwheat Porridge	Miso Caramelized Tofu	Shrimp with Kale	Black Bean Salsa
3.	Salmon & Kale Omelet	Sirtfood Cauliflower Couscous & Turkey Steak	Chicken & Veggies with Buckwheat Noodles	Pumpkin Seeds Bowls
4.	Moroccan Spiced Eggs	Mushroom & Tofu Scramble	Beef & Kale Salad	Eggplant Salsa
5.	Chilaquiles with Gochujang	Prawn & Chili Pak Choi	Prawns with Asparagus	Date Nut Bread
6.	Twice Baked Breakfast Potatoes	Sirtfood Granola	Turkey Satay Skewer	Strawberry Rhubarb Crisp
7.	Sirt Muesli	Tomato Frittata	Salmon & Capers	Avocado Smoothie
8.	Mushroom Scramble Eggs	Horseradish Flaked Salmon Fillet & Kale	Chicken Casserole	Tofu Smoothie
9.	Smoked Salmon Omelets	Indulgent Yoghurt	Veal Cabbage Rolls – Smarter	Carrot Strawberry Smoothie

		with Capers, Garlic and Caraway Seeds	
10.	Date and Walnut Porridge	Tuna Salad	Fragrant Asian Hotspot	Green Smoothie
11.	Beef Stroganoff French Bread Toast	Chicken & Bean Casserole	Tofu Thai Curry	Yoghurt & Fruit Jam Parfait
12.	Classic French Toast	Mussels in Red Wine Sauce	Beans & Kale Soup	Kiwi Smoothie
13.	Avocado and Kale Omelet	Tuna and Kale	Lentils & Greens Soup	Pineapple Kale Smoothie
14.	Easy Egg-White Muffins	Lemongrass Mix	Asian Slaw	Antioxidant Smoothie
15.	Avocado Eggs with Toast	Scallops with Almonds and Mushrooms	Egg Fried Buckwheat	Carrot Beetroot Smoothie
16.	Baked Oatmeal	Scallops and Sweet Potatoes	Aromatic Ginger Turmeric Buckwheat	Black Tea Cake
17.	Sirt cereal	Salmon and Shrimp Salad	Kale and Corn Succotash	Green Tea and Vanilla Cream
18.	Sirt breakfast bar	Shrimp, Tomato and Dates Salad	Asian King Prawn Stir-Fry with Buckwheat Noodles	Cherry Cream

19.	Sirt cocoa pops	Salmon and Watercress Salad	Greek Salad Skewers	Strawberries Cream
20.	Sirt fruit bowl	Tuna and Tomatoes	Sirtfood Couscous	Mozzarella Bars
21.	Grilled sausages with fried Onions and scrambled eggs with herbs	Spinach and Kale Mix	Caramelized Tofu	Baby Spinach Snack

Conclusion

Thank you for making it to the end. Everything you have learned about the Sirtfood Diet, the important question, at least for many people, is whether or not it is worth your time and effort.

Though this trial's findings have proven to be quite promising, other experts have noted certain limitations of the study that could have been improved upon if subsequent follow-up trials had been conducted. Some of the most prominent limitations identified include the following:

- Lack of control group to as serve as baseline and reference point;
- Having 40 participants only, which is a relatively small sample size; and
- Potential bias among the participants since they have been identified as health-conscious individuals.

These limitations, while not conclusive, somehow weaken the foundations of the Sirtfood Diet. Some health experts even argue that much like other types of diets, Sirtfood Diet could help its followers lose weight by imposing caloric limits for a certain period.

While restrictive eating can be helpful and effective to a certain extent, several studies have highlighted the negative impacts that this practice causes. If you have already tried doing diets that are centered on regular fasting, then you would have experienced mood swings, sudden binges to compensate for the lack of food, loss of muscle mass and strength, and even depression.

Granted that you will not be required to undergo special exercise routines or to cut back on different types of food, you would still have to be mindful of what you eat and drink while you are on the Sirtfood diet. Nonetheless, this level of leniency that this diet offers to attract a lot of people who do not want to give up a lot of things for the sake of looking and feeling better.

So, what's the verdict on the Sirtfood Diet?

If you are willing to live through its drawbacks to reap its benefits and enjoy its advantages over other weight loss plans, then go ahead with your plans to follow this diet.

Furthermore, the majority of the top sirtfoods are fruits, vegetables, and plant-based foods. When combined with the right amount of proteins and carbohydrates in your daily meals, then you cannot go wrong by eating more of them than you usually do. Just remember to keep your red wine, caffeine, and dark chocolate in moderation, though, to avoid causing unintentional harm to your body.

Finally, as a rule of thumb, you should not put your 100% trust on a diet that has promises that sound a bit too good to be true. Set realistic expectations based on your current situation in life. Not everyone can live like Adele and the other celebrity endorsers of the Sirtfood Diet. Before you do this diet, think carefully. Chances are it might have a negative effect on your health if you don't follow the diet correctly. Think before you do anything. Sirtfood Diet is not that bad as long as you follow the plan correctly.

I hope you have learned something!

CPSIA information can be obtained
at www.ICGtesting.com
Printed in the USA
LVHW021452090121
676042LV00008B/396

9 781801 327336